Teen Pregnancy and Parenting

Whether glamorized or stigmatized, teenage parenthood is all too often used to stand for a host of social problems, and empirical research results ignored. Identifying core controversies surrounding teen pregnancy and parenting, this book resolves misperceptions using findings from large-scale, longitudinal, and qualitative research studies from the US and other Western countries.

Summarizing the evidence and integrating it with a systems perspective, the authors explore ten prevalent myths about teenage parents, including:

- Teen pregnancy is associated with other behavior problems.
- Children of teen parents will experience cognitive delay, adjustment problems, and will themselves become teen parents.
- Better outcomes are achieved when teen mothers live with their own mothers.
- Teen pregnancy costs taxpayers lots of money.
- Abstinence education is the best way to prevent teen pregnancy.

Teen Pregnancy and Parenting ends by highlighting the prevention and intervention implications for families, practitioners, and policy-makers. It will be of interest to academics and advanced students from a range of disciplines and professions including psychology, public policy, nursing, social work, and sociology.

Keri Weed is Professor in the Department of Psychology at the University of South Carolina Aiken, USA.

Jody S. Nicholson is Assistant Professor in the Department of Psychology at the University of North Florida, USA.

Jaelyn R. Farris is Assistant Professor in the Department of Human Development and Family Studies at Penn State Harrisburg, USA.

Routledge Advances in Health and Social Policy

Teen Pregnancy and Parenting
Rethinking the myths and misperceptions

Keri Weed, Jody S. Nicholson and
Jaelyn R. Farris

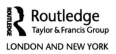
Routledge
Taylor & Francis Group

LONDON AND NEW YORK

X

First published 2015
by Routledge
2 Park Square, Milton Park, Abingdon, Oxon OX14 4RN

and by Routledge
711 Third Avenue, New York, NY 10017

Routledge is an imprint of the Taylor & Francis Group, an informa business

British Library Cataloguing in Publication Data
A catalogue record for this book is available from the British Library

Library of Congress Cataloguing in Publication data
   Weed, Keri, author.
   Teen pregnancy and parenting: rethinking the myths and
   misperceptions / Keri Weed, Jody S. Nicholson, Jaelyn R. Farris.
      p. ; cm. – (Routledge advances in health and social policy)
   I. Nicholson, Jody S., author. II. Farris, Jaelyn Renee.,
   author. III. Title. IV. Series: Routledge advances in health and social policy.
   [DNLM: 1. Pregnancy in Adolescence. 2. Parenting. 3. Social
   Perception. 4. Socioeconomic Factors. WA 310.1]
   RG556.5
   618.200835–dc23
   2014001962

ISBN: 978-0-415-64432-7 (hbk)
ISBN: 978-0-203-07960-7 (ebk)

Typeset in Goudy
by Out of House Publishing

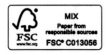

Printed and bound in Great Britain by
TJ International Ltd, Padstow, Cornwall

Dedication

In memory of our friend and colleague Deb Keogh, whose efforts
and passion for the Notre Dame Adolescent Parenting Project made
this book possible, and to John Borkowski and Tom Whitman,
with our utmost gratitude for their leadership and wisdom, whose
quest for the truth inspired us to write this book.

Contents

Figures

Tables

Preface

Our contributions to this book represent nearly 50 years of collective experience studying teen mothers and their children across a variety of basic and applied longitudinal studies. All three of us cut our teeth on research with teen moms with the Notre Dame Adolescent Parenting Project (NDAPP) under the guidance of Drs. John G. Borkowski and Thomas L. Whitman. The NDAPP began in the mid-1980s and followed a sample of over 100 teen mothers and their children for more than 20 years. We have already published two books describing the results of this study; *Interwoven Lives* summarized findings through the first five years of the children's lives (Whitman, Borkowski, Keogh, and Weed, 2001) and *Risk and Resilience* provided an overview of the lives of the mothers and their children across 14 years (Borkowski, Farris, Whitman, Carothers, Weed, and Keogh, 2007).

Like many academics, we see the indelible impression our mentors have left in how we approach our research. We were trained to incorporate all aspects of good science while also recognizing the individual differences of the mothers and children as valuable human beings, and not just participants. Our mentors' personal and professional dedication to social justice and "big picture" thinking continues on in our careers, yet we also bring unique personal strengths and (sometimes contrasting) perspectives. Keri brings the most experience to the group, having been a part of the NDAPP since the beginning and a significant contributor to both previous books from the study. With this experience, she has constructed a deep belief in the importance of viewing teen parenting through a systems perspective that considers all the different influences that must be taken into account when considering human development. Jaelyn's previous background as a clinician has informed her passion about being sure information is relevant and helpful to those directly working with teen mothers and their families. Jody, who was John's final graduate student, has recently started her independent research career, gravitating towards research relevant to public health and how research is (and is not) integrated into public policy. We see our similar training, and different perspectives, as major strengths of this book that will contribute to the existing literature on teen pregnancy and parenting.

Our investigations of the NDAPP data, along with other studies on teen mothers, have been enlightening. What has been even more fulfilling for us, however, have been the interactions we have had with hundreds of pregnant and parenting women and men, both in adolescence and as they have aged, and with their children. These formal and informal experiences in the research setting have helped construct our own beliefs about teen pregnancy and parenting, but have also brought about questions when hypotheses based on our first-hand experiences with our participants were not supported by the results of our analyses. Similarly, we noticed that empirical results from our studies and the general literature sometimes did not match the understanding of teen parenting we heard when discussing our research with friends, family members, and strangers eager to give their opinion. Notably, these points of inconsistency became most obvious following our final NDAPP assessment, which occurred 18–21 years postpartum. At this time, we realized that many of the young mothers and their children had experienced turbulent lives through the 14-year assessment, but their data from the 18–21 year assessment indicated that things had smoothed out dramatically. Mothers had gone on to finish college, were holding down good jobs, and had become advocates in their community; children showed decreases in observed socioemotional and behavioral problems, impressive rates of high-school graduation, and even college attendance (sometimes funded by scholarships for academics or athletics). This level of well-being in our sample went against the "doom and gloom" perspective of teen mothers we found in the general public and in some literature, but was a message that was showing up not only in our own work but also in findings from notable researchers in the field.

Here lies the heart of this book. There is a pressing need to synthesize the inconsistencies between our formal and informal, or professional and personal, observations. We have spent the last few years scrutinizing our own personal beliefs about teen parenting, and considering how others may construct their beliefs, which are often based largely on their personal experiences with pregnant or parenting teens. When beliefs are not properly grounded in truth, there is a great potential for false perceptions that can negatively impact teen mothers in terms of the services they receive, the interactions they have with others, and their children's well-being. Thus was born the current investigation into the myths surrounding teen pregnancy and parenting.

A myth, as defined by Merriam-Webster's dictionary, "serves to unfold part of the world view of a people or explain a practice, belief, or natural phenomenon," and is "a popular belief or tradition that has grown up around something or someone; especially: one embodying the ideals and institutions of a society or segment of society." Myths can also be defined as ideas that are unfounded or false yet perpetuated by specific cultures as truths. However, most myths contain, or are based on, an element of truth. Thus, myths need not be completely false notions. We add the modifier "cultural" to the definition of myths to emphasize that the common beliefs we scrutinize were established within specific cultural contexts and have meaning only within those contexts. Therefore, we have defined cultural myths as generalized beliefs that are shared among people within a culture; these beliefs are based on perceptions that may or may not be entirely accurate.

In preparation for writing the book, we scoured scholarly and popular sources alike in an effort to identify overarching cultural myths about teen pregnancy and teen parenthood. From the beginning, we made a concerted effort to consider the extent to which each of these cultural myths was grounded in truth, and the extent to which each was unfounded and, consequently, detrimental to young mothers and their families. We aimed to objectively synthesize a wealth of data from a variety of fields before determining the validity of the claims. We were able to identify ten cultural myths, which fell into the categories of beliefs about: teen pregnancy, the fate of teen parents, outcomes of children born to teen parents, ways to support teen parents, and the socioeconomic costs of teen pregnancy and teen parenting.

To evaluate the validity of these cultural myths, we utilized our training as developmental psychologists and the subsequent lens with which we view human development. Our approach is best described by what is termed a "systems perspective." This perspective makes an effort to identify all the various factors that influence an individual, including individual characteristics, relationships, societal expectations, and policy and programming. In addition to trying to simultaneously consider how each of these factors impacts an individual, the systems perspective suggests that we must also consider how the factors intertwine, connect with, and impact each other. Throughout the course of the book, we have used this comprehensive perspective to evaluate the cultural myths. Our goal was to conduct an unbiased assessment and, if the cultural myth was not entirely supported, to reword it into a more nuanced truth that can have useful applications.

Over the course of about two years, we compiled evidence from our NDAPP, our other projects on teen parenting, and other teen pregnancy and teen parenting projects in the United States and internationally. Our ultimate conclusion was that all ten of these cultural myths are, at least in large part, founded on false beliefs or misperceptions perpetuated by society and not well grounded in truth or empirical data. In some cases, we arrived at an "it depends" perspective, as there is so much variability between pregnant and parenting teens that it is nearly impossible to draw firm conclusions that generalize to the population. The evaluation of these cultural myths revolves around the general theme that, although teen parenting isn't easy, it's also not a life sentence for negative outcomes. In contrast to much of the literature and general public opinion that touts the detrimental outcomes of teen parenting, and the societal costs of teen pregnancy, we observed that many young parents and their children fare reasonably well when provided with adequate resources and supports.

We begin in Chapter 1 with a focus on the theoretical grounding of our book in systems theory to orient the reader to the importance of considering cultural myths relevant to teen pregnancy and parenting, and their origins. In the next chapter, we summarize our own longitudinal research spanning over 20 years of the lives of teen mothers and their children (Borkowski *et al.*, 2007; Whitman *et al.*, 2001). We also rely on other studies not just from the United States, but from several countries in the EU, Canada, Australia, New Zealand, and South

America. Although our focus is on longitudinal quantitative research, we also include select qualitative research studies that add depth and a more personal touch compared to quantitative findings. Many of the studies that we have relied on during our evaluation of cultural myths are summarized by country of origin in the Appendix. Chapter 2 also compares the types of analyses conducted by researchers, with the intent of putting more weight on findings from studies with more sophisticated and powerful analyses. In some respects, Chapter 2 may be considered a reference chapter that outlines methodological issues in research on teen parenting, allowing us to focus on bigger-picture conclusions as we evaluate cultural myths and misperceptions in later chapters.

Chapter 3 then turns to how pregnant and parenting teens are portrayed in popular culture. Messages about pregnant and parenting teens conveyed by television shows, movies, books, news media, and the Internet are examined, with a focus on reality television. We rely on our own comparative analyses of observable outcomes for characters on MTV's popular reality show *16 and Pregnant* as compared to data drawn from representative samples of teen mothers in the United States. We describe how the conflicting nature of messages in the media has contributed to ongoing cultural myths about teen pregnancy and parenting. Chapter 3 focuses on the cultural myth that *providing media visibility of pregnant or parenting teens will encourage others to become pregnant.*

Chapter 4 provides evidence that counters the cultural myths that *most pregnant teens have behavior problems* and that *all teen pregnancies are unintended and unwanted.* Parents, clergy, and educators alike appeal to teenagers to abstain from sexual intercourse lest they become pregnant. The assumption is that increasing the salience of the likelihood of a pregnancy following sex will deter teens from engaging in behavior that may produce an unwanted consequence. This logic may be flawed if, in fact, some teens are actually engaging in sexual intercourse for the intended purpose of getting pregnant (Dash, 1989). Furthermore, perceptions held by some family members, friends, and broader society that pregnant teens must be delinquent may all too easily be integrated into teens developing personal identities, eventually changing how they perceive themselves. This chapter begins to investigate a series of cultural myths that could result from preconceived notions that are held by society.

Chapter 5 evaluates evidence from our own and other longitudinal studies from the United States and other developed countries that have followed teens into emerging adulthood to investigate the cultural myth that *parenthood derails the trajectories of the teens' lives.* Important social, educational, and economic outcomes are compared for both women and men who began childbearing as teenagers compared to their peers who waited until adulthood to have children. Chapter 6 investigates the outcomes for children of teen mothers, specifically that *teen pregnancies result in poor birth outcomes and that children of teen parents will experience cognitive delay, adjustment problems, and will themselves become teen parents.*

Chapter 7 evaluates cultural myths that are *directly* related to policy and programming relevant to pregnant and parenting teens. The impetus for many of these programs and policies stems from three cultural myths including *abstinence education is the best way to prevent teen pregnancy*, *better outcomes are achieved when teen mothers live with their own mothers*, and *it is better for teens and their babies if biological parents marry*. Acceptance of these, and other, cultural myths has led to policies that provided funds for "abstinence-only" programs, required teen mothers to reside with their parents in order to receive government aid, and have blindly prescribed marriage as the answer to teen pregnancy. In contrast to programs and policies founded on cultural myths and misperceptions, Chapter 7 provides an innovative systems perspective for reworking policy based on an integration of research evidence, program evaluation, and developmental theory.

Chapter 8 begins with the evaluation of the tenth and final cultural myth, *teen pregnancy costs taxpayers lots of money*. We believe this is an overarching cultural myth that drives the relevance of the previous myths to the interest of society. The chapter concludes with an overarching reframing of all ten cultural myths in a way that more accurately captures reality. In doing so, our goal is not to give the impression that we promote teen pregnancy as an ideal pathway. As developmentalists, we value the growth that occurs during adolescence and hope that youths will postpone parenting until they have had an opportunity for experiences and maturation free of the responsibilities of parenting. Our aim is simply to present a realistic perspective in which we advocate for teen pregnancy prevention but recognize that once a teen pregnancy occurs the outcomes are much better if the teens and their children are appropriately supported, rather than discriminated against. We advocate for this by providing recommendations in Chapter 8 for ways that future programs and policies can use evidence to combine teen pregnancy prevention efforts with the provision of appropriate supports for teen parents. Our goal is to shed light on these common beliefs, dispel cultural myths and misperceptions to the extent supported by evidence, and provide as clear a message as possible, so that the field can move ahead in a realistic manner that is informed by evidence rather than by misperceptions.

The preconceived (and often misperceived) notions evidenced in these ten cultural myths, and how they influence what we know about teen mothers, may be best illustrated through the experiences of Leon Dash, a reporter for the *Washington Post* who won a Pulitzer Prize for his series on teen pregnancy. Dash began his investigation of the high rates of pregnancy among urban, Black teens committed to the idea that the pregnancies were unintended and unwanted. His beliefs were initially reinforced as the teens he interviewed shared their personal experiences.

Dash persisted in his investigations through eight months of immersion into the urban ghetto. Over time, he reversed his initial beliefs after the teens shed their "adopted versions" of events they had invented in an attempt to conform to his expectations. Dash writes, "Months after the parents had told me the adopted version [of how they got pregnant], they would contradict themselves, admitting that the first story had been untrue ... In the end, I discovered that not a single one had become pregnant out of ignorance or by accident" (Dash, p. 31). Dash goes on to write convincingly of adolescent males who consider it a "badge of honor" to father one or more children, of girls as young as 13 who believe having a child will give them adult status and respect, and of mothers of older teens who worry that "something may be wrong" with their children who have not yet had children. His experience illustrates our thesis that it is time to take a new look at teen pregnancy and teen parenting by removing the filters through which we have come to view these constructs. Only when we can step aside from cultural myths and misperceptions, and instead acknowledge the lived experiences of these youths, does it become possible to develop and implement relevant and effective ways by which society can help youth avoid unwanted pregnancies and care for the children they create. Our identification and rethinking of the predominant cultural myths surrounding teen pregnancy and teen parenting are an effort to take this step, which can help not only the teens and their families, but also society as a whole.

Acknowledgements

This book would not be possible without the ongoing input of the participants of the NDAPP. We are grateful to the young mothers, their children, and their families who worked with us over the years and taught us about the realities of teen parenthood. The resources and support from the Center for Child and Family Studies at the University of Notre Dame, including the faculty, staff, and students, were invaluable. This project was also made possible by ongoing support from the Eunice Kennedy Shriver National Institute of Child Health and Human Development, which generously supported our study with grant funding over the course of more than two decades.

1 A systems perspective on myths and misperceptions

> With few exceptions, media stories, professional discourse, and advocacy organizations portray teen mothers as irresponsible and inept parents whose lives are forever derailed by parenting.
>
> (SmithBattle, 2013, p. 1)

Controversy exists in both the scientific and popular literature about traits and characteristics possessed by young parents. News articles have portrayed teen parents as selfish, apathetic, and immoral (Bales and O'Neil, 2008), and as welfare dependent and coming from troubled backgrounds (Kelly, 1996). Service providers, the media, and researchers (Breheny & Stephens, 2007a; 2007b) further ascribe traits and characteristics to pregnant and parenting teens that constrain their future potential and the potential of their children. In contrast, popular culture often counters these negative perceptions and depicts teen parents as motivated and resourceful (Murphy, 2012).

In addition to controversy over personal characteristics possessed by teen parents, causes of teen parenthood have also been disputed. News media often imply that teen pregnancies result from poor choices made by teens without consideration of broader social issues that may contribute to early pregnancy (Bales and O'Neil, 2008). Advocacy groups may further reinforce the placing of responsibility for teen pregnancy and its consequences on the teens themselves by decontextualizing informative statistics in their fact sheets and brochures. For example, a recent brochure published by the National Campaign to Prevent Teen and Unplanned Pregnancy stated, "38% of teen girls who have a child before age 18 get a high school diploma by age 22" (Ng and Kaye, 2012). This pronouncement implies that dropping out of school is caused by teen parenthood. Poverty, academic struggles, family instability, and other contextual factors that preceded childbearing are glossed over as contributors to school leaving. Focusing blame on inadequacies in the characters of teen parents diverts attention from the multiple social and cultural contexts that propel teens towards a path of early childbearing (SmithBattle, 2013).

Stereotyped perceptions of pregnant and parenting teens are not limited to media stories and professional discourse. The pervasiveness of negative stereotypes extends to the general public. Our recent survey of undergraduates from two public universities in the southeastern United States, some of whom are contemporaries of teen parents, confirmed that many college students, most under the age of 25, held cold and unfavorable feelings about pregnant and parenting teens. These cold and unfavorable feelings were associated with disparaging attitudes about competencies of teen parents and their children (Weed, Nicholson, and Richter, 2013).

Stereotyped perceptions and misperceptions may lead to more generalized beliefs about the causes and consequences of teen pregnancy and parenting. To the extent that these beliefs are shared among people within a culture they become *cultural myths*. Cultural myths are widely held beliefs that are assumed by many to be true. However, they are unfounded, as they have not been subjected to rigorous scrutiny to determine whether they are based on an objective reality in contrast to their socially constructed meaning.

Through our first-hand experience with teen mothers, and extensive reviews of scholarly and popular literature, we identified ten cultural myths surrounding teen pregnancy and parenting that we have listed in Table 1.1. These cultural myths address the causes and consequences of teen pregnancy for the teens themselves, their children, and society more generally. We do not claim that these are the only cultural myths, or even the most important. Rather, these are cultural myths that have produced considerable discourse and debate in both the popular and scholarly spheres. After carefully subjecting each of these ten cultural myths to rigorous scrutiny, we concluded that many are based on misperceptions with little basis in reality. Some aspects of several myths did stand up to empirical analysis, suggesting that common beliefs may be founded, in part, on the reality of teen pregnancy and parenting. Our overarching goal was not to simply discredit the cultural myths, but rather to reframe each to more closely align with the lived experience of pregnant and parenting teens.

Cultural myths about teen parents have been shaped by multiple, interacting messages accumulated over many years. Although some messages may be consistent with reality, other messages have been exaggerated, or even falsified, perhaps to serve a regulatory function for society. Our purpose in writing this book is to critically evaluate evidence surrounding each of these ten cultural myths to disentangle misperceptions from the reality of teen pregnancy and parenting. Our goal is not to dismiss the idea that teen childbearing should be avoided, but rather to provide a more informed and accurate perspective on issues surrounding teen pregnancy and parenting. Only by separating the misperceptions from the realities will we be able to craft policies and programs that adequately address the underlying causes of teen childbearing and provide appropriate supports for young people who embark on this nonnormative pathway.

In the chapters that follow, we analyze both the process of social construction that frames teen pregnancy and parenting as problematic (Duncan, 2007; Macleod, 2011), and the reality of early childbearing as observed through the lens of scientific methodology. We agree with the following observation that:

It is also possible to point to the ways in which teenage pregnancy has been constructed as a problem while, at the same time, recognizing that it might be a problem but one distorted in everyday representations and magnified out of proportion. Just because something can be seen to be socially constructed as a problem, it does not necessarily mean it does not exist as a problem or cannot be problematic.

(Arai, 2009a, p. 111)

We believe the crux of the problem, and the key to the solution, lies squarely within the interplay between the social construction of teen parenting as problematic and the actual challenges entailed in teen pregnancy. The social construction of teen parenting as problematic perpetuates negative stereotypes and focuses blame on the young people themselves. This negative social construction, in turn, may become a self-fulfilling prophecy if it contributes to additional challenges and consequences for teen parents and their children. A first step towards improving outcomes may be to replace the problematic social construction with one that acknowledges the multiple, interactive contextual forces that lead to teen pregnancy and parenting. Extricating misperceptions from realities requires the consideration of the contextual elements that may be impacting teens on multiple levels. Therefore, we have chosen a systems perspective to approach our discussion of the cultural myths and misperceptions surrounding teen pregnancy and parenting.

We begin by describing the basic assumptions of general systems theory, and then apply one example of a systems perspective, Bronfenbrenner's bioecological systems theory (Bronfenbrenner and Ceci, 1994), to a hypothetical illustration of two teen parents. Bronfenbrenner's theory provides a framework to organize the multiple contextual factors that collectively impact teen pregnancy and parenthood. The developmental status of teens is an important core component of this systems approach, and we provide a brief overview of changes occurring during this time of life. Following our application of a systems perspective to help explain the contexts of teen pregnancy, we recycle general systems theory

Table 1.1 Ten myths about teen pregnancy and parenting

Cultural myths	Chapter
Providing media visibility of pregnant or parenting teens will encourage others to become pregnant.	3
Most pregnant teens have behavior problems.	4
All teen pregnancies are unintended and unwanted.	4
Parenthood derails the trajectories of the teens' lives.	5
Teen pregnancies result in poor birth outcomes.	6
Children of teen parents will experience cognitive delay and adjustment problems, and will themselves become teen parents.	6
Abstinence education is the best way to prevent teen pregnancy.	7
Better outcomes are achieved when teen mothers live with their own mothers.	7
It is better for teens and their babies if biological parents marry.	7
Teen pregnancy costs taxpayers lots of money.	8

as a tool that helps explain the construction of teen pregnancy and parenting as a social problem. Within this systems framework, we summarize potential functions of cultural myths and suggest processes that maintain them despite evidence to the contrary. We end this chapter by explaining the importance of rethinking cultural myths and misperceptions to provide better support for teen parents and their children, with consequences extending to society more generally.

Teen pregnancy and parenting in context: a systems perspective

The word *system* invokes many different images. One may picture physiological systems, weather systems, hydraulic systems, or ecological systems. What these disparate constructs share is a set of interrelated elements that work together to achieve a specific outcome. Although the outcome of a weather system (e.g., a hurricane) may be entirely different from the outcome of a hydraulic system (e.g., deceleration in a vehicle), each outcome only occurs as a result of multiple, interacting elements, each with its own set of properties. The hurricane or deceleration that results from the complex interactive processes of these systems shares few properties with the elements that combined to produce it. A hurricane would not be predicted by examining the isolated characteristics of either warm water or moist warm air, two elements essential to the emergence of a hurricane. Neither element in isolation has much direct impact on the formation of a hurricane; it is only when the two elements interact in a specific manner that a hurricane is created. Therefore, the outcome of any system is conceptualized as an emergent property of elements as they interact. Perhaps Aristotle said it best: "the whole is greater than the sum of its parts."

Societal, family, and individual factors, if considered separately, provide an incomplete and distorted explanation of why teens become parents and how best to prevent or delay teen pregnancies. Despite the value of applying a systems perspective, teen pregnancy and parenting has seldom been examined from a holistic perspective (see Jurich and Myers-Bowman, 1998, and Pedrosa, Pires, Carvalho, Canavarro, and Dattilio, 2011, for exceptions). As an example of how a systems approach may provide a more complete perspective on teen pregnancy, we begin with a hypothetical story of two teen parents, Claire and Jeremy, as viewed through the lens of bioecological systems theory (Bronfenbrenner, 1977; Bronfenbrenner and Ceci, 1994). Their story sheds light on how multiple interacting elements in the lives of any young person may interact to lead to teen pregnancy and parenting, but each provides incomplete information if viewed independently. This conceptualization contrasts sharply from a more traditional, mechanistic perspective that considers teen pregnancy and parenting as a result of character flaws or poor decision-making of individual teens.

Claire was the 14-year-old daughter of a fundamentalist pastor who became pregnant by the 15-year-old "boy next door." Claire and Jeremy were forced by their families into an early marriage so their child would not be born "out-of-wedlock," and Claire moved in with Jeremy's family. It wasn't long before their endearing puppy love turned into frustration and anger, followed by a chilling indifference. Claire's vibrant, outgoing, gentle spirit gradually transformed into one of hostility and bitterness, while Jeremy became increasingly withdrawn from both Claire and the baby. The couple tried to do the best they could for their baby as their marriage crumbled. Their newborn baby was pulled between his teen mom and grandma. Although Jeremy's mother was only trying to help, Claire often felt as though she was not given the chance to be the mother she knew she could be. As relationships with both Jeremy and his mother became increasingly strained, Claire went to live on her own when she turned 18. She took the baby, filed for divorce, and left broken hearts and a broken home behind.

Bioecological systems theory

The curious reader may be interested in the backgrounds of Claire and Jeremy that contributed to their youthful parenthood. Bioecological systems theory (Bronfenbrenner and Ceci, 1994) is a framework that organizes nested causal forces into a series of concentric rings that surround a person. Rings closest to the individual represent proximal or direct influences while rings further away include more distal or indirect influences. The impact of elements with any of the systems may be both *individualistic* and *synergistic*. An individualistic impact occurs when a functional relationship can be identified between any individual element and a specific outcome. For example, accessibility of effective contraception may be related to fewer teen births. Consistent with systems thinking, however, most outcomes result from the synergistic combination of elements. In other words, rates of teen births are seldom attributed to any one factor that acts alone. Accessible contraception may not have much impact if teens lack knowledge about its use or avoid its use due to self-perceptions inconsistent with sexual activity. As this simple example shows, accessibility of contraception interacts synergistically with knowledge and personal beliefs to impact use. This interactive effect may occur within or between any of the nested levels.

The broadest, outermost ring of Bronfenbrenner's model is called the *macrosystem* and includes social and gender norms, cultural expectations, and political and economic trends. Simply put, the macrosystem describes the overarching beliefs and ideals of society. Many aspects of the macrosystem have implications for understanding teen pregnancy and parenting. For example, many cultures hold implicit assumptions that young people will at some point in their lives marry and have children, typically in that order. *Fertility-timing norms* are basic cultural expectations that dictate appropriate ages to begin childbearing that will lead to economic and reproductive success (Geronimus, 2003). Deviation from these social and cultural norms is expected to lead to adverse outcomes, and implies, at best, an attitude of unconventionality and, at worst, lack of adherence to moral standards.

The *macrosystem* surrounding Claire and Jeremy contained some elements that suppressed the likelihood of a teen pregnancy, but other elements that fostered early pregnancy. Although cultural norms for the sequence and timing of role transitions are changing (Billari and Liefbroer, 2010), Claire and Jeremy were both raised with beliefs that marriage should precede pregnancy and that couples should wait until well into their twenties, or at least until their education is complete, to begin childbearing. The expectation of abstinence until marriage was emphasized by their families, church, and school. In addition, Claire was raised to respect her own mother and acknowledged the esteem and value granted by society to mothers more generally. She often empathized with Mary, the young mother of Jesus, and imagined how she must have felt when she realized she was pregnant. Claire's yearning for the prestige associated with being a mother was enhanced by the lack of clarity society affords to teens regarding adult status. Claire and Jeremy had limited access to adult rights and privileges, yet bodies sufficiently mature to allow for reproduction. Finally, a shaky economy left both Claire and Jeremy feeling uncertain about their chances of future career success, diminishing their motivation to continue their education beyond high school. Despite the values instilled in Claire and Jeremy about sexual activity, their high regard for parenthood in combination with their desire to achieve adult status may have created ambiguity about integrating somewhat incongruent macrosystem messages. These elements within the macrosystem of Claire and Jeremy interacted in ways that led to ambivalence about the possibility of pregnancy, and hesitancy to use birth control due to its incompatibility with expectations of abstinence.

Exosystem forces are embedded within the macrosystem and are concrete manifestations of macrosystem ideology (Bronfenbrenner, 1977). For example, macrosystem ideology informs how government dollars are spent, and to what extent provision of birth control, abortion, and sexual health information may be provided to teens. The exosystem includes institutions with which Claire and Jeremy were not directly involved, but that impinged on their lives nonetheless. Exosystem elements included their parents' work environments, and the school board that administered local educational policy, including how to approach sex education and birth control issues. Mass media, in the forms of television shows, videos, and the Internet, as well as community and public health programs, were also important contributors to their exosystem.

Examination of the exosystem of the young couple revealed that both Claire's and Jeremy's parents worked full time, so the teens were often unsupervised after school until their parents arrived home around 5:30 or 6 p.m. The local recreation center offered after-school programming that Claire enjoyed when she was younger, but as she became older she considered the games and crafts too childish, and stopped attending. She typically finished her homework during study hall and preferred to spend time with Jeremy after school, often with the TV tuned to reality shows or dramas about teen parents (e.g., *Teen Mom* and *16 and Pregnant*). Although Claire and Jeremy were curious about sex they were reluctant to bring up the subject with their parents and received little guidance from teachers at school. The school board imposed regulations that schools were to limit sex education to the biological aspects of reproduction and not to provide students information about, or access to, birth control. Finally, the local health department provided an array of reproductive health services to teens, but was only open from 9 to 5 Monday through Friday, making it difficult for Claire and Jeremy to access services without their absences from school being questioned by administration and their parents. Since neither Claire nor Jeremy were old enough to drive, transportation to the health department also made discreet access difficult.

Elements within the exosystem had both individualistic and synergistic impacts. For instance, unstructured and unsupervised time between the end of school and parents' return home from work created opportunities for Claire and Jeremy to engage in sexual activity. In addition, the belief of the school board that abstinence education combined with silence regarding birth control would stop teenagers from thinking about sex or becoming sexually active failed to consider the constant images of teen sexuality portrayed on television and in the movies, and so this philosophy was counterproductive. Unsupervised after-school time may be an important independent risk factor for teen pregnancy, but the availability of private time may also interact synergistically with sexual attitudes informed by media-viewing during this time to impact actual sexual behavior.

The innermost ring of bioecological systems theory is the *microsystem*. This system includes the important settings or contexts that comprise the daily lives of individuals. In contrast to the exosystem, the microsystem includes the settings where lives are lived on a daily basis. Analysis of microsystem elements involves consideration of physical features of the settings, activities, and roles of people within these settings. Microsystems of most teenagers today include their families, peer groups, and schools. Religious settings, sports, and extracurricular activities are also important parts of the micosystem of many teenagers.

An analysis of Claire's microsystem prior to her pregnancy provides a picture of the different settings that may have directly or indirectly impacted her risk for becoming pregnant. Consistent with each systematic level, some elements of the microsystem directly foster teen pregnancy risk, while others suppress risk, and others interact synergistically. Claire lived with her mother, father, and two older sisters in a typical suburban subdivision. As the youngest child she had few responsibilities around the house, and her parents often assumed her older sisters would talk with Claire about boys and the importance of maintaining her virginity until marriage. Claire used to be good friends with three other girls from her school, but stopped spending time with them when Jeremy came into the picture. The school where Claire attended 9th grade had approximately 1,200 students and drew from five different middle schools in the area. She was enrolled in a family life class and was anticipating her turn at caring for a "Baby Think it Over" doll that simulates caring for a real infant. The family attended church regularly where her father was the pastor, and Claire was actively involved with youth group programs. Jeremy started attending church with the family since it was a way to spend more time with Claire. Claire had been a cheerleader in middle school, but didn't make the squad in her new high school.

A similar analysis of Jeremy's microsystem prior to the pregnancy revealed different elements that may have predicted his early parenthood. He lived with his mother, her boyfriend, an older brother and younger sister, and sometimes with two younger step-siblings. His house was in a run-down neighborhood in a poor section of town. Jeremy had a good relationship with his 21-year-old brother and often spent time with him and his friends. When he was with his brother, he sometimes drank beer and smoked marijuana. Sex was a frequent topic of conversation, and Jeremy learned quite a bit about sexual behavior from listening to the exploits of his older brother and his friends. Jeremy worked part time after school and some weekends to get a little extra spending money.

Elements within the microsystems of Claire and Jeremy, including their relationships with their parents and siblings, peer groups, school activities, and church youth group, all exerted powerful forces on their attitudes and behaviors related to sexuality and pregnancy. For example, the anonymity Claire felt at her new high school loosened some of the constraints she had perceived while in middle school where everyone knew her by name and would report her behavior back to her parents. Jeremy felt embarrassed about his lack of sexual experiences or stories to share when he hung out with his older friends.

Connections among elements within the microsystems of the young couple, and between elements in the microsystems and elements from the other systems, constitute what Bronfenbrenner (1977) called the *mesosystem*. This system does not include a new level or ring, but rather encompasses links that exist among elements of the microsystems and exosystems. Systems tend to function more effectively if elements are strongly connected; loosely connected elements are associated with dysfunction and alienation (Bronfenbrenner, 1986). Review of the elements within both Claire's and Jeremy's microsystems and exosystems revealed few and weak connections between elements. Both sets of parents were minimally involved in the educational or social activities of their children. The school was large and generally uninvolved with noneducational aspects of students' lives. The health department provided needed services, but was unconnected to the school. The weak connections among elements in the micro- and exosystems of Claire and Jeremy thereby increased the likelihood of early pregnancy.

Across these different contextual systems, changes over time may also contribute to the risk for teen pregnancy. This element of Bronfenbrenner's model, the *chronosystem*, reflects chronological and historical influences that can have an impact at any or all of the nested levels. For example, the *second demographic transition* refers to the sequence and timing of role transitions that are currently affecting many developed countries (Billari and Liefbroer, 2010; Lesthaeghe, 2010). Examples of the second demographic transition include increased age at first marriage, expectations of cohabitation prior to marriage, increased age at first parenthood, higher rates of parenthood outside of marriage, and greater tolerance of deviations from developmental timing norms. For example, in the United States the age at first childbirth rose from 21.4 years of age in 1970 to 25.6 years in 2011. Perhaps even more striking, in 1980, only 18.4 percent of children were born to unmarried parents, but in 2011, 40.7 percent of all children were born to unmarried parents (Martin, Hamilton, Ventura, Osterman, and Matthews, 2013).

The impact of this chronosystem transition on rates of teen pregnancy and parenting remains to be seen. On one hand, as parenthood outside of marriage becomes more normative, along with reduced pressure to conform to age-related expectations for behavior, stigma associated with teen parenting may diminish.

However, as more young adults postpone parenthood, the age gap between teen parents and the typical parent increases, leading to greater demarcation between teen and adult parents. This later trend may have been reflected in responses to our recent survey in which a sample of college students endorsed negative feelings towards pregnant and parenting teens (Weed *et al.*, 2013).

Individual factors

In his later writing, Bronfenbrenner (Bronfenbrenner and Ceci, 1994) elaborated how individual characteristics, including developmental changes, may interact with system elements to sway attitudes and behaviors. The "bio" component of Bronfenbrenner's bioecological model directs attention to the individual situated at the core of the nested ecological systems. These individual-level influences, including critical developmental processes that occur during the teen years (e.g., puberty) and the mid-twenties, are especially important to consider in the context of teen pregnancy and parenting. Understanding teen pregnancy and parenting from a systems perspective requires integration of these individual developmental factors with other system components, including the micro-, meso-, exo-, macro-, and chronosystems.

Framing issues surrounding early pregnancy and childbearing under the umbrella of *teen* pregnancy and parenting provides a convenient demarcation to differentiate acceptable from unacceptable reproduction (i.e., it is acceptable to have a baby at age 20, but not at age 19), but this distinction between teen and adult is unfounded and does not consider important developmental changes (Rhode and Lawson, 1993). Although chronological age is typically used as a marker for developmental processes, psychosocial maturity or age at puberty may be a more reliable indicator due to the considerable individual differences between young people in maturational processes. Further complexities in defining the boundaries of adolescence arise due to developmental changes within the endocrine system and the central nervous system, and how these biological changes interact with societal expectations based on age. The following section provides a brief review of changes within the endocrine and central nervous systems as well as changes triggered by societal expectations.

Two components of the endocrine system kick-start physiological changes that propel children into adolescence. Physical maturation of the hypothalamic–pituitary–adrenal (HPA) axis results in biochemical changes that lead to feelings of sexual attraction (Dahl, 2004), while maturation of the hypothalamic–pituitary–gonadal (HPG) axis triggers development of primary and secondary sex characteristics associated with puberty that make reproduction possible. Cross-cultural evidence suggests that these hormonal changes are occurring at increasingly earlier ages, referred to as the *secular trend*. For example, the average age that US teens start to menstruate was estimated at 12.43 in 2010, down from 12.77 in 1973, and somewhat earlier than teens in Europe, estimated at age 13 (Chumlea *et al.*, 2003). In the United States, just under 50 percent of Black girls in one study had begun to experience pubertal changes by age 8 and 50 percent of White girls by age 9.5 (Herman-Giddens *et al.*, 1997). This early onset of endocrine maturation implies that the physical changes that transform boys and girls into young men and women capable of reproduction is occurring at younger ages, in turn leading to adult-like appearances, thoughts about sex, and sexualized attention in some pre-teens as young as age 11 or 12, or even earlier.

Important developmental changes are also occurring in the brains of young people (Casey, Jones, and Hare, 2008; Gogtay et al., 2004; Steinberg, 2010). Evidence from neuroimaging studies reveals a time of exuberant neural growth within the cortex of the brain during the early teen years. This initially unrestrained growth gets pruned back over an extended period based on the life experiences of the teen, ending during the mid-twenties. This process is believed to provide an important adaptive function that allows the physical structure of the brain to become fine-tuned to demands of the adult environment, provided that these adult demands are embedded in the activities the youth engages in while the brain is undergoing its remarkable transition (Giedd, 2008).

Related to these neuronal changes, distinct functional parts of the brain are learning to communicate more effectively (Casey et al., 2008). One of the more obvious communication channels is between the limbic system of the brain, which processes emotions, and the prefrontal cortex, involved in logical thought processes. If communication breaks down between these structures, emotions tend to be unrestrained. In addition, the myelination process, which increases the speed and efficiency of neural communication and has been ongoing throughout childhood, nears completion by the mid-twenties. Implications of these maturational changes within the brain include the potential for thinking more logically and abstractly, and applying these abilities to understand oneself, other people, and relationships between people.

In contrast to hormonal systems that have been maturing at increasingly younger ages, there is no evidence that brain maturation has shown a corresponding acceleration. Rather, evidence suggests a gradual strengthening of neural connections that continues well into the twenties. The lack of synchrony in developmental processes among the hormonal and neurological systems may create inconsistencies and confusion for youths and adults. For example, Atwood and Kasindorf (1992) emphasized how messages delivered within the multiple contexts of most adolescents were "full of competing demands, inconsistent expectations, and more messages of don't than do's" (p. 345). When faced with these competing demands about behavior, teens need to integrate thoughts, feelings, values, and actions; however, in many cases teens respond as inconsistently as the messages they receive. From a systems perspective, this inconsistent behavior of teens may trigger a feedback mechanism aimed at achieving homeostasis and regulating behavior (Atwood and Kasindorf, 1992). In other words, inconsistencies in the behavior of teens create social prohibitions against risky behaviors.

The term *teenage* reinforces the idea of an imaginary wall that segregates children from adults (Macleod, 2011), but physiological changes in the endocrine and neurological systems imply that the stage of adolescence is more than just a social construction. Physiological changes combined with social expectations based on age create a unique patterning of thoughts and behaviors that lead to a different experience of parenting at a young age when compared to parenting at an older age. A full understanding of the role transition involved in becoming a parent requires attention to developmental processes and to individual differences in these processes, acknowledging the considerable variability that exists within any developmental process.

Many teens are well aware of a boundary that sets them apart from being adults. In response to survey questions about when people first thought of themselves as adults, some people pointed to specific turning points in their lives, such as becoming a parent, establishing their own residence, or completing their education and beginning a full-time job. Others suggested psychosocial factors such as responsibility for themselves and others, autonomous decision-making, and financial independence (Benson and Elder, 2011; Hartmann and Swartz, 2006). Significant role transitions or turning points may elicit more mature behavior, propelling young people to identify themselves as adults rather than teens or adolescents. Becoming a parent, for example, entails increased responsibility, budgeting skills, and competent decision-making.

Considerable individual differences exist in the age at which people make the transition from perceiving themselves as adolescents to perceiving themselves as adults and taking on adult responsibilities. For example, 31 percent of approximately 7,000 young adults, aged 18 to 22, from a nationally representative sample in the United States were classified as *early adults* based on both a high level of psychosocial maturity and self-perceptions of feeling older than their chronological age (Benson and Elder, 2011). These *early adults* were more likely than other youth to be Black, to come from disadvantaged backgrounds, and to have been raised by a single parent. In addition, *early adults* reached puberty sooner than other youth, took on responsibility for household tasks, and had high self-esteem. Although *early adults* reported somewhat earlier initiation into sexual activity, this was not associated with delinquency or other maladaptive outcomes. Results emphasized that chronological age was an inadequate marker of adult status. Instead, a pattern of characteristics, including early puberty, household responsibilities, and self-perceptions, interacted synergistically to propel some to adulthood while still in their teen years, while other teens persisted in an adolescent stage well into their twenties (Benson and Elder, 2011).

Individual factors in addition to developmental status (e.g., personality, self-regulation) may also interact with other system elements to impact teen pregnancy and parenting. For example, recent genetic research has identified specific genes that mediate how reactive a child is to environmental conditions (Ellis and Boyce, 2011). Additional research is beginning to clarify how adverse environmental conditions may become embedded in the genetic and biological makeup of a child, especially during the prenatal period (Roth and Sweatt, 2011). Models are just beginning to integrate factors within all six systems (i.e., macro-, exo-, micro-, meso-, and chronosystems as well as individual factors) to obtain a more complete understanding of teen pregnancy and parenting (Atwood and Kasindorf, 1992). This integration is essential to understanding the reality of teen pregnancy and parenthood.

Constructing cultural myths

The story of Claire and Jeremy provides one example of how assumptions from a systems perspective may help in conceptualizing the multiple competing factors related to teen pregnancy and parenting. Assumptions of systems theory may also be applied to how teen pregnancy and parenthood have been socially constructed as problematic. Perceptions and misperceptions of pregnant and parenting teens are often a result of a social construction process that can be viewed in terms of systems thinking (Murcott, 1980). Examination of the social construction of myths from a systems perspective requires specification of critical elements and their interaction. Geronimus (2003) specified several of these elements in the following quote:

> Representatives of the dominant group have use of the public stage – through control of the media, advocacy organizations, political campaigns, the legis-lative process, public school curricula, scientific research funding, and pub-lishing – to broadcast the social control message intended for their children that cultural competence requires the postponement of childbearing.
>
> (p. 888)

A systems perspective suggests that multiple sources, including the media, edu-cation, and research, interact in ways that can lead to misperceptions about teen pregnancy and parenting. These misperceptions may then become transformed into broader cultural myths embedded in the macrosystem. Macrosystem beliefs shape policy and practice at the exosystem level, and individual and family atti-tudes at the microsystem level; all of these factors influence the actions and out-comes of individuals. We return to the story of Claire and Jeremy to illustrate how the social construction of cultural myths and misperceptions may influence the reactions of society, friends, and family, and consequently impact outcomes for the young parents and their child.

As we begin, consider the reaction of Jeremy's mother when she discovered the pregnancy. *Wilma was in a state of shock after hearing from her son, Jeremy, that his girlfriend was pregnant. Random thoughts raced through her mind, "But I'm too young to be a grandmother. How could this be? Claire was such a nice girl who came from a good, Christian family. What about their college plans? Their lives will be ruined! They should have known better, they are much too young to be having sex. Is abortion an option? What if the baby is born with disabilities? How can I keep friends and neighbors from finding out?" After a few minutes, Wilma took a couple of deep breaths, steadied herself, and tried to collect her thoughts. She realized that this pregnancy was going to alter not only her life, but the lives of her son, his girlfriend, and their families, friends, and neighbors. She also realized that things had changed since she had her own children. She had a lot to learn about what it was like to be pregnant today, and the type of sup-ports available.*

Wilma's reaction is typical of many parents. Initial thoughts are triggered from beliefs constructed over a lifetime of exposure to information received from many different sources. The family context often provides the foundation for beliefs about many social issues, including teen pregnancy. Portrayals of pregnant and parenting teens on television shows and in the movies are compared and contrasted with messages received from family and social contexts such as church. Observations of, and interactions with, friends, neighbors, and even family members who were pregnant as teens inform perceptions and misperceptions. These experiences create a cognitive template that reflects perceived characteristics of typical pregnant and parenting teens.

This template serves as a filter through which subsequent observations are viewed. New experiences, filtered through existing templates, may be misperceived and misunderstood. Ideally, new exposures and insights gradually broaden and refine initial beliefs, shaping them over time to become closer to an ultimate truth. Rarely is this ideal realized, and more often than not, aspects of new experiences that fail to conform to initial perceptions are simply discarded or discounted, leaving original views intact, a process known as *biased assimilation* (Lord, Ross, and Lepper, 1979; Munro, Stansbury, and Tsai, 2012). As this process is repeated, perceptions gradually become misperceptions. When a sufficient number of others share these misperceptions, they may become cultural myths. Integration over time of verbal and visual messages received from diverse sources may result in strongly held beliefs about the nature of teen pregnancy and parenthood.

As Wilma reacted to Jeremy's news, her thoughts reflected what she believed to be an essential truth about relationships in society. She believed that becoming pregnant as an unmarried teen, or fathering a child as an unmarried teen, violated a critical social convention and would bring embarrassment and disgrace to the young couple, their families, and the unborn child. Instead of a bright future with many opportunities, Wilma believed that early parenthood would doom the young couple to future struggle and hardship. These essential truths that people hold about relationships are considered within a constructivist approach as *social facts* that are generated by societies to establish and maintain the social order (Durkheim, 1960).

A constructivist approach suggests that knowledge is never entirely objective; rather, knowledge is filled with meanings and interpretations derived from social consensus that may be somewhat removed from objective reality (i.e., social facts). For example, a social fact may be the belief that Claire, or any teen who has a child, has ruined her own life and has doomed her child to a life of poverty and hardship. Durkheim (1960) believed that social facts have distinctive characteristics and determinants independent of underlying biological or psychological processes. Once social facts are generated they acquire a degree of substance independent of reality that leads to their perpetuation from generation to generation. Social facts, like cultural myths, are beliefs held by social groups in the absence of evidence attesting to their authenticity. Further, social facts serve as external constraints that channel and direct thoughts and behaviors, and are associated with consequences for violating their expectations. For instance, Geronimus (2003) argued that the provision of social support to new parents is contingent upon meeting culturally derived standards for appropriate ages and circumstances of childbearing. Social facts are used to regulate systems and control behaviors of individuals within groups. For example, the threat of exclusion from family and community provides one mechanism for stigmatizing teen pregnancy as a way to maintain social control.

Functions of cultural myths

Dake (1992) built on the groundwork of Durkheim's approach and suggested that cultural myths are socially constructed and maintained in order to preserve the status quo for society. Situations, events, or relationships that threaten the social order need constraints to curtail their eroding of the social fabric. Societal threats associated with teen parenting may include an undermining of family values, intensification of economic hardships, or shifts in the balance of family and political power to women or minorities. Dake suggested that voicing these fears directly may invoke social or political censure, leading to the establishment of cultural myths that are more acceptable to acknowledge. Thus, cultural myths may be maintained despite contradictory or ambiguous evidence because they serve an important purpose in maintaining or regulating the established social order.

Several recent reviews have been published examining the social construction of teen pregnancy and parenting that are consistent with the work of Durkheim and Dake (Arai, 2009; Luker, 1996; Macleod, 2011; Nathanson, 1991). For instance, Macleod (2011) recently described the social construction process as a reaction to the perceived threat of degeneration in society as a consequence of teen pregnancy and parenting. Although we have tried to synthesize the fundamental assumptions of these works in the sections that follow, the interested reader may wish to peruse the original writings.

Our main proposition, continuing within this social constructivist framework, is that teen parents are perceived as a threat to societies: pregnant teens are perceived as a danger to themselves, their families, and broader society. Prior published support for this proposition is supplemented by our recent survey of undergraduates (Weed *et al.*, 2013). We asked students to "Imagine that the rate of teenage childbearing in the United States doubles in the next 10 years and at the same time the rate of childbearing to adult women decreases significantly." Respondents were then asked to select how likely 25 potential consequences would be, such as "The percentage of children living in poverty will increase." Results from our survey, combined with a review of constructivist publications, provided support for five distinct functions that cultural myths might serve by constraining the reproductive behavior of young men and women. In the section that follows, we briefly describe each of these five functions: provide a moral compass, safeguard the gene pool, sustain power of dominant groups, protect the public health, and bolster the economy. We contend that society is perpetuating these cultural myths, sometimes consciously but often unconsciously, in an effort to maintain the status quo and stabilize the established social order.

A moral compass

Cultural myths related to teen pregnancy and parenting may have been constructed and perpetuated in order to uphold the "moral fabric of society." Teen pregnancy and parenting, along with nonmarital childbearing, has long been credited with causing a moral panic due to the blatant sexuality of teens degrading the moral compass (Cohen, 1972; Nathanson, 1991; Selman, 2003). Historically, one strategy to guard against this moral degradation and restore the moral balance was the establishment of homes for "wayward" or "fallen" women, where pregnant teens could be removed from the attention of polite society. Florence Crittenton Homes were established in 1883 to provide sanctuary for unwed mothers who wanted to avoid public disgrace (Nathanson, 1991). The morality of teen sexuality faded into the background during the 1960s and 1970s, as social sanctions associated with teen sexual behavior waned, but was resurrected in the early 1980s with the passage of the Adolescent Family Life Act. This piece of legislation, referred to as the "chastity bill" (Saul, 1998), encouraged and funded abstinence-only prevention programs. Teen pregnancy was deemed morally offensive because it implied sexual activity of teens outside of a marital relationship. College students today continue to perceive teen childbearing as a threat to morality, with 66 percent of our survey respondents indicating that an increased rate of teen childbearing would be associated with a decline in the moral standards of youth, and 81 percent believing that nonmarital childbearing would become normative should rates of teen childbearing increase (Weed *et al.*, 2013).

Eugenics: safeguarding the gene pool

An equally salient social function, particularly during the end of the nineteenth and first part of the twentieth centuries, was to enhance the fitness of the gene pool (Ladd-Taylor, 2001; Paul, 1968; Ryan, 2007). Eugenics was a new science touted as an answer to the ills of society. Individuals thought to have better genes were encouraged to marry and produce offspring, while checks were put into place to control reproductive behaviors of people perceived as genetically unfit (Luker, 1996). As realization spread that the fertility rate was significantly greater among those living in poverty, social control strategies were enacted to avoid the inferred consequences that children born under these conditions would be genetically less fit and eventually undermine the gene pool, leading to the collapse of society (Ryan, 2007). Reformatories for promiscuous young women were established across the United States to segregate those perceived as less fit, often accompanied by forced sterilization.

During this time period, cultural myths were popularized as a first line of defense to guard against those perceived as less fit having children. For example, in 1920 Paul Popenoe, a noted eugenicist, wrote:

> The typical illegitimate child, then, may be said to be the offspring of a young mother of inferior status mentally, morally and economically; and of a

father who is probably a little superior to the mother in age, mentality, and economic status, if not in morals.

(As cited in Luker, 1996, p. 37)

This cultural myth has continued to infiltrate our beliefs about teen mothers irrespective of lack of evidence. For example, when asked in a 1965 Gallup Poll what should be done about unwed mothers who have more children, about one-half of Americans reportedly said, "stop giving them relief money," and one out of five answered, "sterilize the women" (Paul, 1968). More recently, 58 percent of college students responded that an increased need for special education services in schools would be a consequence of an increased rate of teen childbearing (Weed et al., 2013), implying that increases in teen pregnancy would be associated with the addition of genetically "unfit" children being born into society.

Power: gender and racial inequalities

A third social function served by the establishment of cultural myths surrounding teen pregnancy and childbearing is to maintain the dominant social status of White men (Luker, 1996). A feminist perspective suggests that granting women responsibility for their own sexuality and reproductive behaviors will erode the power base of men (Nathanson, 1991). The establishment of legislation to regulate the sexual and reproductive behavior of teens provides a target that both men and women may be able to agree on. Legislation targeting teens, however, cascades into restrictions on the sexual and reproductive behavior of women of all ages. Current controversies in the United States surrounding women's health in the Patient Protection and Affordable Care Act (ACA) provide a timely example of the tension surrounding controls over women's reproductive behavior.

Provisions of the ACA include mandates that insurance companies cover contraceptive costs, prohibit companies from considering pregnancy as a preexisting condition in order to deny women coverage, and prohibit differential premiums for men and women ("Turning to Fairness," 2012). As these provisions began to go into effect during 2012, a backlash of proposed legislation was generated to counter the changes. Much of this legislation stemmed from long-standing provisions that prohibited public money being used to fund abortions, except in cases of rape or incest. Since the ACA was a government program, it was reasoned that similar restrictive provisions should be applied to all insurance provided under the ACA. Bills were introduced to eliminate public funding for family planning and teen pregnancy prevention, and to restrict funding for contraception and abortion services ("Status of the Lawsuits," 2014).

The contentious debate came to a head during a recent House Oversight Committee hearing on contraception that included only men. Patty Murray, a US Democratic Senator who has become an outspoken advocate for women's reproductive rights, decried the absurdity of limiting the voice of women in the debate. Her response to the Committee hearing included the following comment:

> I'm sure by now many of my colleagues here have seen the picture of this all-male hearing. It's a picture that says a thousand words. And it's one that most women thought they left behind when pictures only came in black and white.
>
> ("Murray on Senate Floor," 2012)

The current debate over public funding for contraception may have roots in the long-standing tensions between men and women over reproductive behavior. An evolutionary perspective suggests that men and women adopt different reproductive strategies (Maccoby, 1991). Men's strategies include having a greater number of partners to increase their chances of passing along their genes. Because women are limited in the number of children they are able to produce, strategies typically involve ensuring high-quality partners. These differences in strategies play out in men's and women's reproductive behaviors, including use of contraception, consideration of abortion, and ultimately mate selection and childbearing. Women can control their reproductive strategy by being selective about their sexual partners, using birth control, and having the ability to choose whether or not to carry a pregnancy to term. Some of these strategies may be unobservable to men, such as use of the birth control pill or having an early abortion. This imperceptible ability to control reproduction may be perceived as a form of power women have over men. Perceived lack of power by men may lead to counterstrategies to gain control. At the extreme, these counterstrategies lead to rape and other forms of sexual abuse. More subtle means of achieving control are to limit access to birth control and abortion, leading to greater visibility of women's reproductive decisions.

Closely related to maintaining the social and political dominance of men is maintaining power to Whites (Luker, 1996). Macleod (2011) made the point that African *culture* is perceived by the dominant group as less desirable than the *way of life* maintained by Whites. Therefore, since rates of teen childbearing to Black teens in the United States are more than double the rates of White teen childbearing (43.9 per 1,000 versus 20.5 per 1,000 in 2012; Hamilton, Martin, and Ventura, 2013), the perceived expansion of the less desirable African culture may lead to degeneration of what is perceived as the more favorable way of life.

Public health

Cultural myths surrounding teen pregnancy and parenting may also have emerged as a response to a perceived threat to public health (Nathanson, 1991). Unprotected sexual activity leads to the spread of sexually transmitted infections (STIs) including HIV/AIDS. Teen pregnancies are the undeniable evidence that teens are sexually active without proper contraception. In addition, early and consistent prenatal care is promoted by public health professionals as the best

strategy to ensure healthy infant and child outcomes, but some teens delay initiation of prenatal care, perhaps out of anxiety about acknowledging the pregnancy
(Hueston, Geesey, and Diaz, 2008). Beliefs that teen pregnancy and parenting are
associated with increased rates of STIs and adverse birth outcomes may have led
to cultural myths designed to regulate the sexual activity of teens through scare
tactics. Ironically, anxieties created by the cultural myths themselves may actually reinforce the reality of these myths (Lawlor and Shaw, 2002). For example,
as we discuss in Chapter 6, high levels of pregnancy anxiety have been associated
with premature births.

Economics

Perhaps the most compelling social function of cultural myths is an economic
function. A stable economy is needed for society to exist harmoniously; anything
that threatens the economy is also a potential threat to the social order. A key
step in the 1960s' War on Poverty was to prevent nonmarital pregnancies. Family
planning was promoted as the single most cost-effective anti-poverty measure
(Luker, 1996). In the United States, teen pregnancy was publicly declared a
social problem in the mid-1970s with debate surrounding the proposed National
School-Age Mother and Child Health Act that stated:

> All of the experts agree that the birth of a child to a school-age parent has
> tremendous consequences to the mother, the father and the child itself.
> Pregnancy among school-age girls is the leading cause of high-school drop-
> out among girls, and imposes a terrible burden on the girl, as well as a social
> burden on society. And for about 60 percent of these girls, the birth of a child
> begins a cycle of dependency upon public welfare.
>
> (As cited in Luker, 1996, p. 71)

Recent campaigns highlighting the "costs of teen pregnancy" attempt to restore
economic and social stability by revealing how provisions and supports for teen
parents and their children are draining economic resources. For instance, the
Counting it Up campaign from the National Campaign to Prevent Teen and
Unplanned Pregnancy specified that national costs in 2010 included "$3.1 bil-
lion in increased child welfare costs" and "$2 billion in increased costs of incar-
ceration" for children born to teen mothers (Counting It Up, 2013). Implied
in these cost figures is the idea that since this money is being spent to address
problems caused by teen parenting, it is unavailable for more constructive uses.
In other words, by highlighting costs attributed to teen pregnancy these campaigns reinforce misperceptions that the teens themselves bear responsibility for
the economy. The cultural myth that teen mothers are a financial burden on
society places responsibility for the economic downturn squarely on the shoulders
of the most vulnerable members of society. This suggests that taxpayers are contributing to the support of pregnant and parenting teens who are in trouble due
to their thoughtlessness or poor choices. We return to the costs of teen pregnancy

in Chapter 8 with an evaluation of evidence related to costs. Perceived threats to the economy by increased teen childbearing were acknowledged by the college students who responded to our survey questions. Close to 75 percent believed that increases in the rate of teen childbearing would be associated with increases in poverty, and 67 percent indicated that increased rates of teen pregnancy would bring about an intensification of the economic downturn (Weed *et al.*, 2013).

Stability of cultural myths

The creation of cultural myths typically does not occur as a result of deliberate, conscious strategizing. Instead, cultural myths, as a means of social control, are more likely to gradually emerge over time due to spontaneous, unconscious processes resulting from the interactions of diverse peoples and social institutions. Once established, these myths take on a life of their own, acquiring a *dynamic stability* that resists day-to-day fluctuations in underlying attitudes, and may continue to exert social influence despite changes in the conditions that gave rise to their initial establishment. Myths are resistant to change, even though they may no longer serve the function for which they were established (Durkheim, 1960). Myths have been maintained in the political arena across changes to dominant political influence, as seen in both the United Kingdom and United States. Teen pregnancy and parenting has maintained its status as an important social issue in the United States since the early 1970s despite other important social, political, and economic issues. Teen pregnancy has remained a point of social concern despite competing issues including the welfare reform movements in 1996, economic downturn that began in 2008, increases in births to unmarried women of all ages, increased impact of terrorism, and exposure of significant corruption among business executives.

Rethinking cultural myths and misperceptions

Pregnant and parenting teens are faced not only with challenges associated with major role changes, but also with challenges due to negative stereotypes, misperceptions, and stigma. Widespread beliefs about pregnant and parenting teens have persisted and taken on the status of cultural myths. Many of these cultural myths and misperceptions have a kernel of truth. Our goal is to critically analyze cultural myths and misperceptions about teen pregnancy and parenting to discern where the kernels of truth lie. As Arai (2009a) stated, "ultimately the myth–reality gap on teenage pregnancy matters" (p. 52). The following chapters consider the gap between cultural myths and the actual experiences of pregnant and parenting teens. We rely on conclusions from empirical research considered in light of a systems perspective to reframe each cultural myth to better reflect actual evidence and experiences. Our intent to is provide useful information to teens, parents, educators, service providers, and policy-makers in identifying meaningful solutions for the challenges that often accompany teen pregnancy and parenting.

Each chapter features a case study of a pregnant or parenting teen. These stories are fictionalized accounts of real teens we have worked with during our own longitudinal research, teens we have known in our personal lives, or accounts of people in popular culture. We emphasize that these fictionalized accounts are not meant to represent typical teen parents. Despite stereotypes of characteristics associated with pregnant and parenting teens, these characteristics are just that: stereotypes. Classifying someone as a *teen parent* provides no information about causes or consequences of getting pregnant, maintaining the pregnancy, giving birth, or choosing to raise a child. Just as there are many reasons adults get pregnant and have children, so are there a myriad of reasons teens get pregnant and give birth, some intentional and some not.

Chapter 2 begins with a look behind the scenes as a teen mother responds to questions posed during a research interview. We revisit Claire and Jeremy in Chapter 3 to emphasize the role of popular culture in contributing to teen pregnancy. Chapter 4 highlights a teen pregnancy due to rape, and Chapter 5 features a teen from a disadvantaged background who has made the best of an unfortunate situation. Chapter 6 documents the contrast between two children born to teen mothers – one who achieved academic and social success while the other was unable to overcome multiple contextual forces. Prevention and intervention needs are showcased in Chapter 7. We will return to the story of Claire and Jeremy in Chapter 8 using our reframed version of each cultural myth to envision more optimal outcomes that may result from replacing myths based on misperceptions with beliefs based on actual experiences.

We believe that a meaningful conceptualization of teen pregnancy and parenting needs to consider developmental processes and specific societal expectations in the lives of young adults, juxtaposed with an in-depth understanding of how becoming a parent has the potential to transform lives. Cultural myths that may have arisen to control or regulate society obscure what may be happening in the lives and families of those who have experienced teen pregnancy and parenting. This tactic may draw attention away from where it needs to be placed and may play a role in the outcomes of a teen pregnancy. In other words, responses to teen pregnancy and parenting are based, in part, on salient cultural myths that may inadvertently perpetuate less than optimal outcomes. Rethinking cultural myths may, therefore, be one method to help design a more effective approach to preventing teen pregnancy or designing appropriate interventions with teen parents. Our goal is to increase attention to the myriad of complex, multi-systemic influences on teen pregnancy and parenting, in order to provide a better understanding of individual, familial, and societal responses to these situations.

2 Myths and misperceptions from research

Adolescent motherhood has been typically framed by social science research as a social problem through an association with psychological dysfunction, poor parenting and socioeconomic disadvantage.

(Breheny and Stephens, 2007b, p. 333)

The role of social science research in advancing our understanding of pregnant and parenting teens is called into question by the above quote. Implied in the quote is a dissociation between the objective reality of adolescent motherhood and how it has been scientifically constructed as problematic. Even a cursory review of published research substantiates negative impacts levied on teen parents and their children. If the research process has been distorted by cultural myths and misperceptions, negative outcomes for teen parents and their children may have been exaggerated or misrepresented entirely. Negative findings from research may then continue to reinforce the maintenance of cultural myths and misperceptions making them even more resistant to disconfirming evidence.

The purpose of this chapter is to critically reflect on how social science research may have contributed to the construction of teen pregnancy and parenting as a social problem, with a goal of redirecting research efforts to more beneficial approaches. We have drawn from over 40 major studies of pregnant and parenting teens, of adolescents and emerging adults, and of adults in later life, some of whom were teen parents. We provide an overview of these studies in the Appendix. Most of the studies were not initiated with a focus on teen pregnancy and parenting, but rather adolescence more generally. Studies are listed in alphabetical order and separated by country. Some readers may find our synopsis of studies interesting in its own right; other readers may prefer to use the Appendix as a reference for information on a specific study.

We begin our critical reflection with a focus on our own longitudinal research study, the Notre Dame Adolescent Parenting Project (NDAPP, see Appendix; Borkowski, Farris, Whitman, Carothers, Weed, and Keogh, 2007; Whitman, Borkowski, Keogh, and Weed, 2001). Following our self-reflection we briefly consider the philosophy of science more generally, and then turn to the functions and stakeholders of the research process from a systems perspective. We then summarize and compare types of research designs and analyses and their implications. We conclude by summarizing five important limitations inherent in the research process. In an effort to make these sections more meaningful, we begin with the illustrative story of Lydia, a teen mother who participated in the NDAPP.

Overlapping images filled Lydia's mind as she contemplated how to answer the question posed during a research assessment: "Has participation in our project had an impact on your parenting or on your life? If yes, in what way(s)?" Lydia recalled the time she had come to the university with Damon when he was just five years old and starting school. She was so scared that Damon's teacher wouldn't take her seriously because she was so young, but the researcher at the university listened attentively to her concerns and she left feeling better just because the researcher had treated her like she knew what she was talking about. Her mind took her back even further to the first time she had come to the university. Damon was just six months old. Lydia was too young to drive, so the researcher, who was a graduate student at the university where the study was being conducted, had come to her house to pick her and Damon up. Lydia felt that she was so young back then, but just reading and answering the questions about parenting and how children grow and change made her think about what others expected of her as a teen mom, and made her aware of things she might need to think about and learn. After she was dropped off back at her house, where she was living with her mom, grandma, and older brother, the questions would pop in her mind and she would think about different ways to respond to Damon when he cried or got upset. Thanks to her participation in this study, Lydia believed that she was better able to think about and do what was best for Damon.

In the current assessment, Lydia started to answer the question posed by the researcher, but then another image from when Damon was around ten years old popped into her head. Lydia had a car and driver's license by then and didn't need to be picked up any more. She had just passed her GED and was so excited to share her news with the researchers. They didn't say much, but Lydia could tell they were proud of her and her accomplishments, and she felt that maybe by sharing what she had been able to accomplish it would help other teen mothers be able to accomplish even more. Her mind finally snapped back to the present. It was hard to believe Damon was now 18 and about ready to graduate from high school. She wondered if she would have been able to survive his teen years without the confidence and security that came from knowing the researchers at the university cared and really understood what she and Damon had worked through together. Finally, Lydia just smiled at the researcher and said she was glad that she and Damon had been able to participate over the years.

The Notre Dame Adolescent Parenting Project (NDAPP)

Lydia and Damon were participants in the Notre Dame Adolescent Parenting Project (NDAPP), a longitudinal research study that began in 1984 (Whitman et al., 2001). The research project, funded by the National Institutes of Health (NIH), was designed to explore early precursors of developmental delay. It was based on a conceptual model that emphasized the importance of maternal learning ability, maternal socioemotional adjustment, and social supports (see Figure 2.1). These three constructs were believed to impact the quality of parenting through

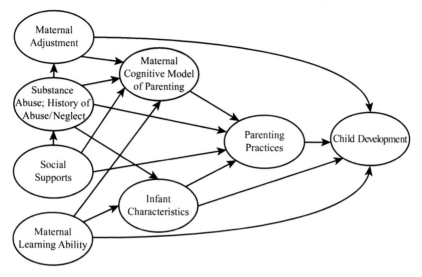

Figure 2.1 Conceptual model of teen parenting and child development proposed by Whitman *et al.* (2001)

how cognitively ready the mother was for her parenting role. Child developmental outcomes were thought to be related directly to maternal parenting ability and indirectly to maternal learning ability, maternal socioemotional adjustment, and social supports (Farris, Borkowski, Lefever, and Whitman, 2013; Whitman et al., 2001). Teen mothers, as a group, were expected to provide a lower quality of parenting than adult mothers. Parenting quality was proposed to depend on being cognitively prepared for the parenting role with appropriate attitudes, beliefs, and knowledge of child development. In addition to being cognitively prepared, better parents were expected to have higher intelligence and fewer adjustment problems. Social support was expected to serve as a buffer for parents who were deficient in these cognitive or psychological areas. These expectations were based on theoretical models and empirical findings from previous research (Belsky, 1984; Broman, 1981; Furstenburg, Brooks-Gunn, and Morgan, 1987; Maynard, 1996). Despite the unidirectional arrows in the NDAPP model, our work has previously documented the interwoven development of teen mothers and their children (Nicholson, Deboeck, Farris, Boker, and Borkowski, 2011; Whitman et al., 2001).

The methods and design of the NDAPP were consistent with three important criticisms levied by Breheny and Stephens (2007b). Our research questions were framed (1) to differentiate teen and adult mothers, (2) to identify individual differences among teen mothers, and (3) to explore factors predictive of more successful outcomes. Our research was based on a model that assumed the typical teen mom was deviant in important ways, but that some resilient mothers would be able to overcome challenges. As Lydia's story illustrates, we were also careful to include the perspectives of the teen moms themselves. Despite the seemingly appropriate focus of our efforts, we were unaware of how we may have been contributing to the maintenance of myths and misperceptions.

Our focus on identifying individual differences presumed that some teens would adapt effectively to the challenges of teen parenting (Weed, Keogh, and Borkowski, 2000). Characteristics of teens who adapted less effectively would be identified and used to develop strategies that could assist these young women as they coped with a major life transition. The flaw in this approach is focusing blame on individual characteristics rather than the many contextual factors that also contributed to maladaptive outcomes. Relatedly, as we attempted to explore factors predictive of more successful outcomes we continued to place responsibility on individual teens as opposed to broader societal factors. For example, consistent with relevant theories our conceptual model proposed that optimal child outcomes would be predicted by optimal parenting attitudes, knowledge, and style. Improving child outcomes consequently necessitated improving the quality of parenting. Ultimately, our attempts to improve child outcomes through parenting intervention were unsuccessful; further, we found few long-term predictive associations between early parenting and emerging adult outcomes for children born to teen mothers.

The conceptual model that guided our investigations was typical of models that guided other longitudinal investigations of teen parents. These models demonstrate how we may have perpetuated misperceptions about teen mothers by how we approached our research questions and the variables we chose to measure, and by how we overlooked the impact of cultural myths themselves in both the questions we asked and on the outcomes for the teen parents and their children. Despite this oversight, results from the NDAPP that were inconsistent with our conceptual model, in combination with a shift in our personal and societal perspectives on teen parenting across the last 30 years, prompted a rethinking of our initial assumptions. We came to realize how our results may have contributed to the social construction of teen parenting as problematic. To understand how this may have happened, a brief overview of assumptions based on the philosophy of science is needed.

Philosophy of science

Scholarly research is grounded in *logical positivism*, a philosophy of science that proclaims an ultimate reality that is knowable and that can be explained using appropriate methodology. Most research addressing issues related to teen pregnancy and parenting is consistent with logical positivism. This perspective implies the existence of a type of person that can be subsumed under the category *teen parent*, and that characteristics of this type of person can be discovered through the research process. In addition to an age between 13 and 19, and the experience of either giving birth to or fathering a child, this label implies other unique and distinctive characteristics and behaviors identifiable through scholarly research (Hacking, 1999). The simple creation of a category (i.e., teen parent) compels a search for characteristics that distinguish exemplars of this category from non-exemplars.

Logical positivism stands in sharp contrast to a constructivist philosophy that posits that knowledge always interacts with characteristics of the knower. The following quote eloquently conveys the essence of the social construction process:

> There are no facts flying around in nature as if they are butterflies that you put into a nice orderly collection. Our cognition is not a mirroring of ultimate reality but rather is an active process, in which we create models of the world. These models direct what we actually see, what we consider as fact.
> (Bertalanffy, as cited by Davidson, 1983, p. 214)

In essence, this quote implies that even researchers who strive to use unbiased designs and offer valid conclusions will be affected by their own beliefs, characteristics, and experiences, which can lead to potentially biased interpretations. Preexisting cultural myths held by researchers, either consciously or unconsciously, may skew perceptions of reality by impacting the questions that are asked, how answers are conceptualized, and how conclusions are conveyed to others.

Finlay's (1996) analysis of research with 62 pregnant teens in Northern Ireland provides a good example of the tension between logical positivism and constructivism. A major goal of the study was to enhance understanding of the extent to which teen pregnancies are planned or unplanned. Semi-structured interviews were conducted with the teens, who were questioned about the strategies they used to avoid pregnancies and, more specifically, about whether or not they had planned to become pregnant. Finlay concluded that the categories *planned* and *unplanned* were based on the researchers' models of the world, and were not relevant from the perspective of the teen respondents. He writes that the study failed to "get beneath the discourse or ideology to the 'reality' of the respondents' emotional experience" (p. 91). Despite this, the teens gave expected answers to the questions posed, thereby enabling the researchers to draw conclusions, however biased, about planned and unplanned teen pregnancies. Finlay's analysis is consistent with reflections of the Pulitzer Prize-winning journalist Leon Dash (1989), who, after living in an urban ghetto for close to one year, realized that his initial round of interviews were cover stories masking the reality of life for the pregnant and parenting teens. We will return to the issue of intended and unintended pregnancies in Chapter 4.

Meckler and Baillie (2003) provided a reconciliation that emphasized the importance of both the social construction process that may lead to the formation of cultural myths as well as the scientific method aimed at discovering objective truths. In part, the reconciliation acknowledged what Hacking (1999) referred to as a *looping effect*, or the bi-directional causal relationships between ideas, people, and practices. This looping effect occurs whenever society generates specific categories in which people might be placed. The category may be teen parent, woman refugee, or something as seemingly vacuous as the child viewer of television. These categories then become infused with meaning that is socially constructed. Characteristics are assigned to people who belong to the categories, expectations for behaviors are anticipated, and strategies are produced to deal with someone who belongs to a category. In other words, a stereotype is created. As people realize they belong to specific categories, and have an awareness of the socially constructed meaning assigned to those categories, a gradual transformation may occur whereby people begin to internalize the socially constructed meaning. As a result of this looping effect, pregnant and parenting teens may acquire behaviors and beliefs consistent with prevailing cultural myths and misperceptions that are then revealed through the process of scientific research and ultimately accorded the status of objective reality (Hacking, 1999).

> Participants in a culture provide and find support for even questionable views through shared inter-subjectivity; the group members concur that the logical or scientific basis for these views is solid … One implication is that conventional wisdom can endure even when it is misleading or false; it can also be generalized to circumstances where it does not apply.
>
> (Geronimus, 2003, p. 884)

Stereotypes of teen parents as immature, clueless, or neglectful may permeate the self-perceptions of teen parents, eventually leading to behaviors consistent with these stereotypes.

Lydia, the teen mother highlighted at the beginning of this chapter, illustrates this looping effect and the motivation to resist succumbing to it. Lydia's participation in the NDAPP crystallized her status as a teen mother. Her awareness of belonging to this category called her attention to beliefs, attitudes, and ways of behaving expected of anyone who belonged to this group. However, a comment made by Lydia and other participants in the NDAPP was, "I don't want to become a statistic." This is a puzzling comment in some ways, but one that implies many teen mothers are well aware of their status and associated expectations, and are intent on defying those expectations by finishing their education, avoiding welfare, and being responsible parents.

To summarize, conclusions from research shape beliefs and attitudes towards identified categories of people. Once this association has been made, some people who belong to a specific category may come to acquire these characteristics despite their motivations to defy the stereotypes. Subsequent research then is even more apt to confirm an association linking undesirable traits to the targeted group. In addition to biases created by how questions are framed, consideration of the research process from a systems perspective sheds light on additional ways that research may be used to reinforce cultural myths and misperceptions of teen pregnancy and parenting.

A systems perspective on the research process

Recall from Chapter 1 that a systems perspective involves a set of elements that combine holistically to produce a specified function or outcome. The specific function or outcome produced from the research process may be conceived of as valid answers to meaningful questions that help illuminate important truths.

Elements involved in this systematic process include governmental agencies, private foundations, advocacy groups, and social scientists. The constituents purported to be the recipients of the knowledge gleaned through the research process (i.e., pregnant and parenting teens and their families) should also be considered important elements involved in the research process. In the following section we touch briefly on the function of the research process, followed by a review of the important stakeholders, or elements, involved in this processes.

Functions of research

Aristotle delineated three functions of scientific research: (1) to generate knowledge for its own sake, (2) to promote goodness in action, at both the individual and societal levels, and (3) for the creation of beautiful or useful objects (Shields, 2008). Although Aristotle's thoughts are over 2,000 years old, these three purposes are as relevant today as they were then. The second function, however, may have the most relevance to research with pregnant and parenting teens. Ultimately, the research process may be used to illuminate important truths that would benefit the development of individuals and of society more generally. At the individual level, knowledge of physiological and psychological development provides strategies that lead to success and that restore optimal development following illness or injury. On a societal level, knowledge of social trends allows disruptions to be caught early so that corrections may be implemented before disasters occur. In other words, knowledge may be used both to regulate individual development and societal development.

A meaningful example of research used to monitor social trends involves tracking rates of childbirth over time. In the United States, the Centers for Disease Control and Prevention's (CDC) National Center for Health Statistics (NCHS), funded by the US Department of Health and Human Services, compiles and disseminates information about birth rates based on information recorded on birth certificates. Most countries have an analogous agency to collect and disseminate these rates. Data collected from birth certificate records, and from participants in the National Survey of Family Growth in the United States (NSFG: 2006–2010, see Appendix), confirmed that the rate of births to teens declined meaningfully since the early 1990s. For example, in 2010, 34 out of every 1,000 women between the ages of 15 and 19 in the United States had a baby; this represents a significant decline from 1992 when 60 out of every 1,000 had a baby. Similar declines were observed for young men between the ages of 15 and 19, from a rate of 57 in 1992 to 29 in 2010 (Martin *et al.*, 2013). The compilation of the important information contained in this and other reports disseminated by the CDC requires contributions from multiple stakeholders, a topic to which we now turn.

System elements – stakeholders

For any system to function effectively, individual elements need to work together in synchrony to achieve the functional goal of generating knowledge that will benefit individuals and society. Within the context of the research process, system elements include both those who have a stake in the process itself, and constituents who may be impacted by the knowledge revealed. Successful collaboration among stakeholders should lead to the generation of knowledge that will optimize developmental processes of the teens themselves and their children, as well as improve conditions on a societal level. However well-meaning this process is, few systems function perfectly at all times, and often dysfunction creeps in, thereby limiting the validity and generalizability of the results. In the sections that follow we describe five types of stakeholders in the research process: governmental agencies, private foundations and companies, advocacy groups, social scientists, and constituent groups. In addition to their primary roles, we highlight areas that may lead to dysfunction.

At the broadest level, governmental agencies (e.g., National Institutes of Health, Centers for Disease Control and Prevention) set research priorities, commission studies, and even establish bureaus and departments to compile statistics and conduct research. However, the government typically comprises elected officials who may want to maintain the status quo or keep their voting constituencies happy. Motivation to conserve their existing power bases may trigger concerns associated with teen pregnancy and parenting that are at odds with motivations to optimize development. These competing interests may be difficult to explicitly acknowledge, leading to the construction and maintenance of cultural myths.

Private foundations and companies also have an important stake in the research process. Similar to government agencies, they set research priorities, provide financial backing, and may even conduct their own studies. Foundations may also introduce competing interests that interfere with the optimal functioning of the system. For example, foundations may endorse specific religious or moral doctrines that governmental agencies are prohibited from endorsing. For example, the Heritage Foundation states that it is "based on the principles of free enterprise, limited government, individual freedom, traditional American values, and a strong national defense" (The Heritage Foundation, n.d.). As a second example, the Guttmacher Institute has close ties with Planned Parenthood and has been a strong advocate for sexual health and reproductive rights. In an attempt to be unbiased, despite its strong political stance, the Guttmacher Institute also clearly states its "commitment to publishing and disseminating results of the Institute's research, regardless of the political or programmatic ramifications" (Mission, n.d.). Motivations of some private foundations to promote specific moral standards of behavior may be at odds with the discovery of an objective reality, leading to funding some research but not others, or to the dissemination of some findings but not others. Although research is expected to provide unbiased results, this process may be subverted in both explicit ways (e.g., when evaluation results that are inconsistent with expectations are discarded and never published) and implicit ways (e.g., providing funding for some types of research, but not others).

Organizations that advocate for pregnant and parenting teens play an important role in how research findings are used to create policy and programs. One influential advocacy group in the United States is the National Campaign to Prevent Teen and Unplanned Pregnancy. This organization was founded in 1996 with goals focused on teens and unplanned pregnancies to women of all ages. Other advocacy groups that include pregnant and parenting teens among their constituent groups include Healthy Teen Network and the Center for Law and Social Policy. These organizations are often involved in translating research findings into policy, although some advocacy groups do initiate and conduct their own research studies. For example, the National Campaign initiated the National Survey of Reproductive and Contraceptive Knowledge (Fog Zone, see Appendix) about sexual attitudes and behaviors of emerging adults, and commissioned the Guttmacher Institute to conduct the study (Kaye, Suellentrop, and Sloup, 2009).

A review of documents disseminated by advocacy groups concluded that the majority of published material contained "long lists of statistics with no interpretive framework," and that little information was provided "within the context of a 'big picture' explanation of teen parenting" (Bales and O'Neil, 2008, p. 21). In other words, conclusions from research that assigned responsibility for teen pregnancy to the teens themselves have been emphasized while community and other contextual factors often have been ignored in materials published by advocacy agencies.

Stakeholders also include the social scientists who coordinate and conduct studies related to teen pregnancy and parenting. These professionals are typically employed by universities that provide additional support and backing for the research endeavors. Untenured faculty are often subjected to considerable pressure to engage in research that will lead to a sufficient quantity of published journal articles in exchange for the granting of tenure after several years. Longitudinal research that takes years to complete, or complex ecological analyses, or even experimental evaluations with random assignment of participants to experimental and control conditions, are not conducive to quick publication. Less rigorous correlational studies relying on self-reported attitudes and behaviors of college students may support tenure goals, but may also provide a less valid representation of the reality of teen pregnancy and parenting. Similarly, comparison between teen and adult parents is a type of study that may be conducted relatively quickly, with the expectation of significant findings leading to almost certain publication. Initiation of research that falls outside of conventional wisdom may be avoided due to the low probability of publication and resulting concerns about tenure.

Teen parents and their children are important stakeholders in the research process. They stand to benefit most directly from well-designed research studies guided by the motivation to improve outcomes. Rarely, however, are these constituents consulted during the research planning stage despite the recognized value of community-based participatory research (Wallerstein and Duran, 2010). Many qualitative studies, however, do include rich narrative descriptions from teen parents and their families in their analyses, which are often used as a foundation for subsequent studies. Whereas quantitative studies have been criticized for ignoring the voice of teen parents and their children, qualitative studies often detail unique and complex experiences of teen parents. In contrast to these qualitative studies that give voice to the actual thoughts and feelings of teens, "experiences of young people are often lost in ... quantitative reviews" (Graham and McDermott, 2006,

p. 22), perhaps perpetuating cultural myths that pertain to some, but not all, teen parents.

In order for the research process to effectively achieve its goal of uncovering important truths about pregnant and parenting teens that can be used to optimize individual and societal development, stakeholders need to work together. Problems arise when stakeholders are motivated by divergent goals or even when motivations are in accord, but the strategies endorsed to meet the goal differ. Bias may be introduced into the research process when stakeholders buy into one or more of the cultural myths identified in this book. Awareness of the social regulating function that cultural myths may be serving may help unmask this systemic dysfunction, and thereby allow for new research agendas that can better elucidate processes that are consistent with the reality experienced by pregnant and parenting teens.

Design and analyses

Scholarly research generates vast amounts of knowledge related to teen pregnancy and parenting. Performing a search on scholar.google.com with the keywords "teen pregnancy parenting" yielded 26,100 hits. The number of published articles on the topic of teen pregnancy and parenting has increased substantially in recent years; there were 4,760 hits between 1990 and 1999, 14,400 between 2000 and 2009, and 5,710 just in 2010 to 2012. Empirical scholarly research is published in journals cutting across disciplinary lines ranging from psychology, sociology, gender studies, and economics, to medicine, nursing, and policy studies. Coming from different disciplinary perspectives, this vast wealth of information on teen pregnancy and parenting is based on diverse research methodologies, both for study design and analytic strategies. Strengths and weaknesses of each methodology must be considered when interpreting empirical results.

Until recently, most statistical methods used to analyze data were linear and reductionist (Urban, Osgood, and Mabry, 2011). Linear relationships exist when one variable is able to be predicted by values of a second variable. For instance, a linear relationship may exist if the educational attainment of a child is predictable by the educational attainment of that child's mother or father. Similarly, the age at which a child became sexually active may be a linear function of the quantity and quality of discussions that parents had with their child about sex. A set of linear relationships that collectively predict an outcome may be described as reductionist. For example, it is unlikely that discussions with parents are the only contributing factor to the age at which a child becomes sexually active. A more accurate prediction would be obtained from an additive combination of factors that may include exposure to sexually explicit media, normative peer and neighborhood influences, and age at puberty.

Reductionist approaches are in conflict with holistic approaches. Consider the proposed relationship between intelligence and teen childbearing from the NDAPP conceptual model noted at the beginning of this chapter and illustrated in Figure 2.1. We proposed a chain of events leading to a higher percentage of pregnancies to young women of low intelligence compared to more intelligent young women. The causal sequence was expected to continue as the pregnant teens became mothers. Teens with low intelligence were expected to be less knowledgeable about child development, less prepared to figure out the complexities of parenting, and more likely to resort to simpler but harsher forms of punishment. As they were less cognitively prepared to become parents, teen mothers, compared to adult mothers, were expected to interact less appropriately with their young children, leading to fewer opportunities for children to develop their own cognitive skills. Children raised by teen mothers were therefore expected to start school less prepared and to eventually fall behind both academically and intellectually, leading to increased risks of dropping out of school and engaging in deviant behavior as they entered adolescence. These reductionist assumptions are inconsistent with basic premises of systems theory that maintain that the whole is greater than the sum of the parts. In the above example, this means that explanations of outcomes for children born to teen parents (the whole) need to consider how multiple interacting contexts, rather than any one factor in the model, work together to impact outcomes.

The distinction between reductionist and holistic perspectives becomes especially meaningful when intervention implications are considered. From a reductionist perspective, interrupting the chain of events at crucial points prevents the disadvantageous outcome from occurring. For example, preventing a woman from becoming pregnant as a teen will stop subsequent links in the chain, leading to the assumption that if she becomes a mother at a later, more mature age, her offspring will experience more advantageous outcomes. In contrast, holistic models consider how the multiple interacting contexts (not just maternal age) that the child is raised in work together to nudge outcomes towards competence or disadvantage, suggesting that even if a woman delayed childbearing for several years the negative outcomes would likely still occur. The advent of more advanced computers and software has allowed analytic techniques to move beyond linear, reductionist explanations to more complex patterns of interrelationships that more closely mirror the real world. Despite these advances, most research designs and analyses continue to be based on more traditional, reductionist approaches.

Study design

Scholarly research on teen pregnancy and parenting has relied on both quantitative and qualitative studies. Qualitative studies are typically initiated to provide a rich descriptive account of targeted behaviors using open-ended questions and observations in real-world environments. Analyses of narratives involve identification of patterns or themes shared by participant accounts. Due to the in-depth nature of the interview process, qualitative studies typically involve small numbers of participants. Although qualitative studies provide invaluable insights, the design is inadequate for testing causal hypotheses about behavior, making quantitative studies necessary. Quantitative studies typically involve more controlled investigations with larger numbers of participants. Hypotheses are generated prior to the study, and designs are invoked to test specific predictions.

Qualitative studies, in contrast to quantitative research, often portray the complexities that surround teen pregnancy and parenting that include concurrent positive and negative components (Clemmens, 2003; Phoenix, 1991). For example, five common themes emerged from a meta-synthesis of 25 studies representing the voices of 257 teen mothers (Clemmens, 2003). Two of these themes conveyed the challenges teens face, such as "the reality of motherhood brings hardship" and "living in the two worlds of adolescence and motherhood"; however, three themes were more positive: "motherhood as positively transforming"; "baby as stabilizing influence"; and "supportive context as turning point for the future." Qualitative researchers criticize quantitative findings for not providing more insight into the processes underlying why teen pregnancy can be connected to poorer outcomes. Qualitative studies match how we hope society would view the adolescent mother – as a process with potential, instead of a product with little hope or future potential.

Many published studies, both qualitative and quantitative, rely on information collected from *longitudinal studies* that have followed the same sample of participants over a period of time, sometimes an entire lifetime. For example, our NDAPP began with a sample of pregnant teens and conducted periodic follow-up interviews and assessments with this same sample for more than two decades. On the other hand, *cross-sectional research designs* collect information from participants of all ages at one point in time. Regardless of design, the number of participants in these studies has varied from small samples of under 100 to large samples of close to 10,000 participants.

One reason for the proliferation of published studies on teen pregnancy and parenting is that the data collected from many of these research projects are in the public domain, meaning that they are available to social scientists who may not have been involved with the actual data collection process. The National Longitudinal Study of Adolescent Health (Add Health; see Appendix), for example, claims to have generated 4,600 "publications, presentations, unpublished manuscripts, and dissertations," with 65 of these directly related to teen pregnancy and parenting. Conflicting results from the same data set may be reported due to reliance on different analytic methods as described below.

Analytic strategies

A major challenge embedded in most social science research is parsing *social selection* effects from *social influence* effects. Social influence effects result *from* early childbearing and suggest that adverse outcomes would be avoided if only teens would wait until their twenties to begin childbearing. These effects are assumed to be caused by factors directly related to the teens' youth. In contrast, social selection effects result from risk factors that exist prior to the pregnancy that may lead to both increased likelihood of teen pregnancy and adverse child outcomes, making maternal age at childbirth irrelevant. Analytic strategies differ in techniques used to disentangle these two types of effects; however, imperfections inherent in each strategy create room for biased interpretation of results.

The estimated impact of teen pregnancy and parenting varies by the type of analytic strategy used. Earlier studies, constrained by limited computational resources, were unable to test complex models. However, as technology has become more advanced so have the models used to understand processes and outcomes related to teen pregnancy and parenting. Fletcher and Wolfe (2009) organized these analytic strategies by "generations," a term we have adopted in our discussion below.

Several early studies, *the first generation*, lacked adequate controls for risk and protective factors (i.e., social selection effects), resulting in simplistic comparisons between pregnant or parenting teens and individuals who postponed childbearing until adulthood (Fletcher and Wolfe, 2009). Perhaps because these conclusions appear straightforward and easy to interpret, they continue to be used, often reinforcing negative views of teen parenthood. For example, a recent fact sheet posted on the website of the World Health Organization proclaimed that "stillbirths and newborn deaths are 50% higher among infants of adolescent mothers than among infants of women aged 20–29 years" (World Health Organization, 2012). Another informational fact sheet from Girls Incorporated asserted that 29.4 percent of teens who had a child while in high school dropped out, compared to only 5.4 percent who had no children (Girls and Sexual Activity, 2007). Although the statistics reported may be true, they promote the misperception that the adverse outcomes are caused by the age of the mother, social influence effect, as opposed to other risk factors that may also have increased the likelihood of a teen birth, a social selection effect.

A *second generation* of studies controls for these risk factors (i.e., selection effects) through regression analyses. Risk and protective factors in the lives of teens prior to the pregnancy are included as control variables in analyses so that the incremental impact of the teen birth can be estimated above and beyond any impact of these background characteristics. These studies attempt to resolve the dilemma between social selection effects and social influence effects, by statistically controlling for *selection effects* through the regression analyses. Therefore, differences between teen and adult mothers that remain after these controls are attributed to the *influence* of maternal age at childbirth. Inclusion of these background characteristics typically reduces the observed impact of teen childbearing as compared to first-generation studies.

Further difficulty arises, even in these second-generation studies, in controlling for all possible risk and protective factors. Some of these factors may be unknown, whereas others may be known but unavailable in the data set. Thus, a *third generation* of studies has attempted to control for these observed and unobserved factors by constructing comparison groups. Three types of comparison groups have been created: teens who became pregnant but miscarried, sister or cousin comparisons (Geronimus, Korenman, and Hillemeier, 1994), and teens who were matched on relevant background characteristics and judged to have equal propensity to become pregnant although they didn't. Since these comparison groups are statistically similar to teen parents on background characteristics, it is assumed that observed differences in outcomes may be attributed to being a teen parent. These approaches have been used to understand outcomes for teen mothers, children of teen parents, and to a lesser extent, teen fathers.

Miscarriage control groups provide an elegant design that relies on a "natural experiment" and provides a glimpse of what the life trajectories of teen mothers may have been if they had delayed parenthood (Hotz, McElroy, and Sanders, 2008). This design compares life outcomes of teen mothers to young women who would have become teen mothers except for the event of a miscarriage. Background characteristics are assumed to be similar between the two groups of young people since they all experienced a teen pregnancy. The miscarriage is considered an event that "randomly assigns" some teens to the early childbearing group and other teens to a delayed childbearing group. Although these studies overcome many of the limitations of regression studies, the possible impact of a miscarriage on a young woman's developmental outcome remains unaccounted for.

Propensity score matching is yet another variation on methods designed to determine the impact of teen parenthood (Rosenbaum and Rubin, 1985). In this procedure, a propensity score is derived for each young person, which estimates the likelihood of becoming a teen parent based on characteristics observed prior to the pregnancy, thereby controlling for social selection effects. The propensity score is used to create a matched comparison group of nonpregnant teens who have similar backgrounds yet delayed childbearing.

Comparison of siblings is an alternative approach used to estimate the impact of teen parenthood; Geronimus and Korenman pioneered this approach in the United States in 1993. This approach uses biological sisters who delayed parenting as a comparison group to their sisters who were teen mothers, as a means of controlling for social selection effects. Similarly, children born to the biological sisters who delayed parenting have been used as a comparison group for their cousins born to teen mothers. The strength of this approach is that it controls for family and socioeconomic factors that are known to impact outcomes. However, criticism has also been levied that the sibling approach fails to account for individual difference factors that may also impact outcomes, over and above the impact of teen childbearing.

Despite the sophistication of these third-generation analytic approaches they remain grounded in a linear, reductionist perspective. Relationships between variables are assumed to operate equally for all individuals subsumed in groupings (e.g., teen mothers). A holistic, systems approach, in contrast acknowledges that the pattern of interrelationships may vary based on individual characteristics. A systems perspective provides a framework to address process-oriented questions (e.g., why, how, for whom, and when) about teen pregnancy and parenthood. For example, instead of asking how teen and adult mothers differ on lifetime earnings, a process-oriented question might seek to discover the most important influences on lifetime earnings, with age at childbirth as only one of several contributors, and then determine why these influences are important. Reframing issues to focus more on answers to process-oriented questions is an important next step that brings researchers closer to their ultimate goal of generating knowledge that will benefit individuals and society.

Some traditional regression approaches address these issues through mediational or moderational analyses. Mediators are variables that explain "why" or "how" relationships between constructs exist. For example, low educational attainment may explain "why" there is a relationship between teen childbearing and lower lifetime earnings. Increased use of condoms may explain "how" comprehensive sex education programs result in reduced pregnancy rates. Although mediational analyses often provide useful information, results can be misleading; once mediators are identified it is all too tempting to infer that changing the mediator will have a positive impact on the outcome (e.g., policies and programs that keep pregnant teens in school will have a positive impact on lifetime earnings). Despite the apparent logic, this reasoning fails to consider the additional influences on lifetime earnings that may alter once the mediator has changed. A systems approach refers to this as homeostasis.

Moderators are variables included in statistical analyses in an effort to answer questions of "for whom" or "when" different outcomes are most likely. For example, Francesconi (2008) answered "for whom" through a study that found psychological distress was only higher in children of teen mothers who also experienced poverty while growing up. The study also demonstrated that family disruption interacted with birth to a teen mother to increase odds of adverse outcomes. These approaches confirm that the impacts of teenage childbearing are not universal and apply only in some situations. Moderational analyses, however, are constrained by the limited number of interactions that it is statistically possible to test; identification of significant moderators typically requires a substantial sample size that is not always feasible in studies of teen pregnancy and parenting. In contrast, newer person-centered approaches are less constrained and provide an analytic alternative consistent with a holistic systems perspective.

Rather than identifying associations between *variables*, person-centered approaches seek to identify patterns among *people*, often conceptualized in terms of identifying subgroups of people with similar characteristics. Person-centered approaches are consistent with systems thinking as they examine

> multiple interacting causal factors rather than attempting to isolate the impact of single factors; this approach views the individual as an organized whole, functioning and developing as a totality that derives its characteristic features and properties from the interaction among the elements involved, not from the effect of an isolated part of the totality.
>
> (Magnusson, 1998, p. 33)

A person-centered approach assumes heterogeneity in any population, which may reflect different vulnerabilities, strengths, and needs. A person-centered approach suggests that not all pregnant teens or teen parents are alike. Some may have considerable vulnerabilities and need targeted supports while others, despite their young age, may view early childbearing as adaptive or already have the necessary development and supports in place for successful outcomes.

Cluster analysis and latent class analysis (LCA) are becoming increasingly popular techniques to identify homogeneous subgroups within a sample or population.

Whereas cluster analysis is based on observable, manifest characteristics of individuals, LCA is a technique based on the assumption that variability in behavior, attitudes, and responses is attributed to "latent," or unobserved, properties of individuals. Identification of subgroups of people that share latent characteristics should reduce the amount of variance within a data set. LCA and cluster analysis do not rely on reductionist assumptions, and are therefore more consistent with systems theory.

Limitations of the research process

Since each type of study design and analytic approach is associated with strengths and weaknesses, revealing important truths related to teen pregnancy and parenting requires converging evidence from different studies, samples, and methodologies. Conclusions drawn from only one study may be biased by any weaknesses inherent in that specific study. Policy and programs will be more effective based on knowledge that has been replicated across different data sets and analytic techniques (Laws, 2013). As we examine specific cultural myths in the chapters that follow, we are careful to synthesize conclusions drawn from studies utilizing different methodologies, designs, samples, and cohorts.

Regardless of methodology, five overarching issues may hinder the effectiveness of the research process in illuminating important truths: (1) reliance on averages, (2) confusion between significant and meaningful findings, (3) the file-drawer problem, (4) how questions are framed, and (5) determinism. The issues are applicable to even third-generation studies and often lead to biased conclusions. Unless these issues are appropriately addressed, the research process may be considered more dysfunctional than functional. We revisit these issues in Chapter 8 with a discussion of policy implications.

Reliance on averages

Results of most quantitative research are reported as averages. In the chapters that follow, findings will often be reported in terms of *average* differences in outcomes between teen and adult parents, or in terms of average rates of behaviors organized by age. For example, reports in declines of births to teens over the past 20 years rely on information averaged over a number of important characteristics, including age, race, socioeconomic status, and geographical area. Investigators make decisions about which of these factors are relevant to report. For instance, birth rates are typically reported by age, race, and State, but not by SES. Considerable differences exist based on age and race even within the United States, with a birth rate of 10.0 of 1,000 for 15- to 17-year-old White teens compared to a rate of 85.6 of 1,000 for 18- to 19-year-old Black women. Striking geographic differences also exist, with the birth rate in several southern States in the United States (e.g., Arkansas, Mississippi, Texas, and New Mexico) being greater than 50 of 1,000 teens, while other States in the northeastern United States (e.g., Connecticut, Massachusetts, New Hampshire, and Vermont) have rates less than 20 of 1,000 teens. Simply citing a birth rate of 34 out of 1,000 provides little information to program- or policy-makers attempting to address teen pregnancy and parenting among high-school or college-aged women in various regions of the United States (Martin *et al.*, 2013). All too often reports that carefully compare outcomes based on multiple characteristics end up collapsed across groups for consumption in the local news media. Complex findings get watered down or oversimplified, and important contextual elements that qualify reported averages may be omitted, leading to false perceptions.

Reports of average rates of anything rarely reflect the reality for any one individual, since approximately 50 percent will always be above this average rate and the other half below. Experts have pointed out the flaws in using averages to make predictions, citing the hypothetical example of a statistician who drowned in a river that was on average three-feet deep (Savage, 2002). As this example humorously illustrates, the average depth of three feet may include a long stretch of one to two feet along with shorter stretches of ten or more feet; the river may not actually be three-feet deep anywhere. Application of this example to estimates of the penalty associated with maternal age at childbirth implies that an estimate may not describe the actual penalty experienced by any particular teen. Instead, steeper penalties experienced by some teens may be offset by gains accrued by others. Inferences about future expectations predicated on averages will be less effective than inferences based on important distinctions that exist within any sample (Savage, 2002). Reports that rely on comparisons between teens and adults on average rates of childbearing, or other important outcomes, may perpetuate cultural myths and misperceptions.

Confusion between significant and meaningful findings

Many professional journals only accept manuscripts with statistically significant results. However, the distinction between *significant* and *meaningful* results is important to keep in mind (Borkowski and Weaver, 2006). Some results may be significant, but not meaningful, while others may be meaningful, although not significant. Significant but nonmeaningful results may be obtained from studies with large samples. A very small difference between teen and adult parents may meet the typically accepted criterion for statistical significance, meaning that there is less than a 5 percent chance that the pattern of results would occur by chance. The age of the parent may, however, account for only a very small percentage of the variance in outcome, perhaps 2–4 percent, indicating that teen and adult parents are much more alike than they are different. Studies with small samples typically have the reverse problem. Even if the age of the parent accounts for 10–15 percent of the variance in outcome, the difference may not be considered significant due to inadequate statistical power associated with small sample sizes. Journal editors and book publishers have begun to consider both the significance and the meaningfulness of the results, but a great deal of inconsistency remains in regards to which studies get published (Kline, 2004). Due to the complexity of this issue, the interpretation of some findings may be ambiguous, thereby allowing preconceived cultural myths and misperceptions to bias conclusions.

The file-drawer problem

The file-drawer problem, also referred to as *publication bias*, refers to the practice of suppressing research findings that fail to substantiate hypothesized differences between groups. These null findings are filed away in the investigator's file drawer rather than disseminated for public consumption (Ferguson and Heene, 2012; Laws, 2013). In relation to teen pregnancy and parenting, this means that some well-designed studies that do not find significant differences between teens and adults may have been rejected for publication. Studies with null findings, therefore, are less likely to be included in literature reviews or evaluations; this omission of unpublished research that may actually contradict published findings leads to a more negative bias towards teen parents. The file-drawer problem may have considerable implications for public policy and advocacy campaigns that rely on results of a single published study from one data set. Our analyses in the chapters that follow attempt to counter the file-drawer problem by including some working papers and technical reports that have not been disseminated through professional journals.

Framing of questions

Framing questions in terms of differences between teen and adult parents, as opposed to numerous other ways questions could be framed, presupposes that at least some of the differences will be significant. Equally significant conclusions may be obtained by looking at differences between teen and adult fathers, or between parents who were abused during childhood compared to those who were not maltreated. An obvious, but misguided, interpretation when differences are found is to infer that adverse outcomes must be caused by teen parent status, leading to the inference that simply postponing childbearing will result in more optimal outcomes. This interpretation fails to consider the multiple, interacting contextual influences that combine to produce the adverse birth and developmental outcomes that are seen among some children born to teen mothers as well as some children born to adults.

Attributions of adverse outcomes to the age of the mother at childbirth may serve an important social regulation function for society, as argued in Chapter 1. Placing responsibility on young mothers, rather than on young fathers or social policies and services, creates a platform to argue against the moral decay of young women, creates a backlash due to fears about social degeneration, and provides fodder to argue about reproductive rights for women (Macleod, 2011). Framing questions in terms of differences between teen and adult mothers allows politicians and service providers to blame "irresponsible" teen moms for increased taxes to cover the billions of dollars in costs that are shouldered by taxpayers.

Determinism

The concept of determinism as applied to the process of research means that all physical, behavioral, and cognitive events have specific, identifiable causes (Hoefer,

2008). Determinism, as applied to pregnant and parenting teens, suggests that causes of teen pregnancy and subsequent outcomes for teen mothers, fathers, and their children are determined by a specific group of causes that may be identified through a systematic research process. In fact, a substantial amount of research related to pregnant and parenting teens is designed to elucidate important causal relationships.

Substantiating causal relationships between variables is tricky. Recall our earlier description of declines in the rate of births to teens over the past 20 years. Curious readers may immediately want to know what has caused the decline in birth rates, and hypothesize various factors as key contributors. However, since data from the NSFG: 2006–2010 was cross-sectional, meaning that it was collected from a group of people who varied in ages, and participants were not followed longitudinally, there is no empirical basis to infer the causes of the decline. Despite this, Martin *et al.* (2012) stated that "The long-term declines in teen birth rates have been linked to the strong pregnancy prevention messages directed to teenagers" (p. 5). Although the authors were careful not to state that the declines were caused by pregnancy prevention campaigns, most readers, including policymakers and frontline service providers who do not have a strong background in critically evaluating research, may not see the difference between these phrases. Martin *et al.* are even bolder when they conclude that increased use of contraception has "likely contributed to the recent birth rate decline" (2012, p. 5).

The implicit message conveyed by Martin *et al.* (2012) – that declines in the teen birth rate may be attributed to pregnancy prevention campaigns and increased use of contraception – is misleading for two reasons. First, the research methodology was inadequate to draw conclusions about cause-and-effect relationships. Second, the implicit message ignores other, and perhaps equally compelling, influences on the decline. For example, the birth rate for women of all ages declined from 15.8 of 1,000 in 1992 to 12.6 of 1,000 in 2012 (Hamilton *et al.*, 2013). It is likely that social and economic factors that impacted the birth rate for women of all ages also impacted birth rates to teens (Kearney and Levine, 2012). Calling attention to some potential influences, while ignoring others that may be equally as important, sets teen parents apart from adult parents and reinforces the cultural myth that they constitute a distinctive type of person. Misinterpretation of data, or lack of attention to consider contextual factors, may further crystallize perceptions and misperceptions into cultural myths and provide an ill-informed foundation for programs and policies.

Summary

Throughout this chapter we have attempted to extol the potential benefits of the research process to generate knowledge in support of pregnant and parenting teens and for society more generally. As is often the case, several important factors constrain research efforts to achieve this potential. We have relied on our involvement in the research process with the NDAPP over the past 30 years as a starting point for our critical rethinking. Our study, similar to many other studies, was based on the belief that teen mothers were a particular type of person, whose traits and characteristics could be uncovered through the research process, a basic tenet of logical positivism. Our assumptions were likely influenced by cultural myths that framed teen pregnancy and parenting as problematic. Research that considers the implications of these cultural myths during the planning phase and also considers how myths may actually impact outcomes has greater ability to fulfill its role in generating important knowledge.

In summary, when the research process functions effectively new knowledge is generated or uncovered that has the potential to improve individual lives and society more generally. However, the research process may become somewhat dysfunctional when:

- results are reported as averages that are assumed to apply equally well to all members of an identified group;
- results that demonstrate significant but not meaningful effects are used to emphasize differences between groups;
- research that fails to find differences between identified groups (e.g., teen and adult parents) remains unpublished and suppressed in the researchers' file drawers;
- the way questions are framed places responsibility on teen mothers rather than alternative factors associated with teen childbearing, and may limit investigations into the processes and mechanisms leading to differential outcomes;
- background characteristics that increase the likelihood of early pregnancy and childbearing, as well as adverse outcomes for teens and their children, aren't fully considered in causal explanations of differences found between teen and adult parents.

We will return to these five issues in subsequent chapters as we attempt to review and integrate research that has been conducted relevant to pregnant and parenting teens.

3 Myths and misperceptions from popular culture

As entertainment programming with an educational mission, *16 and Pregnant* and *Teen Mom* place far less emphasis on birth control and sexual health than they do on the consequences of teen pregnancy. By presenting pregnant teens who are smart, involved, and ambitious, these series may represent a significant intervention into widely held, negative stereotypes that teen mothers are directionless, uneducated, and overly dependent on social welfare programs.

(Murphy, 2012, p. 97)

Popular culture plays an important role in the social construction of teen pregnancy and parenting. Consumers of popular culture, not just children and adolescents, but also parents, scholars, and policy-makers, absorb implicit and explicit messages disseminated by television, movies, the Internet, and other sources. Implicit messages may be conveyed by subtle variations in how teen mothers are portrayed on television programs; explicit messages are evident through more obvious headlines about teen parents on the covers of popular magazines. The opening quote specifically refers to popular culture as represented in television programming, and suggests that these implicit and explicit messages from the media may challenge and inform prevailing cultural myths of pregnant and parenting teens.

Despite depictions of teen mothers that counter some cultural stereotypes, other more subtle stereotypes may be reinforced by popular culture. Alongside the presentation of teen mothers as motivated, independent, and resourceful is the representation of teens as having choice and autonomy while downplaying contributions of social and cultural contexts and the roles and responsibilities of teen fathers (Murphy, 2012). Implicit messages suggesting that teen pregnancies result from lapses in judgment or poor decision-making skills of otherwise responsible young women obscure the roles of social and cultural factors that also contribute to early childbearing. Portrayals of teen mothers as capable and autonomous may also convey the message that social and governmental supports are unnecessary. Relegating fathers to a secondary role reinforces the perception that young women bear primary responsibility for the consequences of early pregnancy and childbearing. We return to the story of Claire and Jeremy, first introduced in Chapter 1, as we consider the potential role of popular culture to shape cultural myths and to impact reproductive behaviors.

Claire and Jeremy used to spend time after school watching reality shows about teen mothers. As she thought back to how they enjoyed rolling their eyes and laughing at the young mothers, Claire felt her stomach turn. She thought of some of the episodes and now saw how these mothers were just like her – a young teen who made some risky decisions about sex among a whole host of good decisions in other aspects of her life. Did this mean she was now like the girls that she had scoffed at – or had she previously been too judgmental about the girls on the reality shows? She overheard one of her classmates saying, "I didn't know Claire was such a slut." How did her classmate get that impression of her? She had only been with Jeremy – her first boyfriend. She also found it strange that her mother actually blamed her pregnancy partly on the TV show – her mom felt that the show made it seem OK to get pregnant. Claire certainly didn't feel the show glamorized her situation – she now knew how the characters felt as their peers and families saw them in a different light. She struggled between how she used to see herself, how others see her now, and how to deal with the discrepancy between the two "Claires."

Since television became popular in the 1950s and 1960s, debates have raged over its potential impact on attitudes and behavior. Initially debates centered on the potential of television to sway children and teens to engage in aggressive and violent behaviors. More recently, attention has turned to the sexual content of television programming. Issues in the debate concern (1) the extent to which television impacts sexual attitudes, values, and behaviors, (2) whether television normalizes behaviors generally considered atypical (e.g., teen parenthood), and (3) how implicit and explicit media messages are integrated with prior attitudes and knowledge. The debate about the impact of television, and popular culture more generally, on the sexual attitudes and behaviors of teens and emerging adults is not easily resolved.

The purpose of the current chapter is to review the content of popular media to more fully understand the implicit and explicit messages conveyed regarding sexuality in general, and teen pregnancy and parenting more specifically. In addition to investigating messages transmitted by popular culture, we also summarize scientific research that has attempted to evaluate the impact of media messages on reproductive behaviors. We begin this chapter with an overview of media usage by children and teens, followed by a summary of sexual content and themes portrayed in popular culture, with a focus on television. Our analysis of the causal role of media consumption is framed by the theoretical foundation of *sexual socialization*, or the process by which people acquire knowledge and attitudes regarding sexuality and sexual behaviors (Ward, 2003). Our focus on television is not meant to imply that other forms of popular culture are unimportant. Music videos, social media, and other popular culture media all have tremendous potential to impact the sexual and reproductive behaviors of youths. Since space limits our ability to address all these important avenues we hope many of the points we raise may have relevance beyond the immediate focus on television.

Following our discussion of the impact of media on the sexual attitudes and behaviors of youths, we turn more specifically to how popular culture portrays pregnant and parenting teens. We focus our investigation on the popular show *16 and Pregnant*, and include results of our own quantitative and qualitative analyses. The chapter ends by rethinking the cultural myth that *providing media visibility of pregnant or parenting teens will encourage others to become pregnant*. We attempt to provide a balanced evaluation of evidence that both supports this cultural myth and refutes it. We conclude with a discussion of potential messages from popular culture that could infiltrate not only the sexual scripts of teens, but may also intrude into cultural myths that shape how society perceives, and often misperceives, pregnant and parenting teens.

Media usage by children and teens

Although controversy lingers on the causal impact of media on reproductive behaviors, few people question the fascination popular culture holds for people of all ages. A comprehensive report, *Generation M²: Media in the Lives of 8- to 18-year-olds*, published by the Kaiser Family Foundation in collaboration with researchers from Stanford University, documented that youths in the United States spent more than 7.5 hours per day with entertainment media (Rideout, Foehr, and Roberts, 2010). The amount of time youths spend with media has increased since 2000, primarily due to the preponderance of mobile devices (e.g., iPods, cell phones). Youths who used smart phones spent more time listening to music, playing games, and watching TV on these devices (49 minutes per day) than they spent actually talking on them (33 minutes per day). Regardless of technology used, television remains the primary source of media consumption among youths in the United States.

Even more notable, youths were found to regularly use more than one media source at a time, with 40 percent of teens reporting that they used another medium most of the time when listening to music, using a computer, or watching television (Rideout *et al.*, 2010). When this *media multitasking* was accounted for, estimates revealed that youths packed 10 hours and 45 minutes-worth of media content into their day, accumulating more than 75 hours of media per week. This staggering amount is nearly equivalent to the time spent working two full-time jobs. About one-half of young people said that they multitasked with media "some" or "most" of the time that they were completing their homework. About two-thirds of the youths said that the TV was usually on during meals, and almost half reported that the TV in their home was left on most of the time even if no one was watching. Youths in these "TV-centric" homes spent an hour and a half more time watching TV per day, and an hour more watching TV in their bedrooms, as compared to youths in homes where the TV was not left on during meals or when no one was watching. The total time devoted to TV viewing is striking, suggesting that the content of what teens are watching has the potential to impact attitudes and behaviors due to the large quantity of time during which teens could be influenced by this medium.

Sexual content on television

Explicit sexual behavior and innuendoes are prominent in television programming, with one analysis revealing that 70 percent of network and cable television shows that aired in 2005 in the United States contained either sexual talk or sexual behavior (Kunkel, Eyal, Finnerty, Biely, and Donnerstein, 2005). Restricting analyses to shows during prime time resulted in an even higher percentage, with sexual content at 77 percent. Even further restrictions to shows marketed to teens revealed that 6.7 scenes involving sexual content were presented each hour. Sexual content appeared consistently across a variety of types of shows including movies, sitcoms, drama, soap operas, news, and talk shows.

The potential impact of story lines with sexual messages may depend on how closely the audience is able to identify with the characters. Teen viewers may be more likely to identify with teen or young adult characters than with older characters. One positive change in the portrayal of sex in the media is that the percentage of characters under the age of 25 portrayed as having sex declined from 27 percent in 1998 to only 11 percent in 2005 (Kunkel *et al.*, 2005, p. 43). Despite fewer portrayals of younger people engaged in sexual relationships, the frequency of sexual behaviors within the context of an established relationship remained unchanged between 1998 and 2005, at 53 percent (Kunkel *et al.*, 2005).

The potential impact of story lines with sexual messages may also depend on the actual content of those messages, including real-life risks and responsibilities. Portrayals of characters engaging in casual sex with little thought given to consequences convey a very different message than portrayals of characters who engage in safe sexual behaviors within the context of close, intimate relationships. Three types of sexual messages were analyzed by Kunkel *et al.* (2005): *sexual patience*, *sexual precaution*, and the *risks and negative consequences* of sexual activity. Sexual patience included messages pertaining to abstinence or postponement of sex, and sexual precaution referred to implicit or explicit messages about the use of contraceptives. Unintended pregnancy, sexually transmitted infections, and negative changes in relationships were coded as risks or negative consequences of sexual activity. Collectively these three themes were coded as *sexual risks and responsibilities*. Among the 20 most highly rated shows targeting teens (e.g., *American Idol*, *The Simpsons*, *Desperate Housewives*, *One Tree Hill*), only 10 percent of those with any sexual content included reference to sexual risks or responsibilities. This rate rose to 25 percent when the sexual content involved actual intercourse. In summary, many teens are spending a significant amount of time watching shows on television that talk about sex and portray characters engaging in sexual behaviors with limited attention to the risks and responsibilities of their actions.

Hetsroni (2007) suggested that public opinion, academic researchers, politicians, and even the TV industry itself have misconstrued media portrayals of the quantity and content of sexual talk and sexual behavior, believing it to be more egregious than the reality suggests. Although this suggestion is worth noting, Hetsroni failed to take into account that the quantity and type of sexual content of television programming differs between cable television and network programming. In the United States, network programming is free of charge and closely monitored for content by the Federal Communications Commission (FCC).

The FCC outlines indecent broadcast restrictions as "language or material that, in context, depicts or describes, in terms of patently offensive as measured by contemporary community standards for the broadcast medium, sexual or excretory organs or activities" (Federal Communications Commission, 2013, p. 1). Due to the First Amendment's right to free speech, broadcast television cannot outright ban indecent material, but restrictions are made between 6 a.m. and 10 p.m. for both indecency and profane speech, to reduce the chance that children would view such material. Sexual content on network TV during prime-time evening hours has actually decreased since the mid-1970s (Hetsroni, 2007); specifically, the frequency of normative sexual content and depictions of sexual intercourse between unmarried partners declined within network programming during this time period. Trends in messages about risks and responsibilities of sexual behavior were less consistent, but fewer safe sex messages were aired during more recent shows.

The preceding analyses of the quantity and content of sexual messages are important to consider only if they actually impact attitudes and behaviors, a presupposition still in need of definitive evidence. Further, potential impacts could be positive with messages advocating for sexual patience, precaution, and risk avoidance; alternatively, viewing sexual content could result in teens normalizing sexual behavior and adopting more permissive attitudes. The potential impact of sexual content may be best understood through the process of sexual socialization.

Sexual socialization

Sexual socialization refers to the ongoing process by which knowledge, attitudes, values, and behaviors about sex and sexuality are developed (Ward, 2003). Children and teens are exposed to sexual information from a variety of sources including parents, friends, extended family, educators, religious institutions, and popular culture (Atwood and Kasindorf, 1992). Some of this information consists of explicit instruction or admonitions of behaviors to avoid (e.g., premarital sex) or to engage in (e.g., contraceptive use), whereas other messages may be transmitted implicitly by how others respond to socially appropriate or inappropriate sexually related behaviors. Integrating sexual information that originates from diverse sources with sometimes conflicting messages makes the process of sexual socialization difficult for many youths.

Wright (2011) proposed a sexual script acquisition, activation, and application model of sexual socialization, termed 3AM. Sexual scripts are used to determine appropriate versus inappropriate sexual behavior, especially in the context of sexual decision-making. Viewing sexually laden content on television can provide consumers with sexual scripts that they were previously unaware of (i.e., acquisition), trigger sexual scripts they were already aware of (i.e., activation), and encourage or discourage the utilization of sexual scripts (i.e., application) by portraying sexual attitudes and behaviors as normative or atypical, acceptable or unacceptable, and rewarding or punishing. Wright's model suggests that existing sexual scripts possessed by viewers may moderate the impact of exposure to sexual media. In other words, existing sexual scripts may affect the particular elements of televised sexual content that viewers attend to and the likelihood that viewers will act on what they observe.

Wright's 3AM model is consistent with a systems perspective. As first explained in Chapter 1, a systems perspective considers how multiple related elements combine to produce a specific outcome or function. This shared process is typically nonlinear, and the function produced is often remarkably resistant to change. Application of general systems theory to sexual socialization views discrete informative sexual messages as the elements that combine interactively to produce one or more sexual script. Some sources of sexual information may exert a more powerful impact on sexual socialization than others. Teens polled in the Annenberg Sex and Media Study (see Appendix) reported they learned about sex from friends most often, followed by teachers, mothers, and the media (Bleakley, Hennessy, Fishbein, Coles, and Jordan, 2009; Hennessy, Bleakley, Fishbein, and Jordan, 2009). Television and movies were reported as the most informative media about sexuality, but individual differences arose in use of media as a source of sexual information; young women reported using media more than young men, Whites more than Blacks, and older teens more than younger teens (Bleakley *et al.*, 2009).

Messages received from these multiple, overlapping sources are filtered by the youth's level of cognitive development and understanding. Exposure to sexually themed media messages while scripts are in the formative stage of acquisition may carry more weight than exposure once scripts have already been established. Once initial scripts are formed, typically in childhood or early adolescence, exposure to new and different sources of sexual information may be compared to existing scripts. Sometimes, the new information will simply be ignored or discarded if perceived as too discrepant from current scripts. Other times, current scripts may be modified to incorporate all, or some, of the new information. Scripts acquired at younger ages are more likely to predict sexual decision making, and may have a more powerful impact on viewers' attitudes and behaviors as compared to later exposure. A critical question pondered by researchers and policy-makers, as well as by concerned parents, is whether sexual messages conveyed by various media sources will distort or alter values and behaviors instilled by family.

Impact of media on sexual behaviors

The crux of the debate over the sexual content in the media centers on whether consuming sexual content actually changes knowledge, values, attitudes, and behaviors, or whether content aired is simply a reflection of the prevailing social and cultural norms that drive youth behavior. Put simply – does viewing sexual content on TV cause teens to engage in sexual behavior? Or does the content they choose to view just reflect how the teens already feel about sexual activity based on their existing sexual scripts? The options in this debate are the same as previously described (see Chapter 2). Recall that a *social selection effect* implies that differences in sexual values, attitudes, and behaviors between groups of teens who are high or low consumers of sexual media may be attributed to personal characteristics. For instance, some teens, perhaps motivated by curiosity, arousal, or confusion about sex *select* to view shows that contain high levels of sexual content. These same motivations may also lead to engaging in sexual behavior. In contrast, a *social influence effect* suggests that media consumption has an *influence* over and above other characteristics that may predispose some teens to spend more time viewing sexual media and subsequently engaging in risky sexual behaviors. Longitudinal and experimental studies have been used to estimate the media influence while controlling for selection effects. Longitudinal studies control selection effects by measuring these factors prior to onset of sexuality; experimental studies control selection effects through random assignment to conditions.

The majority of studies investigating the impact of sexual media has focused on sexual behaviors – including sexual initiation, unprotected sex, or promiscuous sex – rather than on teen pregnancy and childbearing (Aubrey, Harrison, Kramer, and Yellin, 2003; Brown, L'Engle, Pardun, Guo, Kenneavy, and Jackson, 2006; Collins *et al.*, 2003, 2004; Pardun, L'Engle, and Brown, 2005). Two influential longitudinal studies explored relationships between exposure to sexual content through popular culture and actual sexual behavior. One national study, conducted by researchers at the RAND Corporation, concluded that teens who were heavy consumers of sexual content on television were over twice as likely to initiate sex within one year than teens who were low consumers of sexual content (Collins *et al.*, 2004). A social influence effect of TV was supported by controlling for a variety of background characteristics between high and low consumers of sexual content presumed to be associated with sexual initiation.

A second study that focused on popular culture more generally, including consumption of sexual content in television, movies, music, and magazines, reached similar conclusions: young teens who were heavy consumers of sexual content were significantly more likely than low consumers to have become sexually active over the two-year study period (Brown *et al.*, 2006). This social influence effect, however, held only for White teens. The relationship between high consumption of sexual media and sexual behavior was eliminated for Black teens once parental and peer influences were considered (Brown *et al.*, 2006). Studies that substantiate a social influence effect imply that a reduction in the amount of sexual content in the media, or in the amount of time spent consuming sexual media, would result in meaningful postponement of the initiation of sexual activities (Collins *et al.*, 2004).

In contrast to the conclusion that consumption of media with high sexual content has a causal impact on sexual behavior, Steinberg and Monahan (2010) reinterpreted the conclusion reported by Brown *et al.* (2006) as a social selection effect rather than a social influence effect. A sophisticated analytic technique, propensity score matching, was used (see Chapter 2) as opposed to more traditional regression analysis. The propensity score equates groups on background characteristics that are related to the *propensity* to engage in a targeted behavior (i.e., consuming sexually charged media), thus controlling for social selection effects. Once groups were matched by propensity scores, differences attributable to consumption of sexual media were eliminated. Even though the results of this study were questioned due to the inability to completely equate propensity scores between high and low viewers of sexual content, the authors emphasized the importance of using caution in establishing policies based on elusive research results that don't hold up to different analytic techniques.

In addition to these longitudinal studies, experimental studies have also been used to understand how sexual media content changes attitudes towards sex. In one experiment, Taylor (2005) randomly assigned college students to conditions based on the sexual content of TV shows. He concluded that the perception of television as relatively realistic moderated the relationship between viewing sexual content and permissive attitudes towards casual sex. In other words, TV viewing of sexual content was unrelated to attitudes of students who perceived TV as unrealistic, but students who perceived TV as realistic were likely to change their attitudes after watching shows with high sexual content.

Exposure to sexual television content on emerging adults' sexual attitudes and moral judgments was also explored experimentally by Eyal and Kunkel (2008). College freshmen were randomly assigned to view shows that portrayed either positive or negative consequences of sexual intercourse. Results indicated that exposure to shows that portrayed negative consequences of sex led to more negative attitudes towards premarital intercourse and to more negative moral judgments of characters who engaged in this behavior. Results were observed immediately after the viewing and persisted two weeks later. These experimental studies provide strong evidence that consumption of sexual media has an impact on the sexual socialization of young people.

To our knowledge only one study has investigated the causal impact of viewing sexual media on teen pregnancy (Chandra *et al.*, 2008). Youths who participated in this longitudinal study were followed over a three-year period of time. For each of three waves of data collection, teens responded to questions about their television viewing habits, sexual activity, and pregnancy history, as well as measures of sociodemographic variables to control for their influence on pregnancy. Regression models confirmed that the probability of pregnancy, or male responsibility for pregnancy, was higher for teens who were exposed to high levels of televised sexual content, even after controlling for other important factors known to be associated with teen pregnancy. Notably, the risk of pregnancy was over twice as high for teens who viewed shows with high levels of sexual content (Chandra *et al.*, 2008).

The impact of media on sexual and reproductive behaviors may be best explained by the reciprocal, mutually influencing processes of media selectivity and media effects, referred to as a *reinforcing spiral* (Aubrey *et al.*, 2003; Pardun *et al.*, 2005; Slater, 2007). In other words, shows with sexual content are more likely to be viewed by audiences already interested in this content. In turn, the sexual content of the shows is likely to strengthen viewer predispositions. A longitudinal study of teens between 14 and 16 years of age found evidence of this reinforcing spiral; sexually active teens were more likely to expose themselves to sexual content and those who were exposed to more sex in the media were more likely to report more sexual behavior across time (Bleakley, Hennessy, Fishbein, and Jordan, 2008).

Resolution to the debate about the causal impact of sexual media consumption on values, attitudes, and behaviors of youths is hampered by traditional analytic techniques. These techniques typically frame questions in terms of group comparisons – in this case, teens who are high and low consumers of sexual media – on outcomes of interest, with statistical controls for background characteristics. This regression approach is linear and produces statistics that reflect averages assumed to reflect outcomes for everyone that belongs to the identified group. Reframing the important question to understand the process by which popular culture interacts with other sources of sexual information to impact sexual socialization may yield more valuable information than simply comparing reproductive outcomes for high and low media consumers.

Despite a paucity of research, there is some evidence that the impact of sexual media may not be equivalent among all viewers; rather it may be moderated by race, perception of content as realistic, degree of identification with the characters, follow-up discussions of the content, and the meaning attributed to sexual content (Brown *et al.*, 2006; Taylor, 2005). These strong moderating effects may limit the ability of traditional reductionist analyses to provide valid estimates of the impact of sexually laden popular culture on the values, attitudes, and behavior of youths. In contrast, a systems approach suggests that messages teens receive from multiple sources typically combine in complex ways leading to formation of sexual values, attitudes, and behaviors. Unfortunately, little empirical research has examined the complex interactions among the sexual socialization messages targeting youths. Application of a systems approach to integrate personal interests and motivations, cultural and political forces, family factors, and individual developmental status lays an important foundation for understanding the reinforcing spiral of popular culture on the reproductive behavior of teens.

Popular culture representations of teen pregnancy and parenting

Teen pregnancy and parenting have become topics of much interest in popular culture. This trend is seen across all forms of media, with a shift from viewing teen pregnancy as a disgrace, with an emphasis on secrecy and subterfuge, to teen parents being showcased with celebrity status. This shift in the visibility of teen parenthood has implications for how people perceive teen parents, and the potential to impact the sexual socialization process of youth. The following sections provide a brief review of trends in how pregnant and parenting teens have been portrayed on television, in movies, in books and magazines, and on the Internet.

Television shows

American TV in the 1950s generally revolved around artificially positive trad-itional themes, and teens were not portrayed as being sexually active (Boyd, 2011; Sapolsky and Tabarlet, 1991). Portrayals of teen sexuality began to change in the 1960s and 1970s as TV shows began to confront real-life issues, and by the 1980s popular sitcoms such as *Family Ties, Growing Pains, The Cosby Show*, and *Facts of Life* were addressing teen sexuality, sometimes on episodes that were preceded by a public service announcement letting the audience know that the show would contain explicit content. In the 1990s, prime-time soap operas such as *Beverly Hills 90210* and *Melrose Place* frequently portrayed explicit and implicit depic-tions of teen sexuality; *Beverly Hills 90210* tackled the issue of teen pregnancy when one of its key characters became pregnant in real life and the pregnancy was written into the character's story line. This show portrayed the character, Andrea Zuckerman, becoming pregnant in high school after only having unpro-tected sex once with her boyfriend. Andrea considered abortion but ultimately decided to marry her boyfriend and keep the baby.

The 1990s also ushered in the era of "reality TV" that still pervades television today. With the introduction of "real people" as the main characters, shows began to address a variety of topics that had been somewhat glossed over in scripted shows. Teen pregnancy and parenting have been openly discussed on shows such as MTV's *The Real World*, often coupled with discussions about why the couple did not use birth control and whether abortion was a viable option. Two of MTV's most popular current shows, *16 and Pregnant* and *Teen Mom*, portray the lives of real-life pregnant and parenting teens and their children, and began the start of a series of shows whose story lines focused on teen pregnancy. *Underage and Pregnant* follows a similar reality format with teens from the UK. Teen pregnancy and parenting are also commonplace in popular scripted TV shows today, such as *The Secret Life of the American Teenager, One Tree Hill*, and *Pramface*.

Movies

Shifts in portrayals of pregnant and parenting teens have also been seen in mov-ies (Bleakley, Jamieson, and Romer, 2012). Older movies that addressed teen pregnancy were likely to portray the pregnancy as a result of sexual abuse or a first-time sexual encounter, with the couple choosing marriage. More recent movies have provided a more sympathetic portrayal of teen mothers as regular individuals faced with a challenging situation. For example, the 1988 movie *For Keeps* told the story of Darcy, a bright, young woman who was college bound until she got pregnant during her last months of high school. The movie follows the experiences of Darcy and her boyfriend and the pressures they face when their families urge them to have an abortion or place the child for adoption. A similar story line in the 2001 movie *Riding in Cars with Boys* is based on the true story of the author, Beverly D'Onofrio, who in 1965 became pregnant by her boyfriend at the age of 15. The film follows the lives of Beverly, her son, her son's father, and her immediate family as they deal with the consequences of her pregnancy. In 2007, the movie *Juno* switched from the prior movies' focuses on a dramatic portrayal of teen parenting and topped the charts with a comedic drama that portrayed a sassy young woman who became pregnant after her first sexual encounter with her boyfriend. After deliberating about her options, Juno decided to place her baby in an open adoption with a family of her choice. These movies provide a unique and emotional glimpse at how cultural perceptions surrounding teen pregnancy influenced young women during each time period, going from portrayals of the mother as a victim or delinquent to providing a glimpse of regular teens facing nonnormative life circumstances.

The 2009 film *Precious*, based on a true story, provides a less heartwarming tale of teen pregnancy through the story of a troubled teenager who was the victim of sexual abuse by her father that resulted in a first pregnancy at the age of 13. This opened the door for other fictional accounts of real stories, such as the Lifetime network movies *The Pregnancy Pact* in 2010 and *The Pregnancy Project* in 2012. *The Pregnancy Pact* portrayed the experiences of a group of teenage girls who allegedly became pregnant on purpose so they could all have babies together. *The Pregnancy Project* recounted a senior project of a young woman who pretended to be pregnant as a social experiment to expose how peers, teachers, family, and the general public perceive teen parents. The recent proliferation of movies like these illustrates that sex among teens, and its consequence of teen pregnancy, is no longer a hidden or shameful secret. Rather, teen pregnancy is now openly discussed as an outcome of unprotected sex, and in many of the movies the characters are given choices about options to keep the baby, have an abortion, or pursue adoption. Implicit and explicit messages conveyed by some of these recent movies counter negative stereotypes of teen mothers as delinquent and unmotivated, yet reinforce perceptions that decisions that teens make about reproductive behaviors are devoid of social and cultural pressures.

Books and magazines

Teen pregnancy has pervaded other forms of media as well, including print media and the Internet. Many of the movies referenced above (e.g., *Precious*, *Juno*, and *The Pregnancy Project*) were based on top-selling books. Bristol Palin's 2011 memoir, *Not Afraid of Life: My Journey So Far*, provides an open discussion of how teen pregnancy can happen to anyone, including the daughter of a prominent governor and Republican Vice Presidential candidate. In this book, Palin (2011) openly shared the challenges of maintaining a relationship with her baby's father and her struggles to get her life back on track.

Likewise, popular magazines are filled with an abundance of stories about teen pregnancy and parenting. In fact, the stars of the reality shows *16 and Pregnant* and *Teen Mom* frequently appear alongside celebrities on the covers of tabloids. The magazines' headlines sometimes suggest that the teens are in dire straits, yet portray inconsistent images with pictures of flawless-looking teen mothers who are posing happily with their children (e.g., Inside Their Struggle, 2010). This August 2010 issue of *US Weekly* initiated a flood of press coverage in which the supposedly average young women from MTV's reality shows were bolstered to the ranks of high-profile "celebrity" teen parents including Bristol Palin and Jamie Lynn Spears. The implicit message conveyed by many of these magazine stories is one of triumph over adversity (Murphy, 2012).

Internet

Topics focused on teen pregnancy and parenting are also pervasive on the Internet. This can be a positive factor, as opportunities abound for education and support of teens before or after they become pregnant. For example, MTV's *Teen Mom* website features links to websites for organizations such as *It's Your Sex Life* that offers facts about prevention of teen pregnancy and information about sexually transmitted infections and relationships; this website is advertised during episodes of the MTV shows related to teen pregnancy. *Love is Respect* offers information about dealing with teen dating abuse and domestic violence. *Stayteen. org* provides resources offered by The National Campaign to Prevent Teen and Unplanned Pregnancy, and the On Your Feet Foundation is designed to help parents who have placed their children for adoption. Other support sites, including *Young Mommies Homesite* and *Girl-Mom*, are sponsored by individuals rather than corporations. Both of these sites were started by teen mothers with aims to serve as resources and support groups for pregnant and parenting teens. For example, the home page of *Girl-Mom* includes an article that informs pregnant and parenting teens of their rights to stay in school, attend regular classes, and continue to participate in extracurricular activities. Further, information is provided on what to do if teens believe their rights are being violated (www.girlmom.com). Much like the shift in other media outlets, the visibility of teen mothers has increased considerably along with the provision of supports.

Summary of popular culture representations

Clearly, popular culture has opened the doors to discussions that were previously taboo. Honest portrayals of the realities of teen pregnancy and parenthood may begin to counter biased cultural myths. However, emphasizing some aspects of teen pregnancy while selectively ignoring other aspects may also perpetuate misperceptions. In addition, although the acceptance granted to pregnant and parenting teens in much of popular culture has the potential to reduce negative stereotypes, it could also encourage pregnancy by normalizing this typically nonnormative life event. Cultivation theory proposes that people come to accept what they are watching on television as a reflection of real life (Gerbner and Gross, 1976; Shanahan and Morgan, 1999; Shrum and Lee, 2012). According to this proposition, therefore, youths who view television programs showing sexually active teens or pregnant and parenting teens will come to view not only these behaviors as normative, but will absorb implicit and explicit messages about the meanings of these behaviors.

The potential impact, therefore, of how media represents experiences of pregnant and parenting teens is great. We continue by presenting analyses conducted on MTV's *16 and Pregnant* and *Teen Mom*, two related shows which have has become a focal point of attention by advocacy groups, scholars, and the general public. The following sections provide an in-depth examination of how these shows convey the experiences of teen mothers through our own analyses and those of other scholars.

MTV portrayals of pregnant and parenting teens

MTV, a cable network, has developed shows that attempt to include educational messages within entertainment-style programming; this approach is known as "edutainment" (Murphy, 2012). It has been suggested that this approach reflects the influence of the Sabido method innovated at Televisa, a private television network in Mexico, in the mid-1970s (Singhal and Rogers, 2001). During that time, Miguel Sabido, the Vice President of Research at Televisa, incorporated Albert Bandura's social learning theory into the network's popular TV series with the intention of promoting the status of women and family planning efforts by encouraging viewers to learn from the behaviors they watched on television. Working in conjunction with The National Campaign to Prevent Teen and Unplanned Pregnancy, MTV developed *16 and Pregnant* in an effort to expose the reality of teen pregnancy and parenting by being honest and highlighting challenges associated with these experiences, the risk and responsibilities of being sexually active, and a prosocial message for youth (Dolgen, 2011). Lauren Dolgen (2011), creator and developer of MTV's *16 and Pregnant* and *Teen Mom* series, explained:

> Three years ago, I was flipping through a magazine when I read an article that stopped me cold. Jamie Lynn Spears' pregnancy was a lead story in the news, but this piece talked about the 750,000 other teenage girls who get pregnant each year in the US, the ones who were not from wealthy, famous families. This was an issue affecting our audience: something happening to them, their friends and people they knew. I kept thinking about these girls, the ones whose stories weren't being told. The US has the highest rates of teen pregnancy and teen birth in the fully developed world – but at that time, no one was really talking about the harsh reality these young women were facing. I felt like we had to address it. I wanted to help give these teenagers a voice, and to share their stories without passing judgment in a way that could start a real dialogue about the issue.

Based on these beliefs and goals, *16 and Pregnant*, essentially a cross-sectional "reality" show, chronicles the experiences of pregnant teens from approximately the third trimester of pregnancy through the first few months following child-birth. A recent study reflected the pervasive viewership of the program; 84 per-cent of the young women in the sample had viewed *16 and Pregnant*, and most reported that they had seen the shows more than ten times (Wright, Randall, and Arroyo, 2013). Teen and emerging adult viewers were tuning in to the show on a somewhat regular basis, making it even more critical that the show was providing a prosocial message on pregnancy prevention and accurately portraying the chal-lenges of teen motherhood. A recent headline, "MTV's *16 and Pregnant* Credited for Decline in Teen Pregnancy Rates," provides one example that many people believe that Dolgen's show has fulfilled its claim for having prosocial benefits on teen viewers (Dinh, 2010).

Moreover, anecdotal evidence of educators and other professionals using the program with teens reflects the goal of the program creators to intersect sex edu-cation with popular culture (Hoffman, 2011). The program has been integrated into classrooms as a way to develop a discourse on teen pregnancy, sex, and even relationships with parents. This format has the potential to ease the difficult con-versation adults need to have with teens on sexual relationships, and has even been used by parents, in the waiting rooms of reproductive health centers, and in juvenile detention centers in a similar manner. The success of the series has led to the creation of a spin-off show on MTV, *Teen Mom*, as well as television programs in other countries, such as *Underage and Pregnant*, a show with a similar reality format scheduled to air in the UK.

MTV's efforts to show "real" teens navigating their transition into parenthood may have a stronger mark of authenticity than fictional narratives popular in TV and the movies (Murphy, 2012). The show appears to present an accurate version of reality as it unfolds, by documenting the lives of young women and men who are similar to MTV's target demographic in many ways. A report available on the MTV website claimed that 82 percent of teens believed the series helped them understand the trials of parenthood; only 15 percent felt the show glamorized teen pregnancy. The authenticity perceived by viewers of these reality shows may increase the likelihood that messages will impact attitudes and behaviors (Taylor, 2005). Much of society has capitalized on this possibility as well, as evidenced by agencies and foundations such as The National Campaign to Prevent Teen and Unplanned Pregnancy and the Kaiser Foundation including *16 and Pregnant* in their educational materials (Grigsby Bates, 2010).

16 and Pregnant, like other reality shows, is supposedly unscripted. Perusal of a few episodes, however, reveals that, as with all "reality" shows, the content of each episode is carefully formed by editors who condense several months' worth of footage into a single episode that is designed to be convincing, offer a sense of closure on the issues raised in the episode, and educate young view-ers (Murphy, 2012). For example, each episode of *16 and Pregnant* begins with a voice-over narration of the pregnant teen's self-introduction, presented while the teen is engaging in her typical daily activities; these introductions are strik-ingly similar across episodes, indicating that they are more scripted or coached than "real." Starting in the second season, episodes also contain a brief discussion of contraception, usually initiated by a friend or family member who asks the pregnant teen whether she had been using birth control when she conceived. In addition, each show includes the tagline, "Teen pregnancy is 100% preventable," and directs teens to resources that can be found on the show's website.

Despite the network's purported efforts to have a positive impact on adolescent sexual behaviors, many critics have disagreed about the beneficial effects of these shows, accusing them of rewarding teen moms with stardom and glossing over many of the harsh realities of teen motherhood (Bauer, 2011; Marcus, 2011). In fact, the impact of *16 and Pregnant* and the show's spin-off, *Teen Mom*, has been the subject of a heated debate on teen pregnancy and parenting since they debuted (Albert, 2010; Dolgen, 2011; Jonsson, 2010; Marcus, 2011; Roeper, 2011).

MTV's website claims that *16 and Pregnant* "offers a unique look into the wide variety of challenges pregnant teens face: marriage, adoption, religion, gossip, finances, rumors among the community, graduating from high school, getting (or losing) a job." The site goes on to describe the challenges confronting its stars: "Faced with incredibly adult decisions, these girls are forced to sacrifice their teenage years and their high school experiences. But there is an optimism among them; they have the dedication to make their lives work, and to do as they see fit to provide the best for their babies" (About MTV's *16 and Pregnant*, n.d.). Critics who challenge the show's prosocial message, however, believe that an edited representation of teen parenting does not accurately portray the negative consequences of pregnancy or the true depth of the challenges experienced by teen mothers and fathers (Murphy, 2012). In response to the lack of consensus on whether the show is more positive or negative for teens, an entire book, *MTV and Teen Pregnancy: Critical Essays on 16 and Pregnant and Teen Mom*, was penned in 2013 to provide a discourse from individuals in a variety of disciplines arguing both prosocial and antisocial aspects of the show (Guglielmo, 2013). The controversy surrounding the content and influence of portrayals of teen pregnancy and parenting as depicted on *16 and Pregnant* and *Teen Mom* prompted our own investigations into the shows. Our evaluations focused on how closely media portrayals of pregnant and parenting teens matched reality.

Our analyses of MTV's 16 and Pregnant and Teen Mom

We conducted a quantitative and qualitative analysis of all 47 episodes of *16 and Pregnant* from seasons 1 through 4. For the quantitative analysis, careful observations and coding of all 47 episodes of *16 and Pregnant* were conducted, with 20 percent of episodes double-coded to ensure adequate inter-rater reliability (Nicholson *et al.*, 2014). Information was coded that was comparable to national statistics on teen pregnancy and parenting (e.g., variables on the coding sheet assessed portrayals of mother's education and employment, relationships, involvement of the grandmother and child's father, etc.) to allow for an investigation of how generalizable the story lines of the episodes were to typical teen parents.

For the qualitative analysis, we transcribed the final scene of each of the 47 episodes, during which teens provide a brief reflection on their experiences and how their lives changed after the birth of their children. Using a constant-comparative method as outlined by Maykut and Morehouse (1994), and originally introduced by Glauser and Strauss (1967) and Lincoln and Guba (1985), the qualitative study's focus of inquiry was, "What are formative themes young mothers discuss when summarizing their initial experiences of being a teen mother?" Given that the mothers were prompted to summarize their experience for the reality show, it was assumed that the topics they discussed were the ones most pressing or important to their experiences.

Quantitative data indicated that the typical teen mother portrayed on *16 and Pregnant* was 16 or 17 years of age (76 percent) and White (68 percent). The typical dad was 19 years of age or older (64 percent) and White (78 percent). In contrast, in the United States, only 39 percent of all teen moms are White, and only 28 percent of all teen moms are between the ages of 16 and 17, while the majority (66 percent) of teen moms are 18 or 19 years of age. Some of the pregnant teens on this show reportedly considered abortion (16.7 percent) and/ or adoption (13.9 percent); however, none of the mothers on this series chose abortion and only 8.3 percent of mothers chose to place their infants for adoption. These percentages differ from national data, with approximately 25 percent of teen pregnancies ending in abortion and about 3 percent ending in adoption (Curtin, Abma, Ventura, and Henshaw, 2013).

In contrast to biased portrayals of demographic characteristics and choices made by teen mothers related to keeping their children, birth outcomes for teens on *16 and Pregnant* were typical of birth outcomes for teens in the United States. For example, approximately 9.6 percent of babies born to teens between the ages of 15 and 19 in the United States are low birth weight and 13.6 percent are preterm (Martin *et al.*, 2012). Six of the teens (13.3 percent) on *16 and Pregnant* had babies that weighed less than 5.5 pounds, and five (10.6 percent) had preterm babies, rates that did not differ meaningfully from the national data (Smith and Weed, 2013). Teens were not, however, shown as receiving welfare assistance. Only three teen moms on *16 and Pregnant* gave any indication of receiving welfare. This rate of 6.4 percent is somewhat less than the rate of 17 percent found for teen mothers who participated in the Add Health study (Fletcher and Wolfe, 2009). In short, the quantitative analyses indicated that although there is some aspect of "reality" on this show, MTV has chosen to portray a slightly more advantaged group of teen parents than those found in the general population.

Themes that emerged from the qualitative analysis suggested that MTV portrayed a wide range of teen mothers in terms of relationships, attitudes, and beliefs; these themes conveyed real challenges and suggested that the show was not simply glamorizing teen pregnancy. Three dominant themes identified related to: (1) how teens reacted to their status as mothers, (2) how the babies were portrayed as impacting mothers' educations and careers, and (3) social support.

Teens' reactions

How teens processed the fact that they were teen mothers ranged from passive acceptance to making the most out of it. Some teens discussed the need to just *go with the flow* and reported their circumstances in an almost apathetic or passive voice: "I just made a decision to have sex, and it had consequences, and now I'm just living with them" (Samantha, Season 2, Episode 6). Other teens reported being in a state of disbelief on how they ended up as teen mothers, "Sometimes I just look at him and I just think, like, I can't believe I did this. It's so insane, it's so crazy" (Aubrey, Season 2, Episode 15). Others discussed their situation in a more accepting or proactive tone:

> I've had to fight my whole life so I'm just waiting for things to get easier. I think there is a little light at the end of the tunnel, as long as I keep working hard. Probably harder than most teenagers my age, hard work will keep the light coming, keep it shining through.
> (Kailyn, Season 2, Episode 10)

Impact of babies

Similarly, the narratives at the end of the show portrayed a range of education and career goals, with some teens doing better due to their new role while others seemed to perceive that becoming a parent derailed their education and career trajectories. Katie (Season 4, Episode 2) presented the theme of the *baby as a barrier*:

> It's very hard to finish school and continue going with a baby. I am on her schedule. If she is crying and I am in the middle of an exam, I have to figure out how to take this timed exam and get her to stop crying at the same time.

Samantha (Season 2, Episode 6), however, presented the theme of *baby as a drive* for pursuing her education, "College and everything is gonna [*sic*] be so much harder, but I have to do it. I have to for Jordan." Even though some teens reported difficulties with education due to their babies, our descriptive analyses revealed that the majority of the teen mothers on *16 and Pregnant* stayed in high school, worked on their GEDs, or went on to college despite their pregnancies (85 percent). This percentage differs significantly from national data collected from the Add Health study where only 61 percent of pregnant or parenting women stayed in school (Fletcher and Wolfe, 2009), again suggesting that *16 and Pregnant* portrays realistic themes but a generally more advantaged group of teen parents as compared to the general population.

Social support

Themes also emerged related to social support provided by the teens' friends, mothers, and boyfriends. Whereas individual differences were conveyed for the perceived support provided by mothers and boyfriends, a friend shift was consistently discussed in which most teen mothers reported feeling neglected, dropped, or no longer being like their friends. Over half of young mothers on the show did not experience stable friend networks over the course of their pregnancies. The show explicitly and implicitly represented how teen pregnancy can influence peer relationships. Explicitly, teens reported that friendships changed (27.7 percent), friends were lost (17 percent), and they felt betrayed, let down, or hurt (12.8 percent). Even if not explicitly stated, friendships were shown as changing through shifts in the teens' friend network sizes; over one-half showed a decrease in the size of their friendship networks, often dropping to fewer than three friends. These changes in peer networks accompanied changes in schools due to the pregnancy (29.8 percent) and a drastic decrease in extracurricular activities after the pregnancy (26.3 percent). Although friends are often overlooked in the literature on social support for teens (Ensor and Hughes, 2010; Voight, Hans, and Bernstein, 1996), the show depicted how peer relationships may shift based on the different priorities, interests, and activities teen mothers may have in comparison to their friends. Some teens lamented this shift in their summary of their experience; for example, "I feel like I've had to give up my social life. I don't really talk to most of my friends anymore" (Hope, Season 4, Episode 8).

Sixty-eight percent of the teens on *16 and Pregnant* stayed in a relationship with the baby's father throughout the pregnancy. This rate was somewhat greater, but not statistically different, than the 55 percent rate reported for teens from the Add Health study. Most fathers on the show were coded as very involved (63.8 percent) and almost 35 percent lived with the mother after birth. Specific functional aspects of social support from fathers were depicted in terms of financial support (38.3 percent) and help with child care (25 percent), but fathers were also identified by coders as being only somewhat involved (27.7 percent) or not at all involved (6.4 percent) with their babies. Overall, a wide range of levels of support from boyfriends was depicted that likely represents the diversity of relationship outcomes and support that teen mothers experience. The short timeline of the show, however, prevents the audience from seeing if relationships and involvement decrease over the first year of the child's life, a consequence often found in longitudinal studies (Bunting and McAuley, 2004). Even so, themes reflecting how the pregnancy may have negatively impacted the relationship with the child's biological father included:

- *Putting the ball in his court*, where the mother wants the father to be involved, but leaves the responsibility to do so up to the father: "Joey can see Aydenn whenever he wants, but it's up to him if he wants to see Aydenn, not me" (Allie, Season 3, Episode 10).
- *Not stepping up*, where the mother expresses regret and frustration that the baby's father is not involved in their lives, emphasizing a lack of financial contribution and also physical presence: "Andrew's not the person that I would want to have a baby with now that I look back on it, because he's just, he hasn't contributed to any of, anything, nothin'" (Janelle, Season 2, Episode 1).

• *Relationship negatively affected by the baby*, where the mother reports a change in the relationship, either feeling more pressure or more strain, after the baby is born: "We're both moody, we're both tired, we're just, we just want our teen years back so it gets, it just puts a strain on it" (Taylor, Season 3, Episode 9).

In addition to social support from boyfriends, *16 and Pregnant* showed a high number of maternal grandmothers who were involved and supportive both financially and emotionally in the mother's life postpartum: 70 percent of the teen mothers lived with their mothers after the babies were born, 76.6 percent provided some kind of emotional support, and 36 percent helped with child care. Out of maternal and paternal grandparents, maternal grandmothers were the most likely to be shown as being supportive, but these relationships were also more likely to be seen as conflictual (i.e., demonstrating both supportive and unsupportive acts in an episode). Similar to the literature on grandmother involvement, the show depicted how the majority of teen mothers lived with their own mothers and relied heavily on them (Voight *et al.*, 1996).

16 and Pregnant portrayed various ways that living with grandmothers could be beneficial to some young mothers. Teens reported valuing their mothers' emotional support ("Cause if [my mom] wasn't here I wouldn't be able to do half the things I've done" – Briana, Season 3, Episode 4) and functional support ("If my mom wasn't here to take care of the baby I wouldn't have went back to school" – Izabella, Season 3, Episode 7), and ranged from presenting this relationship as essential to reporting it as making life easier. Consistent with prior research, relationships between teen mothers and their own mothers were not without social strain and were not universally helpful (Spieker and Bensley, 1994; Voight *et al.*, 1996). One theme that conveyed this was *trouble with Mom*, either stemming from the relationship, or due to existing strain; teens expressed unfulfilled expectations, not feeling supported, and wanting their mothers to let them be more independent. For example, Catelynn in Season 1, Episode 6, reported, "It hurts my feelings that my mom doesn't support me. It's kind of hard to deal with that because your mom, out of all people, should be like your number one supporter."

Summary: 16 and Pregnant

Overall, findings indicated that *16 and Pregnant* did present some of the challenges and struggles experienced by teen parents, including relationship volatility, financial instability, and life changes required to raise a child. Discrepancies existed, however, in other areas between MTV's portrayals and the actual reality of teen parenting such as maternal age, decisions about whether to keep or terminate the pregnancy or pursue adoption, educational attainment, and the receipt of welfare. To summarize, our findings led to the conclusion that *16 and Pregnant* does not provide a completely realistic representation of the typical teenager; although the show does portray some challenges of teen parenthood, it does not depict the full range of disadvantage faced by some teen mothers nor does it highlight the contextual constraints that may confront some teens. While the show does appear to educate the viewing audience about the struggles faced by many teen mothers, it does not fully inform the audience about resources and options available to pregnant and parenting teens. The incomplete portrayal of reality reflected by *16 and Pregnant* suggests that misperceptions about the ability of the teens to control and manage their situations without institutional supports may be reinforced.

In general, however, we are encouraged by our analyses suggesting that *16 and Pregnant* does not glamorize teen parenting, but provides a somewhat realistic perspective of a topic that, until recently, had been considered taboo. Based on this, it is plausible the show is achieving the goals for which it was originally designed by Dolgen: to give teen mothers a voice. In fact, it is possible that providing this glimpse into the lives of teen mothers could dispel some cultural myths. This notion was conveyed directly in a theme from our qualitative analysis when mothers on *16 and Pregnant* reported their experiences with *negative stereotypes of teen mothers*. Specifically, some teens found that they did not fit into their own or others' previous beliefs about teen mothers. Valeria (Season 2, Episode 3) discussed how facing the negative stereotypes of others changed her own perception:

> I was very judging before, um, I got pregnant. If I saw myself pregnant, and I was 15, so I would've thought, like, she is nasty, she, like, sleeps around with everybody. Like, why else would she get pregnant this young. 'Cause you're just judging from looking, you don't actually know what's going on in their lives.

Samantha (Season 2, Episode 6) discussed how negative stereotypes impacted her own identity development:

> Everybody thought I was like little miss perfect, and then when I got pregnant, everybody's like, "You're pregnant? You don't even do stuff like that. You're a good girl." And it's just like, I am a good girl.

These stereotypes were even reported from close family, as Marai in Season 2, Episode 14 lamented:

> My relationship with my mom has changed as I'm not as open with her as I used to be. Getting pregnant pushed me away. She felt like I was gonna be like those other teenage moms that she's seen and that's just not the way I am.

Narratives from these teen mothers clearly revealed a range of responses in reaction to new responsibilities associated with being teen parents and how these experiences directly changed them. These insights may be informative for both reducing negative stereotypes and preventing pregnancy in young viewers, by providing a realistic understanding of some of the challenges teen parenting entails. In particular, portrayals of teen pregnancy and parenting as seen on reality television may be especially relevant to young women, as identification with the characters in media is a predictor of how much the media will affect the consumer. Thus, we suggest that, despite its lack of attention to broader social and cultural aspects of teen pregnancy and parenthood, MTV's *16 and Pregnant* is a step forward towards increasing dialogue, rethinking cultural myths, and promoting positive behaviors. Our favorable comments towards *16 and Pregnant*, however, do not extend to *Teen Mom*, another show on the same network.

A different portrayal: Teen Mom

A spin-off series using some of the most popular characters of *16 and Pregnant*, *Teen Mom* offers a longitudinal perspective in which the lives of four young women from *16 and Pregnant* are followed through the first three years of motherhood. The popularity of this show led to the 2011 and 2013 debuts of its counterparts, *Teen Mom 2* and *Teen Mom 3*, which present a similar three-year view of eight more teen mothers from *16 and Pregnant*. Preliminary analyses we have conducted on this series suggests it fairs much worse than *16 and Pregnant* in providing a realistic representation of teen parenting (Bamji, Eichelberger, Homick, and Loy, 2013). MTV's *Teen Mom* series shows fewer of the struggles that average teen moms endure on a daily basis, thereby not portraying the life of a typical teen mom. Episodes are more likely to glamorize teen motherhood, and characters undergo life-changing transformations due to their participation on the show. While *16 and Pregnant* chronicled the teens' lives with little evidence of alteration due to its cross-sectional nature, longitudinal participation in *Teen Mom* changes the resources available to the stars of the show and, in turn, their developmental trajectories; this is evidenced by the fact that several of the young mothers have purchased houses, new cars, and expensive wardrobes by the show's later seasons. This portrayal is in sharp contrast to the reality that most teen mothers experience as they struggle to support themselves and their children in the first few years after becoming teen mothers (Whitman *et al.*, 2001). The reality of teen parenthood as viewed through the lens of *Teen Mom* is obviously distorted. Ironically, this distorted perspective has the potential to lessen some of the negative stereotypes associated with pregnant and parenting teens, but at the same time downplays many of the more serious challenges encountered in real life.

Summary: the reality of "reality show" portrayals

The format of reality television may create misperceptions of real life by limiting the mitigating and interacting factors that influence outcomes for teens and their children. Informative details may be left out simply because the show is limited to a one-hour time slot, or perhaps due to the goals and choices of the show's editors and producers. The true experiences of teen mothers cannot be relayed due to the limited time the teens are followed. For example, social support changes the most in the first year of the babies' lives; this change is minimally evident in *16 and Pregnant* episodes that only follow mothers for approximately two to three months postpartum. This somewhat biased portrayal of teen pregnancy and parenting may create norms in the minds of adolescents who may be more susceptible to media influence, especially when the stars are "real people" who are supposedly similar to the teen viewing audience. For example, since few of the mothers were shown receiving any form of government assistance some teen viewers may assume social support was not needed or not understand what type of assistance is available (Shaw, 2010).

Although MTV's reality shows are a step forward in media depictions of teen pregnancy and teen parenting, the shows' effects on teens may be more beneficial if MTV made stronger efforts to provide more specific educational information about sexual health (Smith, 2012). Rather than just using the tagline that teen pregnancy is 100 percent preventable, and having somewhat scripted discussions of whether the teens were using birth control at the time of conception, MTV could make stronger efforts by emphasizing themes of sexual risks and responsibilities (Kunkel *et al.*, 2005). For example, nonpregnant friends or siblings could be shown attending safe-sex classes, while the teen mothers are shown struggling with decisions about sexual activity following birth. Incorporation of discussions among friends of the pregnant teens about successful strategies to avoid pregnancy may also provide new scripts for teens or reinforce activation of scripts already held by teens. Other methods to ensure that the impact is as beneficial as possible may include debriefing (e.g., clarifying to the viewers that the stars of *Teen Mom* are well paid for being on the show), exposure to prosocial or educational media, and parental control of and discussion with their children and adolescents in regards to sexual media consumption (Harris and Barlett, 2009; Wright *et al.*, 2013).

Cultural myth: providing media visibility of pregnant or parenting teens will encourage others to become pregnant

We have presented evidence suggesting that heavy consumption of sexual content in popular culture is associated with sexual attitudes and sexual and reproductive behaviors. This association is perhaps best explained by Slater's (2007) reinforcing spirals approach, which postulates differential attention to sexual content that is based on personal and motivational factors; subsequently, attention to and consumption of sexual media serves to reinforce and strengthen these initial differences. Slater's approach was built on cultivation theory (Shanahan and Morgan, 1999; Shrum and Lee, 2012), which suggests media portrayals shape beliefs about the reality of the social and political world. This theoretical and empirical evidence provides the foundation for the cultural myth that providing media visibility of pregnant or parenting teens will encourage others to become pregnant. Acceptance of this myth may have led to past suppression of pregnant and parenting teens in the media for fear that visibility would normalize teen childbearing. Only a few studies have attempted to empirically evaluate the impact of shows about teen pregnancy, and these have all focused on *16 and Pregnant* (Kearney and Levine, 2014; Suellentrop, Brown, and Ortiz, 2010; Wright *et al.*, 2013).

The National Campaign to Prevent Teen and Unplanned Pregnancy conducted an experimental study to assess the effects of *16 and Pregnant* (Suellentrop *et al.*, 2010). In this study, adolescents between the ages of 10 and 19 were randomly assigned to watch or not watch one episode of *16 and Pregnant* per day for three days and queried on their past sexual experience. Findings indicated that, within the group assigned to watch *16 and Pregnant*, teens who had never had sex were more likely to endorse the opinion that "most teens want to get pregnant," and that if they were to get pregnant or cause a pregnancy, they "will be with the baby's mother/father forever" (Suellentrop *et al.*, 2010, p. 3). Regardless of their own levels of sexual experience, participants in the group assigned to watch the show were more likely to report believing that their peers actually want to get pregnant. The study's authors concluded that viewing *16 and Pregnant* could have an adverse effect; teens who watch the show may come to normalize teen pregnancy believing that other teens may want to become pregnant and overestimating the stability of relationships between the teen parents.

The experimental methodology used by Suellentrop *et al.* (2010) provides evidence of a cultivation effect of viewing *16 and Pregnant* on teen viewers. However, consistent with Slater's (2007) reinforcing spirals approach, how teens process the information is likely informed by their age, experiences, and opportunity to discuss the content with a knowledgeable individual. For example, parent–child sexual communication could be crucial for helping teens process any prosocial messages evident in the show. A recent investigation found the association between exposure to *16 and Pregnant* and *Teen Mom* and college-aged women's recent sexual behavior was contingent upon the degree to which fathers communicated with them about sex while they were growing up (Wright *et al.*, 2013). Specifically, higher levels of exposure to *16 and Pregnant* and its spin-off show, *Teen Mom*, were associated with an increased likelihood of having engaged in recent intercourse for women whose fathers did not communicate with them about sex while they were growing up. Women who had fathers communicate with them about sex often while they were growing up were less likely to have engaged in recent intercourse when they were exposed to higher levels of *16 and Pregnant* and *Teen Mom*.

This moderating effect of father–child sexual communication is consistent with literature on fathers' roles in sexual socialization, the effects of entertainment media on youths' sexual attitudes and behavior, and a theoretical assertion which suggests that previously acquired sexual scripts affect both the acquisition and application of subsequently encountered sexual scripts (Wright, 2009, 2011). Early father–daughter communication about sex has been shown to limit young women's engagement in risky sexual behavior (Wright, 2009), increase their use of contraception (Somers and Paulson, 2000), and postpone the onset of sexual activity (Hutchinson and Montgomery, 2007; Somers and Vollmar, 2006). In accord with their 3AM model (Wright, 2011), the authors suggested that women who receive consistent advisory messages should be especially likely to attend to the negative messages cautioning against becoming a young mother, as portrayed on *16 and Pregnant* and *Teen Mom*. Young women who do not receive these advisory messages should be more likely to attend to the rewarding aspects of teen pregnancy and parenting that are depicted on *16 and Pregnant* and *Teen Mom* (Wright *et al.*, 2013). This study implies that media visibility of pregnant and parenting teens does not directly lead to specific reproductive behaviors; rather, outcomes are attributable to interacting effects with the viewers' personal experiences and characteristics.

While the above studies observed effects of viewing *16 and Pregnant* on attitudes and sexual behavior, evaluating the impact on actual rates of teen pregnancy presents even more challenges. One recent study employed an innovative and sophisticated analytic strategy to assess the causal impact of *16 and Pregnant* on actual rates of teen births (Kearney and Levine, 2014). First, Kearney and Levine (2014) used evidence from spikes in Google Search and Twitter following the release of each new episode of *16 and Pregnant* to substantiate that the content was salient for those who watched. Second, correlations between spikes related to the content of the shows with spikes related to searches on pregnancy avoidance were used to indicate that exposure and salience were associated with teens' interest in sexual activity and contraceptive use. Finally, geographic variations in the popularity of the show were used by the researchers to substantiate that viewing *16 and Pregnant* was responsible for a reduction in teen births by about 5.7% between the period June 2009 and December 2010. The causal interpretation was based on statistically controlling for extraneous variables that may have influenced both viewing behaviors and birth rates.

General summary and reframing

Children and emerging adults are voracious consumers of popular culture. Recent proliferation of electronic media has granted teens an unprecedented access to content previous restricted due to time limitations and parental monitoring. Analyses of the content of video programming targeting youth have revealed high levels of sexual content with limited attention to sexual risks and responsibilities. Not surprisingly, the high consumption of sexual content by young people has sparked vigorous debate about the potential for distorting values, promoting sexual activity, and normalizing teen pregnancy and parenthood.

We have used Wright's 3AM model of sexual socialization to suggest that consumption of sexual content through popular culture may lead to the acquisition of sexual scripts as viewers acquire knowledge about sexual activities, may activate existing scripts, and may prompt the application of scripts. Scientific evidence attesting to the impact of sexual media on attitudes and behaviors has been inconclusive, fueling both sides of the debate. A major challenge for social scientists is to show that media influences attitudes and behaviors over and above selection effects that occur when teens who have more interest in and curiosity about sex are more prone to consume sexual media and to have more liberal attitudes about sexual behavior. We endorse the conceptual framework of Slater

(2007), who refers to reinforcing spirals, which acknowledges the reciprocal nature of selectivity and media effects that have implications on both the individual and societal levels.

Teen pregnancy and parenting have become increasingly salient within popular culture, as represented in television, movies, books, magazines, song lyrics, and on the Internet. In contrast to much of the debate on the impact of sexual content, proponents of MTV's representation of teen parenting suggest that these portrayals may have a prosocial message that may actually discourage sexual activity that may lead to pregnancy. We have used our own quantitative and qualitative analyses to show that portrayals of teen parents on the popular show *16 and Pregnant*, in many ways, represent the true struggles and realities that accompany early childbearing. Further, the diversity of responses to these challenges counter many of the prevailing negative stereotypes of teen mothers.

In summary, we found little evidence that supported the cultural myth that providing media visibility of pregnant or parenting teens will encourage others to become pregnant. Alternatively, we suggest that *providing media visibility that emphasizes sexual risks and responsibilities and the challenges resulting from teen parenting can help prevent teen pregnancy*. We were unable to completely reject the common belief that media visibility may encourage pregnancy, however, since some evidence suggested young adolescents were more likely to perceive teen childbearing as normative after viewing episodes from *16 and Pregnant*. More generally, however, the impact of media visibility is likely to depend on a variety of personal, familial, and sociocultural factors. Messages from popular culture are only a fraction of messages children and youths use to construct sexual scripts. The impact of messages from popular culture depends to a large extent on their integration with other messages.

Media portrayals of adolescent pregnancy and parenthood have the potential to affect common beliefs of society, making it essential that representations reflect the diversity of experiences and responses to early pregnancy. The impact of popular culture may be more subtle, however, by neglecting the important roles of poverty and sexual abuse in rates of teen pregnancy. Omitted information may be as influential as what is included in television programs. Portrayals showing teens who make autonomous choices about contraception, birth outcomes, relationships, and parenting could negate the importance of contextual forces in these behaviors. This omission may lead parents, taxpayers, and policy-makers to place sole responsibility for teen pregnancy and parenting on the shoulders of the teens themselves, while ignoring society's contribution to these life-changing experiences. Consequently, MTV's lack of attention to these contextual factors means that the network is missing some of the valuable educational opportunities that they are aiming to provide through their programs.

4 Myths and misperceptions about teen pregnancy

In the UK, public perceptions about the kinds of women who experience pregnancy and motherhood in their adolescence often combine elements of truth ... and also aspects of the worst prejudices ... In contemporary British society, negative stereotypes about young mothers dominate the popular imagination and teenage mothers are generally considered to be young women deficient in morals and conduct, and even appearance.

(Arai, 2009a, p. 19)

The negative perceptions of teen pregnancy portrayed in the above quote are not limited to the UK, but are echoed in similar sentiments from around the globe. College students in our own research ascribed traits of delinquent, immoral, irresponsible, foolish, and clueless to pregnant teens and teen mothers; teen fathers were rated even more negatively than teen mothers (Weed et al., 2013). Further, a review by Bales and O'Neil (2008) found that US news articles published between 2006 and 2008 framed "teen pregnancy as a result of immoral cultural values, poor decision-making, misguided mindsets, apathy, and personal moral failings" (p. 6). Stereotypes derived from these negative perceptions have the potential to create additional challenges for pregnant and parenting teens as they face major role transitions in their lives.

Negative perceptions and stereotypes may provide convenient explanations of behavior that may mask more uncomfortable, but also more valid, explanations. Consider the case of a child born to an unmarried, 18-year-old woman in the southern United States. *The little girl was raised by her grandmother while her teenage mother left home to find work in the city. A few years later, the grandmother became ill so the girl was reunited with her mother in a poverty-stricken inner-city area. Despite her chaotic and neglectful upbringing, the girl was academically gifted and excelled in school. Tragically, at the age of nine, she was raped by a male relative and experienced ongoing sexual abuse from that point forward. Feelings of shame and fear resulted in the abuse being kept a secret. Soon however, the girl began skipping school, stealing, and running away from home. By the age of 14, her mother labeled her as a "bad" child and tried to put her in a home for wayward girls. The home was not accepting new residents, so the girl went to live with her father. She was already pregnant when she moved in with her father and stepmother, but she kept the pregnancy secret. The secret was revealed nearly seven months later when she went into premature labor and delivered a baby who did not survive. Despite many challenges faced as a child and adolescent, this child of a teenage mother went on to become a well-known, wealthy, and highly respected woman who has made many positive contributions to society: Oprah Winfrey* (Krone, 2005).

Winfrey's story highlights the complexity surrounding beliefs about teen pregnancy and depicts the first cultural myth we address in this chapter: *that most pregnant teens have behavior problems.* This common belief is fueled by stereotypes that characterize pregnant and parenting teens as delinquent, promiscuous, and irresponsible. The tendency to attribute teen pregnancy to internal traits and characteristics rather than external circumstance is consistent with a well-known concept in the field of psychology known as the *fundamental attribution error* (Ross, 1977). This error may underlie common beliefs that pregnant teens are rebellious and troubled. An example of this tendency to attribute behaviors to internal characteristics is found in Jessor and Jessor's (1975, 1977) problem-behavior theory that places teen pregnancy alongside delinquency and substance abuse.

The first part of this chapter provides a brief overview of problem-behavior theory and the fundamental attribution error, followed by an analysis of evidence that counters this perspective and confirms that the majority of teen pregnancies occur to teens without a history of problem behaviors. We then review additional evidence of a contextual factor – a history of sexual abuse – that significantly increases the likelihood of early pregnancies for both women and men. Our objective is to rethink the common belief that teen pregnancy only happens to certain types of young people; that only teens who are rebellious, delinquent, and irresponsible end up pregnant or causing a pregnancy, while teens who are conscientious, obedient, and competent avoid pregnancy. As demonstrated in the brief biography of Winfrey, external circumstances are often a more powerful influence on behavior than internal traits and characteristics.

The second part of this chapter explores the cultural myth that *all teen pregnancies are unintended and unwanted.* As we examine this common belief, we highlight the ambiguity that many teens feel about pregnancy and childbirth. Accumulating evidence suggests that framing the issue as a dichotomy (i.e., intended or unintended) may constrain efforts to further understand the complexities of how multiple influences combine to result in teen pregnancy (Phipps and Nunes, 2012). In this portion of the chapter, we review some of the motivations that compel young people into wanting a child as well as motivations that curtail their desire. Our objective is to remove the artificial distinctions between teen and adult pregnancies and to propose that teens become pregnant for many of the same reasons as adults. Motivations of both teens and adults contain elements of both wantedness and unintendedness.

We end the chapter by considering how we need to move beyond a narrow focus on attitudes and behaviors of youth to fully account for teen pregnancy. Consistent with a systems perspective, we emphasize that teen pregnancy is embedded within multiple interacting personal and sociocultural contexts (e.g., the respect and esteem that typically accompany motherhood, and cultural views of when it is appropriate to begin motherhood). To address this socio-cultural embeddedness, we draw on research conducted in several countries; we also maintain a multidisciplinary focus by including evidence from diverse fields that include psychology, sociology, economics, communications, public health, and nursing. In addition, we rely on data collected from the Notre Dame Adolescent Parenting Project (NDAPP; Whitman *et al.*, 2001) to inform our discussion. Further, a full understanding of the complexity that underlies these beliefs on teen pregnancy requires consideration of the developmental context of adolescence (see Chapter 1). Our goal in this chapter is to rethink two cultural myths about teen pregnancy using evidence conceptualized through a systems perspective.

Rates of teen pregnancy and teen births

Within the United States, rates of teen pregnancy have declined significantly from a high of 111 out of 1,000 women during the years 1988 through 1992, to 68 out of 1,000 for the period 2005 to 2008; the rate fell even further to 29.4 out of 1,000 in 2012 (Curtin, Abma, Ventura, and Henshaw, 2013; Kost and Henshaw, 2013). Corresponding declines were observed in rates of abortions and births to teens in the United States, and in other developed countries during this time period (Singh, Wulf, Hussain, Bankole, and Sedgh, 2009). Estimating the number of youths who experience a pregnancy during the teen years is difficult since pregnancies that do not result in either a birth or an abortion (i.e., miscarriages) often go unreported. Since pregnancies are not observed directly, rates must be inferred using data from births, abortions, and fetal deaths. The striking declines in births to teen mothers, used as a proxy for pregnancies, between 1991 and 2011 in the United States and the United Kingdom, are shown in Figure 4.1.

A review of trends in pregnancies and births to teens raises two important issues. The first issue concerns identifying differences between teens who become pregnant from those who postpone pregnancy until adulthood. A second issue relates to causes of the declines in rates of teen pregnancy since the early 1990s. Consistent with the fundamental attribution error, a common tendency is to blame an off-timed pregnancy on character flaws within the teens. However, placing responsibility on personal attributes of the teens fails to consider broader social and cultural conditions that also shape reproductive behaviors. The rest of this chapter will address these two important issues. Our review of evidence surrounding these two issues begins with a cultural myth that answers the question of who becomes pregnant as a teen by suggesting that pregnancies only happen to teens with a history of serious behavior problems. Serious behavior problems refers to problems that go beyond the occasional disobedience and limit pushing that may be associated with typical teenage behavior, and includes substance

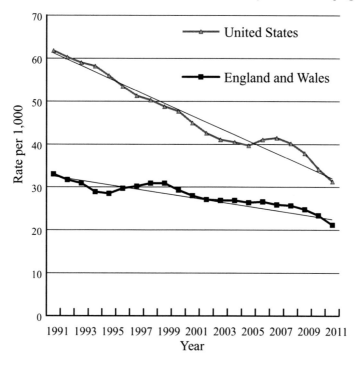

Figure 4.1 Teen birth rates in the United States and England and Wales from 1991 through 2011

Source (US): Hamilton, Martin, and Ventura, 2013. Source (UK): Office for National Statistics.

abuse, delinquency, and aggression, often collectively referred to as externalizing behaviors.

Cultural myth: most pregnant teens have behavior problems

Oprah Winfrey's mother was not the only parent who sought to reform her daughter by placing her in an institution for troubled youths. During the late 1800s and continuing throughout most of the 1900s, sexuality and childbearing among young women, but not young men, was attributed to a general pattern of problem behavior (Kennedy, 2008; Lesko, 2002; Schlossman and Wallach, 1978). During this time period, young women were labeled wayward, promiscuous, or degenerate if they engaged in, or gave the appearance of engaging in, sexual behavior outside of marriage. A typical solution was to banish these women to institutions. Segregating young women in this way minimized their perceived threat to society. As a further precaution, institutionalization was often accompanied by sterilization to ensure that people with undesirable traits did not pass on these characteristics genetically to their offspring (Kennedy, 2008).

Strategies to reduce the prevalence of undesirable behavior by segregating the perceived offenders are consistent with the fundamental attribution error that blames other people's problem behaviors on internal and unchangeable characteristics or personal flaws. Explanations for our own rude behavior, however, are often attributed to situational constraints (Ross, 1977). Many engage in the fundamental attribution error on a daily basis, typically without conscious awareness. Consider the following example: on the drive to work you get cut off by another driver and immediately think, "what a jerk!" However, on the way home, late for an important social engagement, you cut off another driver; you do not think that you are a jerk but rather attribute your poor driving to being late for an appointment. In the context of teen pregnancy, the fundamental attribution error leads to the assumption that teens who engage in sex and become pregnant must also be generally rebellious and troubled. An example of this tendency is found in Jessor and Jessor's (1975, 1977) problem-behavior theory.

Problem-behavior theory proposes that internal characteristics increase the likelihood of some teens engaging in behaviors viewed by society as problematic. Specifically, the behavior of these teens may be driven by an *unconventional* personality. This attribution implies that pregnant teens reject conventional societal norms and values and have a tendency to engage in behavior that does not conform to society's standards (Costa, Jessor, Donovan, and Fortenberry, 1995; Donovan, Jessor, and Costa, 1991; Jessor and Jessor, 1975, 1977). Since behaviors stem from internal characteristics, problem-behavior theory implies that teens who engage in one type of nonnormative behavior will be more likely to engage in other types of nonnormative behaviors. Consequently, delinquency, substance abuse, and sexual activity constitute a pattern of behaviors exhibited by a certain type of teen. In contrast, teens with a more conventional personality are viewed as being more likely to abstain from behaviors seen as problematic.

Problem-behavior theorists acknowledge that internal characteristics may not be solely responsible for the tendency of teens who exhibit one problem behavior to also exhibit other problem behaviors. In addition, the theory refers to the *social ecology of youth* to explain how the unconventional personalities of some teens interact with risk and protective factors in their social environments, leading to the expression of problem behaviors (Costa *et al.*, 1995). Within this social ecology, problem behaviors may acquire specific culturally laden meanings, distinct from more general meanings. For example, sexual activity of married adults may be interpreted as a symbol of intimacy and affection. However, within the social ecology of youth, this same sexual behavior may be interpreted as an overt violation of societal norms or as an effort to express independence from parents.

Once culturally laden meanings are acquired then the youths' environments may be transformed. Youths perceived by others as unconventional and rebellious may attract other unconventional peers and be provided new opportunities to engage in additional problem behaviors that are also in opposition to conventional norms. Similar to a self-fulfilling prophecy, the attributions society makes may end up being expressed, regardless of whether the youth actually possessed those characteristics prior to engaging in the behavior. These linkages or cascading effects within the social ecology provide a pathway for the initiation of any one behavior to lead to engagement with other problem behaviors.

Problem-behavior theory also introduced the concept of *transition proneness*, which refers to the tendency to engage in behaviors considered normative for adults but which contain social sanctions when engaged in by underage youths (i.e., drinking, sexual activity; Donovan *et al.*, 1991). Some teens may come to think of themselves as adults at relatively young ages and correspondingly view sexual activity as a normative behavior consistent with their perceived maturity. Although the concept of transition proneness may consider the teens' perceptions of themselves as adults rather than adolescents, it fails to take into account their actual levels of psychosocial development (Benson and Elder, 2011). In other words, not all teens who think of themselves as adults actually display the maturity and responsibility that accompanies adult status.

In summary, the cultural myth that most pregnant teens have behavior problems has been reinforced by problem-behavior theory. Consistent with the fundamental attribution error, problem-behavior theory explains that teens with an unconventional personality type or those who perceive themselves as adults are more likely to be sexually active and, therefore, at risk for early pregnancy. Well-behaved teens who conform to social expectations are not considered to be at risk. Although problem-behavior theory was developed in the 1970s it remains highly influential today; a search on Google Scholar revealed over 700 publications based on problem-behavior theory since 2009. The next section scrutinizes three scientific studies that represent current applications of problem-behavior theory to teen pregnancy, with a goal of providing an objective evaluation of the extent to which this cultural myth is consistent with scientific evidence.

Research evidence

At first glance, some empirical evidence appears to support an association between problem behavior and teen pregnancy. For example, data collected from the Western Australia Child Health Survey (WACHS, see Appendix) revealed that 40 percent of women who had been classified as both aggressive and delinquent during childhood, based on reports by their primary caregivers, had experienced a teen pregnancy (Gaudie, Mitrou, Lawrence, Stanley, Silburn, and Zubrick, 2010). In contrast, less than 10 percent of the teens who were neither aggressive nor delinquent experienced pregnancy. Data from the Christchurch Health and Development Study (CHDS, see Appendix) in New Zealand also suggested that behavior problems reported during middle childhood were a significant risk factor for early pregnancy. This relationship was consistent for both girls and boys, and remained even after controlling for other important family and socioeconomic influences (Woodward, Fergusson, and Horwood, 2006). This longitudinal data provides some credence to the belief that having a general pattern of serious behavioral problems is a precursor to teen pregnancy.

In contrast, results of a study examining patterns of risk among teen mothers provide evidence that contradicts the cultural myth that most pregnant teens have behavior problems (Oxford, Gilchrist, Lohr, Gillmore, Morrison, and Spieker, 2005). In this study, eight aspects of teen mothers' lives were used to create risk profiles: criminal involvement, illicit drug use, alcohol use, mental health problems, intimate partner violence, risky sexual practices, public assistance, and stressful life events. Three distinct patterns emerged: *normative, psychologically vulnerable*, and *problem-prone*. Youths classified as *normative* (43 percent) had low levels on all risk factors except for receipt of public assistance, implying that even this well-functioning group of teen mothers had low incomes. Another 42 percent were considered *psychologically vulnerable* due to relatively high reports of depression, anxiety, alcohol use, stressful life events, and exposure to intimate partner violence. Only 15 percent of the sample was identified as *problem-prone*, based primarily on the combination of illicit drug use, criminal involvement, and risky sexual behaviors. In other words, only a small minority (15 percent) of teen mothers had a pattern of serious problem behaviors, while close to one-half (43 percent) of the teen mothers refrained from behaviors considered problematic.

The apparent discrepancies between conclusions drawn from the Australian and New Zealand studies with results from Oxford *et al.* (2005) are superficial. Interpretations of the data have exaggerated the strength of the relationship between problem behaviors and teen pregnancy. For example, Gaudie *et al.* (2010) began their discussion with the conclusion that delinquent behavior (including breaking rules and norms set by parents and communities) and aggressive behavior (including bullying, teasing, temper tantrums, arguing, fighting, and threatening) were strongly associated with teenage pregnancy in their Australian sample. However, since very few children engaged in high levels of both aggressive and delinquent behaviors, this predictive relationship accounted for only a small percentage of pregnant teens. We provide further details below to illustrate how findings of these three studies may actually converge.

The Australian sample was divided into three groups: (1) teens who had a history of both delinquency and aggression, (2) teens who had a history of either delinquency or aggression, but not both, and (3) teens without a history of either delinquency or aggression (Gaudie *et al.*, 2010). Approximately 39.5 percent of the teens who exhibited delinquency and aggressive behavior became pregnant as a teen, whereas 17.5 percent of those with only one type of behavior problem, and only 9.4 percent of teens without any behavior problems, became pregnant. At first glance, this seems like compelling evidence to show that teens who became pregnant had a prior history of behavior problems. It is important to note, however, that only 2.3 percent of their entire sample of young women exhibited a history of delinquent and aggressive behaviors, accounting for 12 or 13 of the pregnancies in this WACHS sample. An additional 15 pregnancies occurred to teens with a history of either delinquent or aggressive behaviors, but not both. On the other hand, the vast majority of pregnancies in this Australian sample (approximately 117) occurred to teens with no history of behavior problems. Reframing the results in this way reveals that over four times as many teen pregnancies in this sample (117 compared to 27 or 28) occurred to teenagers without a history of any behavior problems. Therefore, while delinquent and aggressive teens were more likely to get pregnant than teens without a history of delinquency and aggression (i.e., 39.5 percent versus 9.4 percent), most pregnant teens had no history of either delinquent or aggressive behaviors. Results from this Australian study, therefore, are quite consistent with conclusions by Oxford *et al.* (2005) that most of the teen mothers did not have behavior problems.

Pregnancy and problem behaviors within the NDAPP

Additional evidence from our own research bolsters the conclusion that most pregnant teens do not have a history of serious behavior problems. The NDAPP is a 20-year longitudinal study of adolescent mothers and their children, who have been followed since the prenatal period (Borkowski *et al.*, 2007; Whitman *et al.*, 2001). At the time of our final assessment, when the youths were between 18 and 21 years of age, approximately 35 percent of the

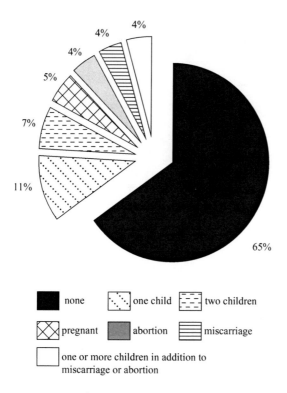

Figure 4.2a Reported pregnancy status and outcomes of young women from the NDAPP at 18 years of age

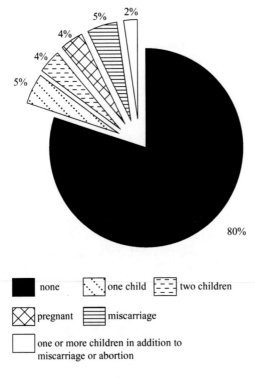

5%   2%

4%

4%

5%

80%

◼ none   ⬚ one child   ⬚ two children

⬚ pregnant   ⬚ miscarriage

⬚ one or more children in addition to
miscarriage or abortion

Figure 4.2b Reported pregnancy status and outcomes of young men from the NDAPP at
18 years of age

young women in our sample reported having been pregnant by age 18, and
20 percent of the young men reported having caused a pregnancy by age 18.
Figure 4.2a summarizes the pregnancy status of young women from the NDAPP
and Figure 4.2b summarizes the pregnancy outcomes of the young men. The
critical question was whether the youths who had experienced an early pregnancy were more likely to exhibit serious problem behaviors than the teens
who avoided pregnancy.

To answer this question, we first used latent class analysis (LCA; see Chapter 2)
to sort the 113 young women and men from our sample into relatively similar
subgroups based on patterns of behaviors (Weed and Noria, 2011). Eight indicators within the domains of academics, substance use, health, risky behaviors, and
psychological functioning were used to identify these subgroups. Approximately
56 percent of the sample was classified in a *normative* category because they had
optimal values on all measures of functioning. In other words, the majority of
teens had no serious problems in academics, substance use, health, risky behaviors, or psychological functioning. Another 22 percent was classified in a *delinquent* category; almost all of the youth in this category had been arrested and

reported significant substance use prior to age 18. Despite these negatives, most had held paying jobs and none had serious psychiatric disorders. A third category included 18 percent of the sample; all of these *maladjusted* youths reported a history of adjustment problems (e.g., depression, anxiety, ADHD, eating disorders) and over one-half reported significant substance use prior to age 18. Youths in the maladjusted category tended to have problems in school, as indicated by below-average functional academic scores and high rates of grade repeats. The smallest category included only 4 percent of the sample and was labeled *misfits*. These youths were all obese and had repeated grades in school, but had not used substances or been involved with juvenile justice.

After verifying that these four categories described patterns of behavior among the young men and women in our sample, we examined pregnancy status in relation to group membership (Weed and Noria, 2011). The percentage of young men from the normative group who reported having caused a pregnancy was not very different from the percentage of pregnancies reported by young men from the delinquent group (21 percent versus 25 percent). For young women, pregnancy was somewhat related to patterns of problem behaviors, as more youths in the delinquent group reported pregnancy (60 percent) compared to those in the normative group (38 percent).

Consistent with our reframing of results reported by Gaudie *et al.* (2010), however, examination of percentages without looking at actual numbers of pregnancies would result in misleading conclusions. Since the normative pattern of outcomes was most frequent in the NDAPP sample, far more pregnancies occurred to young women without behavior problems than to young women with behavior problems. In fact, 11 of the pregnancies among young women in our sample were to teens in the normative group, whereas only six pregnancies were to teens with a delinquent pattern. This data confirms that teens who struggle with behavior problems may be more likely to become pregnant or cause a pregnancy, but the reverse cannot be assumed; most teens who become pregnant do not have serious behavioral problems.

Summary and reframing

Attempts to explain the occurrence of teen pregnancy based on problem-behavior theory fall short. Empirical evidence confirms that most pregnant teens do not have an overall pattern and history of behavior problems (Gaudie *et al.*, 2010; Oxford *et al.*, 2005; Weed and Noria, 2011). Although some evidence suggests that teens with a history of behavior problems may be somewhat more likely to engage in risky behaviors and become pregnant, there is little to no evidence to suggest that when teens become sexually active they also get involved with other unconventional behaviors. We conclude that the cultural myth that most pregnant teens have behavior problems is largely based on misperception. Reframing this myth consistently with the evidence we have reviewed suggests the alternative perspective that *the majority of teen pregnancies occur to, or are caused by, young women and men without a history of behavior problems.* Stripping the explanatory power for pregnancy from behavior problems leads to the search for alternative explanations to account for which teens get pregnant and why. Contextual influences in the lives of teens may provide additional predictive value. One of these contextual influences is the experience of childhood sexual abuse (CSA).

Childhood sexual abuse increases risk of teen pregnancy

In 2010, the movie *Precious* highlighted a pregnant teen who struggled against stereotypes. In this popular movie, Precious became pregnant at the age of 13 after being raped repeatedly by her father. Although she was unable to read, grossly overweight, and even rejected by her own mother, eventually an alternative school teacher was able to make a connection with Precious. The relationship Precious developed with her teacher unlocked her world through words and allowed her to confront many of the negative stereotypes she faced due to her pregnancy. Sapphire, the author of the book on which *Precious* was based, reflected on misperceptions held about young pregnant teens similar to Precious with the statement, "we brought up a stereotype, and we cracked it open, and a human being comes forth" (Sapphire's Story, 2009).

Scientific research has confirmed that youths who experienced CSA are at heightened risk for teen pregnancy. Findings from 21 studies within the United States, Canada, and New Zealand were reviewed to determine the relationship between pregnancy status of young women and a history of CSA (Noll, Shenk, and Putnam, 2009). After combining information from all studies, the authors concluded that 45 out of every 100 pregnant teens had a history of CSA. A similar study of more than 40,000 high-school students in the United States and Canada reported the same pattern among boys; boys who experienced CSA were more likely than other boys to cause a pregnancy as teens (Homma, Wang, Saewyc, and Kishor, 2012). Teens with a history of CSA were observed to be more preoccupied with sex, as evidenced by reports of a higher frequency of sexual thoughts and feelings, having more ambivalent sexual attitudes, and expressing a heightened desire to become pregnant (Noll *et al.*, 2009). The young men who experienced CSA were five times more likely to cause a teen pregnancy, three times more likely to have multiple sexual partners, and two times more likely to have unprotected sex, when compared to boys without a history of sexual abuse (Homma *et al.*, 2012).

A history of CSA is therefore a strong predictor that distinguishes teens who become pregnant from those who delay pregnancy. This contextual factor challenges the assumption that internal traits and characteristics are responsible for the majority of teen pregnancies. A comparison of the strength of the predictive relationships from the studies we have reviewed suggests that although 45 out of 100 pregnancies may be attributed to CSA (Noll *et al.*, 2009), less than 25 out of 100 are explainable by serious problem behaviors (Gaudie *et al.*, 2010; Weed and Noria, 2011). It is likely that CSA and serious problem behaviors are not entirely independent, however, since a history of abuse may lead to externalizing problems. Acting out through substance abuse or delinquency may be understandable reactions to the betrayal and harm caused by adults in positions of authority (Jones *et al.*, 2013). Associations between risky sexual behavior, substance abuse, and delinquency may all be partially due to an underlying history of CSA. Additional personal and societal influences that may impact teen pregnancy are reviewed in the sections that follow, in which we review a second cultural myth surrounding teen pregnancy.

Cultural myth: all teen pregnancies are unintended and unwanted

The search for answers to the question of why some teens become pregnant and have children is often based on the assumption that teen pregnancies are not planned or wanted. This assumption has recently been challenged by the realization that some teen pregnancies are intentional. It is important to rethink the cultural myth that all teen pregnancies are unintended and unwanted because teens who have conscious or unconscious desires to bear children may be less receptive to standard teen pregnancy prevention strategies. For example, campaigns that focus on the benefits of sexual abstinence or how to use contraception to prevent pregnancy will not be as effective for teens who want to become pregnant.

Since the 1960s, the United States and many countries in Europe have collected information at the time of birth to classify pregnancies as intended, unwanted, or mistimed. Recent definitions of *mistimed* differentiate births to parents who wanted a child sometime within the subsequent two years from those who wanted a child but expected to wait more than two years before having children (Mosher, Jones, and Abma, 2012). To classify pregnancies into these categories, women respond to questions about use of contraception, and about whether and when they wanted to become pregnant. Birth data from the United States in 2008 revealed that approximately 63 percent of all births (i.e., teen and adult mothers combined) were intended. This rate was similar to rates in Australia and New Zealand, but less than many countries in the European Union (Singh, Sedgh, and Hussain, 2010).

Pregnancies to adult women were more likely to be reported as intended than pregnancies to teens and emerging adults (Mosher *et al.*, 2012). Approximately 75 percent of pregnancies to mothers between 25 and 44 years of age were reported as intended, but only 23 percent of pregnancies to mothers between the ages of 15 and 19 were reported as intended. Pregnancies to married women were more likely to be intended than pregnancies to single women, with only 33 percent of births to women of any age who were not married or cohabiting intentional. These data indicate that even though teen mothers report a much lower rate of intended pregnancies compared to adult mothers, there is clearly a consciousness of becoming pregnant for close to one-fourth of teen mothers. These data need to be interpreted with caution; rates of intended pregnancies to teens may be underreported due to the perception that admitting to wanting a baby as a teen, or as a single parent, violates strong cultural norms and should not be voiced (Dash, 1989; Kearney and Levine, 2012).

The reluctance of teens to admit to wanting a pregnancy was portrayed in the writings of a journalist, Leon Dash, who relocated to an impoverished area of Washington, DC, to more fully understand the experiences of the residents, with a focus on teen mothers (Dash, 1989). Dash recounted the story of Tauscha Vaughn, a 16-year-old, who he referred to as the most perceptive young adult that he had ever interviewed. During their interviews, Tauscha had convinced Dash that she was committed to staying in school and avoiding pregnancy. Months later, when Tauscha admitted she had become pregnant only days after speaking with Dash, he was forced to reevaluate his long-held assumptions about the unintentional nature of teen pregnancy. Tauscha's pregnancy made Dash realize that the motivations behind many teen pregnancies were much more complicated than they appeared, and might not be openly expressed by teens. Dash's experiences with teen parents and their families resonate with conclusions from empirical research suggesting that the reality of teen pregnancy is more complex than initially perceived. Social and cultural expectations interact with personal characteristics and contextual influences to impact the likelihood of a teen pregnancy.

Fertility-timing norms

Acceptable ages for women to bear children vary by country and by culture, and even by subcultures within countries. These expectations about reproductive behaviors are referred to as *fertility-timing norms* (Geronimus, 2003). Figure 4.3 shows the percentages of all births to women aged 15 through 19 in comparison to women aged 25 through 29 by country for the period 2005 to 2010 (United Nations, 2013). This comparison provides a visual estimate of differences between countries in fertility-timing norms. In Brazil and Mexico almost as many births are to women aged 15 to 19 as to those aged 25 to 29, suggesting younger fertility-timing norms. In contrast, rates of childbearing to French and Swedish women in their late twenties are over ten times greater than rates to teens. In terms of fertility-timing norms, teen pregnancies may be considered more normative in Brazil and Mexico, compared to France and Sweden. Fertility-timing norms are important macrosystem elements that impact the likelihood of youths becoming pregnant, or causing a pregnancy, during the teen years.

Just as fertility-timing norms influence differences in maternal age at childbirth between countries, they also have the potential to impact maternal age at childbirth between cultures within countries or even between communities (Geronimus, 2003; Warner, Giordano, Manning, and Longmore, 2011; Witt, 2012). Cultural groups within countries have differing norms that drive the timing of reproductive behavior (Geronimus, 2003; Henly, 1997; Witt, 2012). Geronimus (2003) provided a convincing comparison of timing of first birth by neighborhood, indicating that considerable variability existed within race based on more local norms within neighborhoods. Postponement of childbearing was more normative for non-Latina Whites, especially in neighborhoods within higher median incomes. Although earlier childbearing was more normative

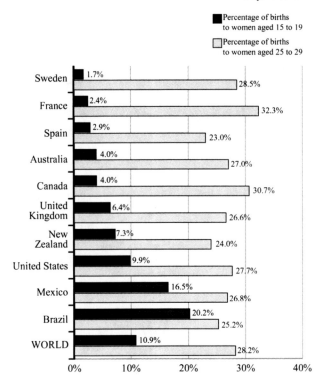

Figure 4.3 Percentage of all births to women aged 15 to 19 compared to adult women aged 25 to 29, by country

Source: United Nations, Department of Economic and Social Affairs, Population Division.

for Blacks, this was especially true in the most economically disadvantaged neighborhoods.

Similar differences in fertility-timing norms were found between cultures in New Zealand. Data from the Christchurch Health and Development Study (CHDS) confirmed that cultural groups differed in the optimum timing of human reproduction (Marie, Fergusson, and Boden, 2011). The CHDS sample was split into three groups based on their identification with the native culture of New Zealand, the Maori: sole Maori, mixed Maori, and non-Maori. After controlling for important socioeconomic and family functioning influences, sole Maori young people had significantly higher rates of pregnancy and parenthood than those who had mixed identity or non-Maori identity. In fact, the rate of parenthood was almost twice that of young people in the other groups (Marie *et al.*, 2011).

Fertility-timing norms may impact both the likelihood of a teen pregnancy and the willingness to confess to wanting a baby during the teen years (Dash, 1989; Kearney and Levine, 2012). Bearing children within socially appropriate ages confers acceptance and approval, whereas beginning childbearing either too early or too late may result in ostracism or other social censures. The powerful impact of fertility-timing norms was confirmed by several of the teen mothers from the NDAPP. For example, when questioned about her family's response to learning of her pregnancy, one young woman responded, "My mother was relieved – she was beginning to wonder if something was wrong with me since I was almost 20 and hadn't had a child yet." This teen, and others like her, was aware of early fertility-timing norms, which may have consciously or unconsciously impacted her reproductive behaviors.

Several studies have confirmed that perceptions of teen pregnancy as more normative, and therefore less embarrassing, were associated with a greater likelihood of an early pregnancy (Afable-Munsuz, Speizer, Magnus, and Kendall, 2006; Jaccard, Dodge, and Dittus, 2003; Mollborn, 2010). Positive pregnancy attitudes were stronger for Black and Latino youths, compared to Whites, and for young women living with single or less-educated parents. Older teens in close romantic relationships also held more accepting attitudes towards teen pregnancy (Jaccard et al., 2003).

Ambivalent attitudes

Skeptics have questioned the validity of traditional surveys to adequately capture the ambiguity felt by many women about their pregnancies (Finlay, 1996; Phipps and Nunes, 2012; Santelli, Lindberg, Orr, Finer, and Speizer, 2009). Ambivalent attitudes are feelings of both wanting and not wanting aspects of pregnancy and motherhood. Ambivalent feelings are often present even in pregnancies to adult women and pregnancies that are planned (Higgins, Popkin, and Santelli, 2012; Yoo, Hayford, and Guzzo, 2012). Women of all ages may look forward to pregnancy and motherhood but lament how it will impact other aspects of their lives. These conflicting feelings may sometimes be misinterpreted as an unintended or unwanted pregnancy. Although only 23 percent of teens admitted that their pregnancies were intended at the time of conception (Mosher et al., 2012), if ambivalence was interpreted as lack of intent, the rates could actually be much higher. One recent survey of unmarried and childless emerging adults between the ages of 18 and 29 observed that over 36 percent of the women and 50 percent of the men had ambivalent attitudes about pregnancy (Fog Zone; Higgins et al., 2012; Yoo et al., 2012).

Typical survey instruments used to measure pregnancy intentions have women respond to questions about their thoughts and feelings regarding the impact of pregnancy, for example, "I think I would be happier if I got pregnant now," or "I think it would be good for me to get pregnant at this time in my life" (Sheeder, Teal, Crane, and Stevens-Simon, 2010). Ambivalent attitudes are inferred from either inconsistent responses (i.e., a strong "yes" to becoming happier, but a strong "no" to pregnancy being a good thing) or to responses indicating indifference to pregnancy (i.e., neither a strong "yes" nor a strong "no"). However, averaging positive and negative scores obscures the reality that some women hold simultaneous positive and negative feelings about pregnancy. Strong opposing responses may actually reflect a different type of ambivalence than indifference, and these varieties of ambivalence may have distinct implications for contraceptive use and pregnancy. Consistent with systems thinking, Sheeder *et al.* (2010) acknowledged that contraceptive use and, indirectly, pregnancy are not predicted from simply adding up or averaging the pros and cons about wanting to become pregnant; attitudes, feelings, and intentions interact in complex ways to predict contraceptive use and pregnancy. For example, declines in both contraceptive use and birth rates may stem from changes in the economy.

Ambivalence has been reported in several studies about pregnancy intentions from sexually active teens (Drebitko, Sadler, Leventhal, Daley, and Reynolds, 2005; Rosengard, Pollock, Weitzen, Meers, and Phipps, 2006; Sheeder *et al.*, 2010). Younger teens were more likely than older teens to express strong opposing views about both wanting and not wanting to become pregnant (Sheeder *et al.*, 2010). Developmental considerations of younger teens, as discussed in Chapter 1, suggest that they may integrate feelings and thoughts differently than older teens, due to ongoing brain development. Specifically, the less sophisticated cognitive development of younger teens, coupled with their ambivalent views about pregnancy, raises serious concerns about the utility of standard pregnancy prevention programming with young teens.

Acceptance of the stipulation that some teens hold ambivalent attitudes, or unvoiced pro-pregnancy attitudes, raises the additional questions of what motivates teens towards pregnancy and parenting, and what factors inhibit the desire for early childbearing. Although it may be tempting to suggest teens are motivated by anticipation of welfare support (as noted in the quote at the beginning of this chapter), there is little evidence to support this conclusion. In contrast, motivations and desires towards childbearing are likely to result from a complex combination of feelings, thoughts, and behaviors (Miller, Barber, and Gatny, 2013).

Conceptual model of reproductive behavior

The quest to discover causes of teen pregnancy might appropriately begin with an understanding of forces that cause men and women of all ages to desire pregnancy and childbearing. Although skeptics may suggest that pregnancy and childbearing are the inevitable, and often unintentional, consequences of responses to a biologically based sex drive (Basten, 2009), recent studies suggest the sex drive may have distinct physiological underpinnings and different behavioral associations from a drive to bear children. For example, both the number of children *desired* and the number of children *intended* were found to have strong genetic components leading to intergenerational similarities in family size among youths who participated in the National Longitudinal Study of Youth (see Appendix; Miller, Bard, Pasta, and Rodgers, 2010). This biological drive for children has been integrated with motivational forces in a conceptual model of pregnancy intentions, by Miller and his colleagues, referred to as the Traits, Desire, Intentions, Behavior

(TDIB) model (Miller *et al.*, 2013). The TDIB model is a predictive model of pregnancy that integrates positive and negative motivations towards childbearing (*traits*), *desires* related to the number and timing of childbearing, *intentions* about childbearing, and contraceptive *behavior*. The TDIB model acknowledges that men and women may hold simultaneous positive and negative motivations for pregnancy.

A desire to have children, or *baby longing*, is an important component of the TDIB model that may vary by age and by gender. Although both men and women reported experiencing a desire for children (Brase and Brase, 2012; Rotkirch, Basten, Väisänen, and Jokela, 2011), women reported a stronger and more frequently felt desire than men. In one study, baby longing was predicted by both more positive and less negative feelings and attitudes towards infant cues (e.g., baby smells or sounds, baby crying, dirty diapers; Brase and Brase, 2012). These visceral reactions to cues combined with cognitive responses to survey questions to explain the degree of baby longing. Results were consistent with the TDIB model that the desire for a baby may have a physiological basis that is influenced by sociocultural expectations, and that these factors may interact throughout the life span to regulate reproductive behavior (Brase and Brase, 2012; Miller *et al.*, 2013). Most of the adults in the study reported that baby longing had preceded childbearing and culminated in actually having a child. Typically, this desire for children tended to peak in the early to mid-twenties and then decline, but close to 20 percent of women and over 10 percent of men reported being aware of this longing since youth. Baby longing may precipitate ambivalence in some young men and women who feel strong desires towards having a baby despite awareness of social prohibitions against early childbearing.

The TDIB conceptual model proposes that contraceptive behavior is dependent on both positive and negative motivations and desires for children. Feelings of shame, guilt, or embarrassment associated with early pregnancy may serve as deterrents for teens, even those who experience baby longing (Jaccard *et al.*, 2003; Mollborn, 2010). However, the relationship between negative feelings about pregnancy and actual pregnancy may be considerably weaker among samples that include only sexually active teens. For instance, Brückner, Martin, and Bearman (2004) reported that pregnancy attitudes were unrelated to either contraceptive use or actual pregnancy, using a sample of close to 5,000 sexually experienced unmarried young women between the ages of 15 and 19 from the Add Health study.

Acceptance of the cultural myth that all teen pregnancies are unintended and unwanted leads to the assumption that most pregnancies could be prevented by increasing knowledge of and access to contraception (Zolna and Lindberg, 2012). Reports of both increased contraceptive use and declines in rates of teen pregnancy make it tempting to infer that increased access to contraception is responsible for the observed declines in teen pregnancies. For example, a recent news article began with the statement, "More teenage girls are using contraception, which may explain part of the dramatic drop in the US teen pregnancy rate, federal health officials reported Thursday" (Reinberg, 2012). Careful reading of the CDC report on which the news article was based, however, failed to substantiate remarks about a causal connection between contraceptive use and teen pregnancy (Centers for Disease Control and Prevention, 2012). Instead, the CDC report carefully documented the rates of both behaviors, and the journalist drew his own oversimplified conclusions. Parallel patterns of change in contraceptive behavior and rates of teen pregnancies may be due to broader social and cultural forces that have similar impacts on both use of contraception and pregnancy, rather than one factor causing the other.

Obviously, effective use of birth control prevents pregnancies. However, arguments that knowledge of and access to contraception will continue to decrease rates of teen pregnancies lack conviction. For instance, consider a teen with strong normative values to avoid pregnancy who therefore decided to use a highly effective birth control patch. However, when the time came for the patch to be replaced, she was filled with baby longing, and so delayed making the appointment. She may have only let the time slip by a week or two before making the appointment, but even a couple of weeks could result in pregnancy. Inconsistent use of contraception was linked to pregnancy intentions in one study of Canadian teen mothers (Kives and Jamieson, 2001). Close to 38 percent of the teens reported that they had "sort of" or "really wanted" to be pregnant, and 72 percent reported being happy about their pregnancy. Resolving how knowledge of and access to contraception is related to pregnancy prevention may entail looking more closely at teens' attitudes about pregnancy, intentions towards parenthood, and their past sexual experience. Contraception use may be more consistent if the tension between positive and negative motivations associated with childbearing shifts so that intentions to avoid pregnancy become stronger. In other words, both contraceptive use and more general pregnancy avoidance may result from changes in attitudes or motivations, not from improved knowledge and access alone.

Summary and reframing

To what extent are teen pregnancies unintended and unwanted? Although less than one-fourth of teens explicitly admit that their pregnancies are intended (Mosher *et al.*, 2012), many teens endorse attitudes and emotions consistent with the desire for a pregnancy, suggesting that the true rate for pregnancy intention is likely underreported. The willingness of teens to admit to wanting a pregnancy appears to depend to some extent on cultural norms, with Black and Latina teens in the United States more likely to report intentionality. Competing motivations, ambivalent attitudes, and mistaken perceptions of responses by intimate partners and family all play out in the actions taken by young men and women towards sexual activity, contraception, and response to pregnancy. In summary, the cultural myth that all teen pregnancies are unintended and unwanted appears to be based largely on misperceptions. In contrast, we propose that *many teen pregnancies occur to youths who have conflicting feelings and attitudes about becoming parents.* Acknowledgement of these conflicting feelings and attitudes, and how they interact with developmental status and social context, may provide a more meaningful foundation for prevention efforts.

A systems approach to understanding teen pregnancy

Despite decades of research focused on unraveling the complexities that contribute to teen pregnancy and parenthood, questions about who gets pregnant or causes a pregnancy during the teen years, and why the pregnancies occur, remain largely unanswered. Although many predictive relationships have been identified (e.g., CSA predicts early pregnancy), explanations of how influences interactively combine to increase risk remain limited. Models that integrate chronological age, along with other important contributing factors, to explain pregnancies in women of all ages would provide better direction for further research than models that assume that influences on teens are different than influences on adults.

Although the TDIB conceptual model of pregnancy considers multiple factors that may account for pregnancies in both teens and adults, its focus remains centered on the individual. In contrast, a systems perspective suggests that a more holistic approach is needed in order to consider multiple interacting contexts of teens' lives and the meaning of a teen pregnancy within these contexts. In this final section of the chapter we review work that has focused on macro-level influences between States and cities within the United States to explain variations in the teen birth rate (Kearney and Levine, 2011; Males, 2006). Results from this research may lead to alternative ways to conceptualize teen pregnancy, allowing the cultural myths that most pregnant teens have behavior problems and all teen pregnancies are unintended and unwanted to be discarded.

Data from the National Survey of Family Growth (NSFG) and the Fertility and Family Surveys (FFS; see Appendix) were used by Kearney and Levine (2011) to investigate the roles of social and economic constraints in teen parenthood. The researchers believed that young women would be more likely to postpone childbearing if they perceived opportunities for personal or professional advancement through successful marriages or through careers. If these options appeared limited then the immediate benefits of having a baby may outweigh potential long-term losses (e.g., unrealized educational and economic opportunities). The NSFG allowed investigation of State-level differences in both potential for economic improvement and fertility rates in the United States. The FFS provided the opportunity for the same type of comparative analysis across countries. Conducting analyses that considered differences in socioeconomic policies by State and by country is consistent with a systems approach that embeds individual and family attitudes and behaviors towards early childbearing within the broader exo- and macrosystems.

Comparative data across States in the United States led to the conclusion that rates of childbearing did not differ for adolescents from higher socioeconomic backgrounds, regardless of economic opportunities normative for their State

(Kearney and Levine, 2011). However, among teens from lower socioeconomic backgrounds, childbearing was higher in States with fewer economic opportunities compared to States with greater opportunities. In contrast, abortion rates showed an opposite pattern, with higher rates of abortion among teens from lower socioeconomic backgrounds from States with greater economic opportunities. To avoid the criticism that unmeasured influences may be associated with variations between States in economic opportunities, the authors controlled for differences among States in poverty concentration, incarceration rates, absolute levels of deprivation, religiosity, political preferences, and social capital. None of these additional variables altered the estimated relationship between inequality and teen pregnancy among women from low socioeconomic status backgrounds. Conclusions from this study provide further substance to the questions of who become pregnant as teens and why the pregnancies occur. Put simply, teens with fewer economic and social opportunities are more likely to become pregnant because there are fewer incentives to postpone childbearing.

Similar conclusions were reached in a comparison of teen birth rates among 55 cities in California (Males, 2006). The author stressed a fairly obvious, but often forgotten, point: to a large extent teen birth rates are strongly correlated with the same economic circumstances that affect adult birth rates. Poverty, household income, educational attainment, and labor-force participation affect teen and adult birth rates in a similar fashion. Declines in the teen birth rate from 1990 to 2002 paralleled declines in the adult birth rate in the locations studied. Further, the declining teen birth rate was predicted by both the adult birth rate and increases in overall educational attainment within the specific region, together explaining nearly two-thirds of the decline in the teen birth rate over the 12-year span.

Findings from these studies highlight the importance of acknowledging that teen pregnancy and parenting need to be considered within the context of more general pregnancy and parenting. In contrast to explanations consistent with the fundamental attribution error, which place primary responsibility on internal and unchangeable characteristics of young women and men, evidence suggests that social and economic contexts contribute substantially to rates of teen pregnancy. Consequently, efforts to further reduce rates of teen pregnancy need to target not only attitudes and behaviors of youths, but also more general societal factors. Conceptual models, based on systems thinking, that integrate exo- and macro-level political, social, and economic factors with micro-level neighborhood and family influences, along with individual differences in physiological maturation and childbearing feelings, motivations, and intentions, are needed to more fully explain who becomes pregnant, or causes a pregnancy, during the teen years, and why the pregnancies occur.

General summary and reframing

In this chapter we examined two related cultural myths about teen pregnancy. The first suggests that most pregnant teens have behavior problems, and the second maintains that all teen pregnancies are unintended and unwanted. Public perception tends to view pregnant and parenting teens as rebellious and troubled young women and men who are likely to abuse alcohol and other drugs, and whose pregnancies may be related to a broader pattern of promiscuous or reckless behaviors. When pregnancies occur, they are likely to be perceived as mistakes or errors in judgment. We have reviewed ample empirical evidence that largely rejects these common beliefs.

Most importantly, evidence contradicts stereotypes suggesting that teen parents have identifiable traits and characteristics that set them apart from teens who delay childbearing. Teens become pregnant for diverse reasons. Some pregnancies do occur to teens with a history of aggressive and delinquent behavior, consistent with problem-behavior theory, while others become pregnant subsequent to sexual abuse. Yet other teens experience feelings of longing for a baby. Additional contextual influences include fertility-timing norms and future opportunities that are dependent on delayed childbearing. The diversity in explanations for teen pregnancy parallels the diversity of explanations for pregnancies to adults.

The evidence that we have reviewed leads to the conclusion that the majority of teen pregnancies occur to, or are caused by, young women and men without a history of behavior problems, and that many teen pregnancies occur to youths who have conflicting feelings and attitudes about becoming parents. Given all of the evidence to contradict the two cultural myths presented in this chapter, the question remains why they remain so ingrained in our belief system. Successful reframing of cultural myths requires an understanding of the regulating functions that cultural myths serve for society. Both the myth that most pregnant teens have behavior problems and the myth that all teen pregnancies are unintended and unwanted divert attention away from deeper social issues. Instead of acknowledging that teen pregnancy and parenting may sometimes be an adaptive response to unequal social conditions, acceptance of these beliefs places the problem on the teens themselves and their families. Interventions targeted to specific types of people may be perceived as more manageable than interventions designed to rectify unequal social conditions. Countries with low rates of teen pregnancy have shown that solutions are available, but implementing these solutions in the United States and other countries with high rates of teen pregnancy would require rethinking deep-seated cultural myths. We return to this issue in Chapters 7 and 8 with a cross-national review of social policy followed by recommendations for more effective strategies to prevent unintended teen pregnancies and to support pregnant and parenting teens.

5 Myths and misperceptions about teen parents

One of America's national myths has been that if teenage mothers simply postponed childbearing until they were more mature, their lives would improve substantially and the costs to society of early childbearing would decline dramatically. Such mothers would be more affluent, more likely to be married (and stably married), and more likely to bear healthy babies – babies who as adults would be well prepared to compete in the new global economy. But this myth is exactly that – a myth.

(Luker, 1996, p. 41)

Affluence, stable marriages, and healthy babies are lofty goals. These goals are not just part of the "American dream," but ideals that youth aspire to worldwide. From early childhood, youths are guided towards pathways that lead to achievement of socially valued outcomes, and admonished to avoid situations that may constrain attainment of these markers of success. Teen pregnancy and parenting is included among the situations that are believed to derail or disrupt progress towards wealth, family stability, and life satisfaction. However, pathways available to youth may begin to diverge even prior to the pregnancy, setting a course towards success for some while leading to poverty, instability, and frustration for others. Just as an early pregnancy has the potential to derail a pathway headed towards success, youths following less optimal pathways may experience life-altering boosts in their trajectories as a result of early parenthood. We explore these alternative scenarios using the following hypothetical case study of Darcy.

As 17-year-old Darcy walked home from the street corner where the school bus dropped her and the other students who lived in "New Hope," she felt her spirits sink. She pictured the mess awaiting her inside the dingy apartment she shared with her mom, her mom's boyfriend Mac, her older brother, and younger twin sisters. Her mom and Mac had scored some meth a couple of days ago and had been too high to care about doing dishes, laundry, or even getting the little ones ready for school. Darcy had been the one to make sure her little sisters were fed and looked after as long as she could remember. She sighed with the weight of responsibility seeming almost unbearable. For a moment she wondered how she would ever be able to handle the additional responsibility of the new baby she was carrying inside her. She soon smiled, however, with the *thought that J'nice would be hers, and neither her mom nor Mac would be able to take her away.*

Although Darcy is only 17, she is healthy and has not yet developed high blood pressure, diabetes, or the thyroid problems that plagued her mother when she was pregnant with the twins six years ago. After the twins were born, her mother's sister moved in for a while to help, since the pregnancy and birth took their toll on her mother's body. Her aunt taught Darcy how to feed and care for the babies, gradually turning their care over to her, even though she was only 11 years old at the time.

Despite Darcy's struggles to keep up with her schoolwork that sometimes makes her doubt her abilities, at home when her sisters look up to her it makes her feel that at least she is good at something. As Darcy thinks about her future she recalls her brother's girlfriend's offer to share child care responsibilities so that Darcy can finish school, and hopes that she was sincere since she knows she can't rely on her own mother for help. She would rather move in with Michael, her baby's daddy, but he just graduated from high school and hasn't managed to find a job that pays well enough to get his own place yet. She knows better than to count on Michael for help and promises herself that she will find a way to provide for her and for her baby.

Projections for Darcy's future as early as age 11 appear to leave little hope for wealth, family stability, or even life satisfaction. The struggles she had to endure as a child typically leave scars that are difficult to overcome. We will review evidence in this chapter that explores the impact of teen parenthood for youths from disadvantaged backgrounds as well as youths who begin life with more social and cultural resources. As we rethink the cultural myth that *parenthood derails the trajectories of teens' lives* we use data collected from both quantitative and qualitative research studies, and consider both objective reports and the teens' own perspectives. We further consider individual differences that may have already nudged teens similar to Darcy and her boyfriend, Michael – who entered adolescence already facing serious challenges due to low socioeconomic status, inadequate parenting, and academic struggles – towards one trajectory; teens with greater personal and social resources have embarked on quite different trajectories leading to adulthood. Although our focus is on teen mothers, we also examine the impact of early parenthood for teen fathers. We suggest that teen parenthood may be an adaptive response within some sociocultural contexts (Geronimus, 2003); the presumed benefit of delayed parenthood might not apply universally. We begin with an overview of the normative transition from adolescence to adulthood.

Transition to adulthood

Understanding the impact of early parenthood and its potential derailing effect relies on a solid grasp of normative transitions from adolescence into adulthood. This poses a challenge since what is considered normative is constantly in flux depending on individual, societal, and historical factors. For example, demographic transitions begun during the early part of the twenty-first century in many countries include increased age at first marriage, expectations of cohabitation prior to marriage, increased age at first parenthood, higher rates of parenthood outside of marriage, and greater tolerance of deviations from developmental tim-ing norms, collectively referred to as the *second demographic transition* (Billari and Liefbroer, 2010). These demographic changes suggest that the impact of teen pregnancy and parenting may vary by cohort, and that evidence based on earlier cohorts may not be valid predictors of consequences for teen parents today.

The transition from adolescence to adulthood may be viewed from two dis-tinct perspectives. One perspective, *emerging adulthood*, which has recently been proposed, encompasses the span from 18 to 25 years of age (Arnett, 2000, 2007). Important aspects of this period of life include identity exploration, a focus on the self, along with awareness of future possibilities (Arnett, 2007). Emerging adulthood is seen as a time period for the young person to figure out who they are and where they are heading in life. A second perspective suggests that becoming an adult involves self-perceptions of an adult identity combined with the assump-tion of adult roles and responsibilities (Benson, Johnson, and Elder, 2012). This perspective focuses on both *subjective age* and *psychosocial maturity* as markers of the transition to adulthood. Subjective age considers how youths compare their levels of maturation to same-age peers and their identification with specific age groups. Psychosocial maturity involves autonomy and social responsibility. Although chronological age is often considered a marker for normative expecta-tions of when this transition in self-perceptions and adoption of adult roles occur, individual variations in the timing of these processes negate the usefulness of chronological age per se in marking this important transition.

Within the nationally representative Add Health sample, the combination of higher and lower subjective age and psychosocial maturity resulted in four types of youth: (1) *early adults*, who had both older subjective ages and higher levels of psychosocial maturity, (2) *pseudo-adults*, who had older subjective ages but lacked psychosocial maturity, (3) *anticipatory adults*, who had young subject-ive ages but high levels of psychosocial maturity, and (4) *late adults*, who had both young subjective ages and low levels of psychosocial maturity. Pathways to adulthood varied for youths from each of these four categories (Benson *et al.*, 2012). By age 25 to 29, early adults, compared to pseudo-adults, were more suc-cessful in terms of occupation and earnings, despite lower educational attain-ment. Early assumption of an adult identity was only problematic for youths who lacked psychosocial maturity, but growing up quickly did not appear to derail youths who were independent, self-reliant, and who possessed a sense of social responsibility.

Conceptualizing the transition to adulthood based on identity profiles in con-trast to chronological age may provide a more meaningful understanding of the impact of teen parenthood on important outcomes. In other words, the impact of becoming a mother at age 17 may be quite different for a teen similar to Darcy, who had been forced to take on adult responsibilities at an early age and already considered herself an adult, than for other teens who envisioned many years ahead of themselves before becoming adults. Darcy's early acquisition of adult roles and responsibilities precluded an extended period of time to explore her identity, a defining feature of the period of emerging adulthood.

It is likely that demographic transitions, including completion of schooling, forming romantic partnerships, and becoming a parent, may provide the contexts to acquire self-perceptions of an adult identity (Andrew, Eggerling-Boeck, Sandefur, and Smith, 2006). Role changes provide the context to acquire new skills and further develop nascent abilities. Thus, acquisition of adult roles and self-perceptions of an adult identity go hand in hand. Youths who perceive themselves as adults may be more likely to adopt adult roles, and youths who adopt adult roles lacking this self-perception may quickly acquire it consistent with the psychosocial maturity demanded by their new responsibilities.

The perceived significance of demographic markers of adulthood was studied by Aronson (2008) in the context of the Youth Development Study (YDS, see Appendix). Young women between 23 and 24 years of age responded to in-depth interview questions about the meanings that they attached to: completing schooling, beginning full-time work, becoming financially independent, getting married, and becoming a parent. Within the sample, women had followed diverse pathways to adulthood, with some focusing on education, some on careers, and some on early motherhood. Despite the different pathways chosen, most young women agreed that financial independence and becoming a parent were the two most important markers of adult status. Financial independence was associated with being responsible for past debt (e.g., from student loans) and current bills, as well as being able to live independently from parents. Working was perceived as a means to achieve financial independence but not as a direct marker of adult status. In contrast, becoming a parent was perceived by both mothers and those who delayed childbearing as an important turning point signifying adulthood. Marriage, traditionally perceived as a demarcation between adolescence and adulthood, was not considered necessary for adult status, and many of the women indicated that marriage may pose challenges to further personal and identity development thought to provide the foundation for adulthood.

Young women from working-class backgrounds responded similarly to those from middle-class backgrounds on meanings attached to full-time work, becoming financially independent, getting married, and becoming a parent, but had different perspectives on the meaning of completing their education (Aronson, 2008). Young women from working-class backgrounds tended to enroll in postsecondary education that would prepare them for specific careers (e.g., nursing, administration, child care) and perceived graduation as an important transition into the adult world. In contrast, women from middle-class backgrounds who had attended four-year colleges tended to focus more on identity exploration and self-growth during college. Consequently, they expressed more feelings of being unprepared to enter the world of work upon graduation. Meanings expressed by women from middle-class backgrounds reflect an emerging adulthood perspective in which extended education provides a time of self-exploration. In contrast, women from working-class backgrounds were more focused on developing skills consistent with their perceived adult identities.

Although the study by Aronson (2008) included only young women, a similar study by Furstenberg and his colleagues included both men and women

(Furstenberg, Kennedy, McCloyd, Rumbaut, and Settersten, 2003). In response to survey questions about the importance of accomplishing specific life events for attainment of adult status, the majority of both men and women included financial independence, completing education, working full-time, and ability to support a family. In contrast, having a child and getting married were only endorsed by slightly over one-half of the respondents. Although these results differed somewhat from those of Aronson, the differences may be attributed to how questions were framed. For example, while having a child may provide a definitive transition to adulthood, it is not a necessary requirement for being considered an adult as is financial independence. In other words, childbearing may initiate the transition to adulthood regardless of age, but having a child is not a requirement for being perceived as an adult.

Childbearing is, thus, one of several life events that signifies adult status. Teens who embark on a path towards early parenthood do so from diverse routes. Some teens, similar to Darcy, may have already acquired the psychosocial maturity and self-perceptions consistent with adulthood. Other teens may lack these characteristics, but gain them quickly as a consequence of the demands of their new role. Still others may view the demands of adult responsibilities as inconsistent with their self-perceptions and resist adopting a firm identity as a parent while still exploring alternative future options. In rethinking the cultural myth that parenthood derails the trajectories of teens' lives it is imperative to acknowledge these diverse trajectories teens' lives took even before pregnancy occurred.

Cultural myth: parenthood derails the trajectories of teens' lives

The common belief that becoming a parent during the teenage years disrupts the goals and aspirations of young people is largely unsubstantiated. Although parenthood requires adjustments at any age, the question of how these events impact life outcomes needs further scrutiny. Our intent in the sections that follow is to objectively evaluate evidence from scientific research that has attempted to answer questions about the impact of teen parenthood on the transition to adulthood and beyond. We have omitted details of the actual studies to better focus on the evidence. However, the interested reader can refer to the Appendix for further information about the studies we cite in the following review.

Our conclusions are limited by constraints inherent in the research process. As discussed in Chapter 2, research results are typically presented as average effects that may not be an accurate representation for individual teens in the sample. In addition, studies that fail to find significant differences between teen and adult parents may be less likely to be disseminated. Further, studies that frame questions as differences between teen and adult parents may obscure effects actually caused by nonmarital or unintended parenting. The majority of these studies were based on expectations that teen parents will be deficient when compared to adult parents and failed to look for ways in which teen parents may have advantages. Finally, the underlying assumption that the category of "teen parent" represents a type of person with characteristics that can be identified through the research process may not be valid. Our conclusions are tempered by these constraints.

The impact of teen parenthood on life pathways also depends on important contextual factors that include nationality, government welfare policies, cultural norms, family support, and individual motivations (Billari and Philipov, 2004). As we have explained in prior chapters, the objective of much of this research is to differentiate the causal impact of maternal age at childbirth from the impact of background characteristics that may affect outcomes independent of early parenthood. Overall, evidence suggests that forces present in the lives of youths prior to pregnancy were the best predictors of outcomes, implying that social selection effects account for more of the variations in outcomes than social influence effects. The following sections consider the impact of teen parenthood on educational attainment, employment and financial status, romantic relationships, quality of parenting, and mental and physical well-being.

Educational attainment

Educational attainment refers to the level of schooling completed and is typically measured using one or more indices that include the probability of completing high school or secondary qualification (UK), receiving a General Educational Development (GED) certificate, and the number of years of postsecondary schooling. Alternatively, the school dropout rate is a measure of the lack of educational attainment. An important trend during the early part of the twenty-first century across countries is a decline in the percentage of young people who have not attained an upper secondary education and an increase in the proportion of young people going on to higher education. Overall, educational attainment of emerging adults has increased in recent years across a number of developed countries (OECD, 2011).

One of the most consistently reported conclusions from research investigating the impact of teen parenthood is an association between early childbearing and low educational attainment. For example, a recent cross-national comparative study confirmed that early childbearing was more concentrated among those with low levels of education across 12 countries and within three cohorts that included women born as early as 1955 and as late as 1984. The association between teen parenting and low educational attainment was maintained despite overall trends indicating later cohorts attained higher levels of education and had lower rates of teen childbearing (Raymo, Lim, Perelli-Harris, Carlson, and Iwasawa, 2011). Even though these findings appear straightforward, they may provide misleading messages about the consequences of teen parenting. All too often readers misguidedly assume that if only teens had delayed childbearing they would have gone on to finish high school and perhaps even enrolled in college, rather than dropping out. Descriptive studies like this cross-national comparative study provide valuable information about patterns of outcomes but are not intended to provide causal explanations about the influence of teen parenthood on educational attainment.

To determine the extent to which parenthood derails the trajectories of the teens' lives by decreasing educational attainment it is important to understand how likely high-school completion would have been if a pregnancy had not occurred. Consider the story of Darcy at the beginning of this chapter. What would Darcy's chances be of graduating high school and continuing her education, either in college or through a vocational program, if she had not become pregnant? Growing up in poverty, having an unstable family life, and living in a disadvantaged community are all risk factors associated with low educational attainment (Fletcher and Wolfe, 2009; Hoffman, 2008). Alternatively, good physical health, a history of school success (Heilborn and Cabral, 2011), and support from extended family may allow Darcy to continue her education despite concomitant risk factors. The critical question addressed by multidisciplinary research is to estimate the incremental impact of teen childbearing on educational attainment, over and above the impact of other risk and protective factors.

Recent sophisticated research designs have allowed investigators to tease apart these background influences, or selection effects, from age at childbirth on educational outcomes. By taking these contextual factors into account, newer analytic methods have provided a more nuanced explanation for the association between early childbearing and low educational attainment. Several research studies have used samples from the Add Health and NLSY data sets to compare the educational attainment of teens who delayed childbearing due to miscarriage to teens who became parents (see Appendix; Hoffman, 2008; Hotz, McElroy, and Sanders, 2008; Fletcher and Wolfe, 2009). In general, these studies concluded that the impact of early childbearing on the probability of graduating high school, attaining a GED, and total years of education was slight and nonsignificant. These conclusions were reinforced by data from the National Education Longitudinal Study (NELS, see Appendix), using a comparison sample who were deemed to have an equivalent propensity to become parents (Levine and Painter, 2003; Strange, 2011). However, a study of Swedish women that compared educational attainment of sisters, some of whom become mothers before age 20, found that controlling for familial and sociocultural factors reduced, but did not eliminate, the educational disadvantage attributed to teen childbearing (Holmlund, 2005).

Despite the elegance of these techniques, results still provided an estimate of the *average* educational penalty attributed to maternal age at childbirth, which may not describe the actual penalty experienced by any teen. Instead, steeper penalties experienced by some teens may be offset by educational gains accrued by others. A few studies have attempted to delineate these important distinctions and have found that, in general, steeper educational penalties accrued to women who perceived greater future opportunities prior to pregnancy. For example, women actively trying to avoid pregnancy by using birth control were impacted more negatively than women who were not trying to avoid pregnancy (Fletcher and Wolfe, 2009). Similarly, early parenthood was less disruptive for teens from more disadvantaged situations (Levine and Painter, 2003). Race has also been found to moderate the educational penalty, with greater estimated penalty for White teens compared to Black teens (Casares, Lahiff, Eskenazi, and

Halpern-Felsher, 2010). It appears that teens who are more entrenched in poverty, who are not actively trying to prevent pregnancy by using birth control, and who are from cultures more accepting of early childbearing may actually benefit educationally from teen parenthood, whereas, more negative educational effects accrue for teens from more advantaged backgrounds and who are actively trying to prevent pregnancy by using birth control.

Only recently has the impact of becoming a father on educational attainment been considered. Several newer studies, however, have explored this question using a variety of methodologies that mirror those used with teen mothers (Brien and Willis, 2008; Covington, Peters, Sabia, and Price, 2011; Sigle-Rushton, 2005; Taylor, 2009). Similar to results of studies on young women, men who fathered children as teens had lower educational attainment than men who delayed parenthood (Fletcher and Wolfe, 2012; Taylor, 2009). However, the magnitude of this educational penalty was reduced substantially when contextual factors were considered, suggesting that much, but not all, of the differences in outcomes between teen and adult fathers were due to selection effects. In other words, prior to pregnancy, men who became fathers as teens differed from men who delayed fatherhood. These preexisting differences were considered differences in *economic potential* defined in terms of intelligence, educational level of parents, and literacy resources in the home (e.g., magazines, newspapers, and library cards; Brien and Willis, 2008).

The impact of teen fatherhood on the trajectories of men's educational attainment may depend on several factors including relationship status, economic potential, child support policies, race, and personal motivation. For example, teen fathers who marry or cohabit in households with their children may complete less education, as they are required to work more hours to support their children (Covington *et al.*, 2011). Alternatively, unmarried teen fathers who fail to acknowledge their paternity escape a rather substantial educational penalty (Brien and Willis, 2008). Personal motivations may also moderate the association between teen fatherhood and educational outcomes. For example, men in the Add Health study who had been motivated to avoid pregnancy by using birth control were less impacted than men who had not been using birth control (Fletcher and Wolfe, 2012), presumably due to the implication that these men possessed greater social responsibility. Although the processes by which teen fatherhood impacts educational attainment are not clearly delineated by these studies, results strongly suggest that it is inappropriate to refer to an *average* educational penalty for either teen mothers or teen fathers.

Completion of high school is an important step along a life journey towards financial sufficiency. Adults who lack either a high-school diploma or GED are more likely to be unemployed and to earn significantly less throughout their lifetimes. Educational attainment, although important in its own right, is especially critical due to its link with attainment of better jobs, higher wages, and job satisfaction (Carnevale, Jayasundera, and Hanson, 2012). Regardless of status as a teen parent, teens who limit their education may also be constraining the types of job they are able to get and ultimately their ability to earn sufficient wages to provide for themselves and their families.

Employment and financial status

Financial independence from parents was perceived by both men and women as a necessary and sufficient marker of adult status (Aronson, 2008; Furstenberg *et al.*, 2003). Annual earnings, lifetime earnings, reliance on governmental support, and length of time unemployed are influenced by both childbearing and marriage, but the impact of these life events is different for men and women. Regardless of age at childbirth, married men typically earn more than never married men, and women with children earn considerably less than women without children. However, both men and women benefit financially from delaying marriage and childbearing, since even small decreases in wage growth at relatively young ages can lead to substantial decreases in lifetime earnings (Loughran and Zissimopoulos, 2007). Evaluation of the extent to which parenthood derails the trajectories of the teens' lives by reducing financial independence needs to consider that parenthood at any age causes financial disruption for women.

Much like educational attainment, a complicated pattern emerges in estimating the impact of teen parenthood on employment and financial status. Estimates vary depending on the timing of measurement (i.e., short- or long-term consequences), sample selection, cohort effects, changes in welfare policies over time and between countries, gender, and analytic techniques used. Conclusions from several studies have indicated that once appropriate controls are included for selection characteristics, differences between teen and adult parents on measures of financial status are greatly attenuated (Boden, Fergusson, and Horwood, 2008; Chevalier and Viitanen, 2003; Fletcher and Wolfe, 2009, 2012; Goodman, Kaplan, and Walker, 2004; Hobcraft and Kiernan, 2001; Hoffman, 2008; Jacobsen, 2011; Jaffee, 2002; Walker and Zhu, 2009). In other words, although some studies have found slight financial penalties associated with early childbearing, others have found small positive effects, while most studies have concluded that differences between teen and adult parents are negligible once appropriate controls are included.

While financial status may depend, in part, on the age that a young person begins childbearing, background characteristics in the lives of young people prior to childbearing may explain even more of the differences in financial outcomes between teen and adult parents. For instance, much of the association between maternal age at childbirth and financial outcomes in one study was actually attributed to conduct disorders, intelligence, educational attainment, and childhood SES. Preexisting differences in these characteristics intensified the impact of teen motherhood, suggesting that many financial difficulties faced by young mothers are not due solely to age at childbirth (Jaffee, 2002). Further, community-level factors including median income and, to a lesser extent, the unemployment rate and welfare benefits, have also been shown to impact both financial outcomes and rates of teen parenting (Fletcher and Wolfe, 2009). Some of the negative impact of teen childbearing on financial status also depends on subsequent fertility, as having more children without simultaneous increases in income results in a lower estimate of income per family size (Goodman *et al.*, 2004). Subsequent fertility may also further constrain women's return to work by limiting affordable child care.

Teen parenthood may impact the financial status of young men in different ways than the impact on young women. For example, *short-term* financial outcomes for teen fathers from the Add Health study were not significantly different from outcomes of fathers who avoided early childbearing due to miscarriages by their partners (Fletcher and Wolfe, 2012). In contrast, teen fathers from the NLSY had lower *lifetime incomes* than men who delayed fatherhood even when controlling for economic potential (Brien and Willis, 2008). Within a UK sample from the British Cohort Study (see Appendix), young fathers were more likely to receive government benefits compared to a matched sample with a similar propensity to become fathers, although differences in productive employment were not found (Sigle-Rushton, 2005). Apparent inconsistences may be explained, in part, by differences in the contexts of fatherhood. Reflecting the idea of a *marriage premium*, marriage may provide an important incentive for young fathers to achieve financial stability compared to men who reject the traditional fatherhood role (Sigle-Rushton, 2005; Tuffin, Rouch, and Frewin, 2010). Thus, the impact of teen parenthood on financial status may be influenced, in part, by the relationship status between young couples.

Romantic relationships

Establishment of long-term romantic relationships through marriage or nonmarital commitments is no longer viewed as a requirement for adult status (Aronson, 2008; Furstenberg *et al.*, 2003). Although intimate romantic relationships are desired by young people, they are becoming increasingly dissociated from childbearing, with many women choosing to have children as single mothers. These cohort changes pose challenges to evaluating the extent to which early parenthood disrupts the formation of stable intimate relationships, as conclusions from past studies may not generalize to current cohorts of teen parents.

In contrast to misperceptions that romantic relationships among teens are temporary infatuations or simply the result of raging hormones, many romantic relationships among teens are surprisingly long lasting (Collins, 2003; East and Felice, 1996). Most teen pregnancies occur in the context of these close romantic relationships. For example, data from the UCSD Teen Obstetric Follow-up Study indicated that close to 75 percent of teen mothers had known their partners for at least six months before becoming pregnant. Three years following the birth, 36 percent of the teens were living with the father of the baby (27 percent were married), and 61 percent reported that the father had a warm and loving relationship with his child (East and Felice, 1996).

Data from a more recent cohort confirmed that many pregnancies occurred in the context of ongoing romantic relationships, although few of these relationships lasted more than a few years (Oberlander, Agostini, Houston, and Black, 2010). This sample included only Black teen mothers who were all under 18 at the time of childbirth and who lived with their own mothers at the time of delivery. Fathers ranged in age from 15 to 31, but were on average only two years older than the teen mothers. Within three weeks following delivery, 66 percent of this sample reported that they were in romantic relationships with the fathers of their babies. The percentage declined to 34 percent two years later and only 10 percent remained involved by the time the children were age seven. Despite the value placed on marriage by these young mothers, seven years after giving birth only 14 percent had married, and of those who married only 23.5 percent were married to their children's fathers. Rates of ongoing romantic relationships were somewhat higher in a slightly older sample of young mothers who participated in the Fragile Families and Child Wellbeing study (see Appendix). In this study, 84.1 percent of the mothers reported that they were in romantic relationships with the babies's fathers at the time of childbirth, although only 11 percent were married to them (Gee, McNerney, Reiter, and Leaman, 2007).

In addition to the descriptive studies reviewed above, a few studies have attempted to disentangle the causal influence of maternal age at childbirth from background characteristics that are related to the formation of stable relationships (Ermisch, 2003; La Taillade, Hofferth and Wight, 2010; Sigle-Rushton, 2005). In general, conclusions confirm that background characteristics including educational level, nonmarital childbearing, and psychosocial characteristics were responsible for more of the relationship outcomes than maternal age at childbirth. Consistent with other outcomes, the impact of a teen birth on relationship stability is different for men and women.

Women in the UK who began childbearing before age 18 were less likely to be living with a romantic partner during midlife (British Household Panel Survey, see Appendix; Ermisch, 2003). However, it appears that nonmarital childbearing was a more important influence than maternal age at childbearing on this relationship outcome. Maternal age at childbearing was associated with having an unemployed, or underemployed, partner for women who were living with a partner. These results suggest that having a teen birth, particularly when aged under 18, constrains a woman's opportunities in the "marriage market" in the sense that she finds it more difficult to find and retain a partner, and she partners with more unemployment-prone and lower-earning men (Ermisch, 2003).

In contrast to the somewhat negative relationship outcomes found for young women, becoming a father prior to age 20 was found to increase the likelihood of being in a later romantic relationship (La Taillade *et al.*, 2010). Fathers from the NLSY79 cohort who were living with the biological mothers of their children at the time of childbirth were likely to continue to cohabit with or marry them. However, if the father was not in residence when the child was born, it increased the likelihood of greater conflict in the romantic relationship. The authors suggested that balancing parenting and romantic responsibilities may have required more skills, creating increased dissatisfaction with the relationships.

Characteristics in the backgrounds of men who become fathers as teens, including family disruption, childhood poverty, low academic achievement, and delinquency, all increase the likelihood of both teen fatherhood and subsequent relationship problems. One study of men from the British Cohort Study (BCS)

concluded that the relationship differences between men who fathered children before age 22 and those who delayed parenting were reduced substantially
following control of these background characteristics through propensity score
matching (Sigle-Rushton, 2005). Men who fathered children as teens were only
somewhat more likely to have three or more partnerships and reported somewhat lower levels of life satisfaction. Childhood characteristics of both women
and men that impact the stability of romantic relationships may also impact the
quality of parenting.

Quality of parenting

The ability of teens to be good parents has garnered much attention from researchers, the media, and policy-makers, with most forming the conclusion that teen
parenthood is inconsistent with characteristics of a good parent (Breheny and
Stephens, 2007a; Whitman *et al.*, 2001). Traditionally, the answer to the question
of what it means to be a good parent has been an authoritative parent who provides a warm, but firm, child-rearing environment (Baumrind, 1966). However,
some experts argue that other parenting styles may be equally effective within
some cultural contexts (Horn, Joseph, and Cheng, 2004). In consideration of the
potential diversity in definitions of good parenting, we have chosen to focus our
investigation on parental maltreatment, an unequivocal manifestation of poor
parenting.

Studies of teen parents published between 1970 and 2000 provided a clear
and consistent message that teen parents were at increased risk to maltreat their
children, and if they had only waited until after age 20 to begin childbearing, the
likelihood of maltreatment would diminish significantly (Connelly and Strauss,
1992; Maynard, 1997). Whitman *et al.* (2001) proposed that maltreatment was
partially a consequence of teen mothers' lack of cognitive readiness, or their
knowledge and skills regarding parenting. In general, the message received from
the scientific community was that teen parents were more likely to abuse their
children than were adult mothers, and if they had only waited a few years to
begin childbearing this abuse potential would diminish, perhaps as teens became
more cognitively prepared for their parenting roles. Geronimus (2003) dismissed
this message, stating, "that adolescent parents are more likely to maltreat their
children than are older parents appears to be a myth entrenched in the popular
culture" (p. 883), a perspective that appears at odds with conclusions drawn from
scientific observations.

Despite the apparent inconsistencies of the above perspectives, both may be
correct – just for different teen parents. Sufficient evidence has accumulated
that some teen parents are more likely than adult parents to maltreat their
children. Children from these homes are at risk for removal and may spend
time in foster care (Goerge, Harden, and Lee, 2008). Alternatively, most teen
parents do not maltreat their children, supporting the quote by Geronimus
(2003). Further, even though many teens may be cognitively unprepared for
parenting, their early role transition may lead to resilience (Arai, 2009b; Breen,

2010; Butler, Winkworth, McArthur, and Smyth, 2010; Courtney, Dworsky, Brown, Cary, Love, and Vorhies, 2011; Hunt, Joe-Laidler, and MacKenzie, 2005; SmithBattle, 2007).

Diversity of parenting within a sample of teen mothers was clearly demonstrated in an evaluation study of a home-visiting program available to first-time parents under the age of 21 (Easterbrooks, Chaudhuri, Bartlett, and Copeman, 2011). Three categories of parents were identified: (1) 73 percent were classified as *typical* parents who came from low-risk backgrounds and who did not maltreat their children; (2) 10 percent were classified as *vulnerable* who came from high-risk backgrounds and who tended to maltreat their children; and (3) 17 percent were considered *resilient*, as they came from high-risk backgrounds but did not maltreat their children. Resilient mothers were more likely to live independently with their children or with romantic partners compared to mothers in the other groups. They also received the least amount of caregiving and emotional support from their own parents, although they reported frequent social contacts with persons from their broader social networks. Easterbrooks *et al.* suggested that "young mothers' independence from their parents may contribute to the establishment of autonomy and to feelings of self-efficacy during the transition to adulthood" (2001, p. 48). Further, and similar to conclusions from Tuffin *et al.* (2010), these resilient mothers may consciously be involved in a process of intergenerational repair. Meaningful role transitions, including parenthood, may create particularly fruitful opportunities to work through issues from the past.

Observations of teen parents who participated in the New York Study prompted Leadbeater and Way (2001) to conclude that "Parenting at a young age did not derail these young women. Indeed, some were motivated to improve their own lives because their children added meaning and purpose to their young lives" (p. 26). These observations, combined with conclusions from a synthesis of qualitative studies of teen parents in the UK (McDermott, Graham, and Hamilton, 2004), imply that it is inappropriate to make generalizations about the quality of parenting provided by teens compared to adult parents. A more appropriate conceptualization may be to work at understanding how to promote resilient parenting at any age. McDermott *et al.* concluded that:

> Having the support of kin, and of their mothers in particular, and being able to maintain a strong and positive identity as a good mother were the pivots around which their relationship with, and care for, their children were built.
>
> (2004, p. 38)

Mental and physical well-being

Common perceptions are that teen parenthood not only disrupts educational, financial, and relationship outcomes, but may also lead to impaired mental and physical well-being. Substantiation of this belief implies that teen parents may have difficulty in achieving the psychosocial maturity to successfully cope with the challenges of being a parent. An extensive body of research has addressed the impact of teen parenthood on internalizing problems (including depression and anxiety), externalizing problems (including delinquency and aggression), and substance abuse problems. It has also been suggested that teen parenthood may jeopardize the physical health and well-being of both young men and women (Hardy, Lawlor, Black, Mishra, and Kuh, 2009).

Studies that have relied on simple comparisons or regression techniques to control for background factors in the lives of teen and adult women have typically reported that teen parents are more likely to engage in risky behaviors and report more symptoms of depression and anxiety compared to teens who delay childbearing (Biello, Sipsma, and Kershaw, 2010; Falci, Mortimer, and Noel, 2010; Henretta, Grundy, Okell, and Wadsworth, 2008; Lanzi, Bert, Jacobs, and the Centers for the Prevention of Child Neglect, 2009; Spence, 2008). Although some of these studies found mental health differences between teen and adult mothers to dissipate with the inclusion of appropriate controls (Boden *et al.*, 2008; Spence, 2008), other studies reported more negative mental health for teens despite these controls (Biello *et al.*, 2010; Falci *et al.*, 2010; Henretta *et al.*, 2008).

In one study, Australian women who had their first child before age 20 were compared to their twin sisters (a subsample were identical) who delayed childbearing to after age 20 (Webbink, Martin, and Visscher, 2008). Women who became mothers before age 20 smoked cigarettes for more years than their sisters, were less likely to quit smoking, and were more likely to be overweight. Webbink *et al.* (2008) suggested the spouses of teen childbearers were more likely to smoke and drink, and that the poorer outcomes for the teen mothers may be attributed to the behavior of their spouses. Although using twins as a comparison group controls for many important genetic, family, socioeconomic, and cultural factors, even twins may be exposed to different life events during childhood that may also account for differential outcomes. Childhood sexual abuse (CSA), for example, may be experienced by one twin but not the other.

Despite the strong associations between childhood sexual abuse, adjustment problems, and teen parenthood (see Chapter 4), few studies of mental and physical well-being have included adequate controls for CSA. However, relationships between CSA and health outcomes were investigated in a three-generation longitudinal study that compared multiple outcomes between women who had experienced CSA to a matched comparison group of young women (Trickett, Noll, and Putnam, 2011). Women who had experienced CSA were more likely to be obese, begin puberty earlier, have cognitive deficits, report more symptoms of depression and PTSD, to be involved in abusive romantic relationships, to engage in self-mutilation and risky sexual activities, abuse alcohol and other drugs, and to meet criteria for at least one psychiatric diagnosis. Associations between adverse physical and mental health outcomes and teen parenthood may therefore be partially explained by a history of CSA. Studies that fail to include controls for CSA may mistakenly attribute negative mental and physical health outcomes to maternal age at childbirth rather than to abuse history.

Another factor often omitted in studies investigating the impact of teen parenting on health outcomes is fertility-timing norms. However, evidence suggests that this macro-level factor may moderate the relationship between teen parenting and adverse health outcomes. For example, teen motherhood was only associated with distress for Brazilian teens who felt the pressures of and strived to comply with normative values (Béhague, Gonçalves, Gigante, and Kirkwood, 2012). This conclusion implies that negative outcomes may be magnified by a role transition that deviates from culturally accepted timing norms.

In contrast to expectations that teen pregnancy and parenting lead to risky behaviors and poor mental health, however, some evidence suggests that the transition to parenthood provides some young people with new meaning for their lives and a sense of purpose that inspires them to make positive changes (Fergusson, Boden, and Horwood, 2012; Fletcher, 2012; Hunt, Joe-Laidler, and MacKenzie, 2005; Leadbeater and Way, 2001; Tuffin *et al.*, 2010). Sophisticated analyses of data from the Add Health study led to the conclusion that teen child-bearing had negligible effects on smoking or obesity and also suggested that there were protective effects for drug use and binge drinking in the short term (Fletcher, 2012). Fletcher also used data from the Midlife Development in the US study of adults at mid-life (MIDUS, see Appendix), concluding that teen parenthood had resulted in some long-term benefits and enabled some teens to reorient their priorities away from risky and unhealthy activities.

Positive mental health benefits of teen parenthood were also observed in smaller studies in the United States (Hunt *et al.*, 2005), Australia (Butler *et al.*, 2010), Canada (Breen, 2010), and the UK (Arai, 2009b). Hunt's provocative study of female gang members revealed that despite living in environments that condoned or even promoted participation in substance use and gang-related activities, 85 percent of the teens modified their risky behaviors, including abstinence from substance use, when they discovered their pregnancies (Hunt *et al.*, 2005). Based on qualitative analyses of in-depth interviews with teen mothers, Arai (2009b) concluded that:

> Early motherhood was reported, then, to have had a positive impact on the respondents' lives and the lives of those around them, even when pregnancy was unplanned. For those young women who had previously had fraught relationships with parents, birth transformed family dynamics and healed breaches.
>
> (p. 175)

Breen (2010) suggested that, for some young women, the transition to motherhood encouraged active engagement in self-reflection in an effort to construct meaning from this life experience. Positive changes were attributed to the realization of the consequences of engaging in antisocial behavior, and fear of how disruptive behavior would impact their children and their own ability to provide for the children. Breen also suggested that having a child provided an opportunity for the young mother to see herself in a new light – the child may become an extension of the self. Granting value to the child enabled the mother to also believe in her own value.

In a departure from traditional quantitative analyses that search for relationships between variables (e.g., timing of parenthood and health), person-centered approaches seek to identify patterns that represent subgroups within a more het-erogeneous sample. From this perspective, mental and physical health outcomes are attributed to not just individual characteristics (e.g., age at childbirth), but rather to a composite of characteristics that interact in a predictable, but compli-cated, fashion. A person-centered approach was used by Amato and Kane (2011) to investigate the extent to which physical health and psychosocial adjustment of young women at ages 23 to 25 from the Add Health study were associated with choices made at the end of high school.

Instead of a simple comparison between emerging adult women with and without children, Amato and Kane (2011) identified different patterns among choices made by the women regarding school completion, employment, cohabit-ation, marriage, and parenthood. Amato and Kane concluded that although young mothers, especially single young mothers, tended to have more physical and mental health problems and lower self-esteem than women who postponed childbearing, the differences were due to a *selection effect* since the differences were apparent prior to becoming parents. Their results suggested that levels of well-being in early adolescence led women to select different life course path-ways; the pathways, once selected, had no consequences of their own for subse-quent levels of well-being. The authors concluded that well-being in adolescence largely determines well-being in early adulthood, irrespective of what people choose to do with their lives following the high-school years. Person-centered approaches such as this one are consistent with systems thinking since they con-ceptualize outcomes as a result of multiple, interacting influences.

A systems perspective on the impact of teen parenting

As we have seen, teen parenthood does not confer the same impact upon all teens who become parents; rather, there is considerable variation, with some teens using the role transition to make positive changes in their lives, while other teens may find themselves overwhelmed, with few resources and options. Additionally, impacts may not be consistent across divergent domains of teens' lives. While one teen may be able to stay on track educationally and vocationally after giving birth, the stress may have a negative impact on her mental health. Another teen may handle her own personal responsibilities of school, work, and stress, but at the expense of attention to her child, and become a neglectful par-ent. Prior chapters have described results of studies by Benson and Elder (2011) and by Oxford *et al.* (2005), who used person-centered approaches to identify the multiple pathways youths travel on the road to adulthood. The next section reviews two additional studies that used person-centered approaches to under-stand consequences more generally in the lives of teen parents.

Recall the dilemma of Lydia (see Chapter 2) in responding to questions posed by researchers from the NDAPP; she has now been asked to evaluate how being a young mother has affected her life. *She's not sure she understood completely, so asked the researcher to explain. In other words, the researcher was asking her to think about how her life might have been different if she would have delayed having a child until she was older, say 22 or 23, instead of 17. So, what do you think the impact was of having a child at 17 on your ability to get an education, get along with your family, be a good parent, or be satisfied with your life? Lydia thinks it is an odd question, how would she even know if things would have been different if she would have waited to have a child? Her thoughts start to drift as she imagines a very different future for herself – a future where she finishes her teen years without a child, maybe going to college in a different state, like her friend Madison, and a future where she never has to see Macaijah, Damon's father, again. She smiles briefly at that image of the future, but then imagines the hole that would be ripped in her heart to have lived those years without Damon in them. She can't even imagine life without Damon. Her thoughts return to the present, as the experimenter calls her name and asks her again to circle a number on the survey form.*

Data accumulated from Lydia and over 100 other young mothers who gave birth as teenagers confirmed that reliable patterns could be identified in how women perceived the impact of their early transition to motherhood. Weed and LeMay (2012) used latent class analysis to identify potential patterns of perceptions. Five patterns emerged: overall positive, overall negative, neutral, and two mixed classes with women reporting positive perceptions in some, but not all, domains. Close to 26 percent of the women from the NDAPP expressed the belief that being a teen mom had made a positive impact on their ability to stay in school, finish their education, and get a good job. Eighteen years after becoming a teen mother, women with positive perceptions of achievement-related outcomes, compared to those with neutral or negative perceptions, were less likely to drop out of high school (3.3 percent versus 15.1 percent), more likely to have attained a baccalaureate or graduate degree (33.3 percent versus 17.4 percent), had more consistent employment, and attained higher socioeconomic status. Consistent with theories of Geronimous (2003), Black women (33 percent) and Latina women (38 percent) were more likely to report a positive impact of teen motherhood, compared to White women (11 percent).

A second study investigated relationships between patterns of role transitions during emerging adulthood, and circumstances during late childhood and early adolescence (Seattle Social Development Project, see Appendix; Oesterle, Hawkins, Hill, and Bailey, 2010). Young men and young women were followed longitudinally beginning at age ten. Youths in this study were later categorized based on four indicators (school attendance, employment status, marital status, and living with children) assessed at five times from ages 18 through 30. Three distinct pathways to adulthood were identified. Just over 26 percent of men and women traveled a pathway that involved neither marriage nor postsecondary education. Women in this classification tended to be early childbearers. Approximately 31 percent followed a pathway that involved marriage and living with children but little postsecondary education. Investment in postsecondary education and postponement of family formation characterized a third pathway, followed by approximately 43 percent of the sample. Early adult profiles were reliably predicted by variables measured during high-school. Participants with higher high-school grade point averages and those whose parents had relatively higher educational levels were more likely to postpone family formation and continue their investment in postsecondary education. Black youths and those who had experienced family disruption during adolescence were more likely to be classified in the early childbearing group.

Conclusions from these person-centered studies dovetail nicely with conclusions derived from more traditional types of analyses, but also emphasize the diversity of life courses for teen parents. Most identified a "normative" group of teen mothers that appeared to adapt effectively to the demands of early childbearing, while acknowledging that other teen parents struggled to meet their adult responsibilities. Evidence from each of the studies, along with research by Amato and Kane (2011), confirmed that parenthood did little to derail trajectories of teens' lives, and may actually have provided incentives for some to decrease their involvement with alcohol or other drug use and with delinquent behaviors.

General summary and reframing

Not quite ten years after the quote by Luker at the beginning of this chapter, Oxford and her colleagues agreed that:

> Lingering stereotypes based on early research (e.g., Hofferth & Hayes, 1987) suggest that the lives of girls who give birth as unmarried adolescents follow a typically challenging and largely negative course, characterized by school dropout, long-term welfare dependence, mental health problems, and unstable interpersonal relationships. The public image persists that adolescent mothers are unable or unwilling to complete school, enter a stable marriage, or become financially and residentially independent – achievements that are typical markers of adult status.
>
> (Oxford *et al.*, 2005, p. 480)

Early studies that lacked adequate controls for risk and protective factors resulted in simplistic conclusions from comparisons of parenting teens to teens who postponed childbearing. Perhaps because these conclusions are straightforward and easy to interpret, they continue to be used to reinforce cultural myths, despite ample evidence suggesting a much more complex picture.

Evidence we have reviewed leads to the conclusion that age at childbirth may alter the life pathways of some teens. Becoming a parent during the teen years may directly impact educational attainment, financial status, romantic relationships, parenting, and mental and physical well-being. However, the assumption that this impact will be negative is clearly a misperception. Much of apparent advantages associated with postponement of parenthood may be attributed to selection effects that place some teens on more optimal pathways beginning in childhood.

Low educational attainment for some teen parents may be traced to academic problems that begin as early as primary school. Unemployment, welfare dependence, and low wages are predicted by childhood socioeconomic status and community disadvantage more than by teen parenthood. Relationship disruption may be a continuation of an intergenerational pattern begun by the teen parents' own parents. Associations between teen parenthood and well-being may be due to a history of childhood sexual abuse. Inadequate parenting by some teen parents may be a collective result of the interaction of all of these factors. Qualitative and person-centered approaches, in contrast to more traditional analytical techniques, allow investigation of patterns of outcomes that may be obscured by reductionist analyses that investigate each outcome independently. Results of these more appropriate analyses suggest that many teens appear capable of responding with resilience and using their new roles as the motivation to make positive changes in their lives.

Conclusions drawn from empirical research studies have several implications. First and foremost, there is clearly insufficient evidence to confirm that parenthood derails the trajectories of the teens' lives. Instead, robust evidence suggests that growing up with few economic advantages sets a course that leads to both early parenthood as well as a continuation of the original low economic trajectory. A second implication is that more and better quality research is needed to resolve conflicting findings. Aside from appropriate formation of comparison groups, studies on the impact of parenthood need to consider gender differences, national welfare policies, cohort effects, educational attainment, intelligence, emotional adjustment, and other relevant individual differences. A systems perspective that uses a person-centered approach may be called for to account for multiple, interacting influences on the life trajectories of teen parents.

A third, and related, implication is that research needs to move beyond comparisons of teen and adult parents, instead investigating the processes by which age moderates the impact of parenthood. Finally, since results are often reported as "average" effects, it implies that some participants will accrue more negative impacts and some will accrue positive impacts, meaning that early childbearing may actually lead to more optimal outcomes for some teens. For instance, young men interviewed by Tuffin *et al.* (2010) reported that becoming fathers motivated them to get better jobs so that they could contribute to the development of their children. This potential for positive changes triggered by teen parenting leads to a reframing of the cultural myth suggesting that *becoming a parent has the potential to transform lives for men and women of all ages.* Whether the transformation triggered by parenthood is positive, negative, or neutral depends on a variety of past and present contextual factors including socioeconomic status, culture, motivation, and relationship status.

A systems approach suggests that cultural myths may be maintained because they serve a regulatory function for society. The belief that becoming a teen parent derails lives serves as a warning to teens that may be used by parents, religious leaders, and educators to urge teens towards abstinence, or if not, towards using contraception. Take away the myth, and admonitions to avoid pregnancy lose some of their urgency. Belief in a future where teen parents can go on to complete their education may be perceived by some as acceptance of early pregnancy and parenthood. Becoming a parent at any age, however, has the potential to transform lives.

6 Myths and misperceptions about children of teen parents

Babies born in the US to teenage mothers are at risk for long-term problems in many major areas of life, including school failure, poverty, and physical or mental illness.

(When Children Have Children, 2012)

The above quote was disseminated by a professional organization involved with advocacy and education on issues related to children and adolescents to the general public as part of a series called *Facts for Families*. The endorsement by a professional medical association in a document labeled as *Facts* provides convincing evidence of the validity of the claim. The widely held belief regarding negative consequences for children born to teen parents has been reinforced by the "Counting It Up" strategy of The National Campaign to Prevent Teen and Unplanned Pregnancy announcing that "Teen Childbearing Cost Taxpayers $9.4 Billion in 2010." The report stated that most of the public costs were attributed to negative consequences for children born to teen mothers. The majority of these expenses were due to health care, child welfare, and incarcerations (Counting It Up, 2013). The common beliefs that children born to teen parents, or more specifically teen mothers, will experience a variety of problems throughout their development and that these problems entail economic burdens to society will be investigated in this chapter, along with the belief that babies born to teen mothers are likely to have birth complications, be born prematurely, or have low birth weights. Although there is no doubt that some teen pregnancies do result in poor birth outcomes and that some children of teen parents do experience problems throughout their development, and that these scenarios can contribute to economic burdens to society, the majority of recent research has contradicted prior findings that emphasized negative outcomes for children of teen parents. In other words, although the undesirable consequences of teen pregnancy and parenting can have a negative impact on individuals, families, and societies, most young women who become pregnant, most teens who choose to parent, and most of their children escape these hardships and do not contribute to economic or societal strains. An example from the Notre Dame Adolescent Parenting

Project, fictionalized only to the extent to maintain confidentiality, highlights the fallacy of these common beliefs:

Amanda was 17 years old, a junior in high school, when she found out that she was pregnant. Her mother had been a teen mom and, although the family was doing OK, Amanda's mother was disappointed and concerned that her daughter was repeating the cycle of becoming a young mother. Amanda was disappointed in herself too, but determined that she would not let this experience harm her own or her child's development. Amanda discussed the situation and her goals with her mother and boyfriend in an effort to try and plan ahead and not let this pregnancy derail her life. Both were supportive. She stayed in school and her boyfriend, who was a high-school senior at the time of pregnancy, graduated and secured a job with a stable income. Keith was born into a stable and loving home with parents and a grandma, who were all determined to work together to provide the best life for him. Amanda graduated from high school, married Keith's father and had two more children over the next seven years, although there was a four-year gap between Keith and his next sibling. Keith did well in school; he got involved in sports and found his niche in basketball. At age 18, Keith graduated from high school and went to a nationally acclaimed university on a full scholarship for basketball. Keith is now 20 years old and on track to graduate with a bachelor's degree in engineering. He maintains a GPA of 3.5 and will be a strong candidate for a successful career. He hopes to get married and have children of his own someday, but he has chosen to delay having a family until he finishes college, starts his career, and finds himself in a stable living situation.

Amanda and Keith are prime examples of how the choices that a teen makes during and after her pregnancy, and the support she receives from others including her parents and the child's father, interact in determining the child's outcomes. This chapter will focus on the development of children born to teen mothers using empirical evidence from scholarly research, including the NDAPP, to rethink two cultural myths. The first cultural myth we evaluate is that *teen pregnancies result in poor birth outcomes,* and the second suggests that *children of teen parents will experience cognitive delay, adjustment problems, and will themselves become teen parents.*

In this chapter, we use data from our own and other longitudinal projects to describe, explain, and emphasize the competence and adaptability of children born to teen parents. The overarching conclusion of this chapter is that children born to teen parents are a diverse group, with the majority being born healthy and going on to cope effectively with environmental hardships, while only a subset succumbs to more negative outcomes that may place burdens on their families or society. The first part of the chapter focuses on the cultural myth suggesting that teen pregnancies result in poor birth outcomes. We begin by reviewing birth outcome data on infant mortality, low birth weight, and prematurity. Subsequently, summarize studies that have attempted to explain variations in birth outcomes based on maternal age at childbirth. Differences in adequacy of prenatal care between teen and adult mothers is one factor that may be more important than age of mother in explaining adverse outcomes; teens sometimes delay entry into prenatal care in attempts to hide their pregnancies. We conclude our evaluation of this myth with one model, consistent with a systems perspective, that explains how high levels of anxiety over the pregnancies could eventuate in a premature birth.

The chapter then turns to evidence associated with the common belief that children born to teen mothers will experience a wide variety of problems that begin in childhood and persist throughout the life course. We organize the evidence by domain, specifically addressing cognitive and academic; behavioral and psychosocial; early pregnancy and parenthood; employment, nonproductive activity, and earning; and arrests and incarcerations. Our aim is to provide a balanced, nonbiased perspective of research in each of these domains. Despite several well-designed studies, we conclude that results remain inconclusive due to important limitations. For example, research often minimizes fathers' contributions to outcomes as well as the contributions of influences from the broader exo- or macro-systems of families headed by teen mothers. Stereotypes and resulting stigma due to inaccurate cultural myths are often overlooked as factors associated with adverse outcomes. We end the chapter by revisiting Bronfenbrenner's bioecological systems theory as an alternative way to understand the multiple, interacting influences on children born to teen parents.

Cultural myth: teen pregnancies result in poor birth outcomes

In the early part of the twentieth century in the United States as many as 140 out of 1,000 babies died before their first birthday. The majority of infant deaths were attributed to congenital malformations and perinatal conditions, followed closely by diarrheal diseases (Wegman, 2001). The advent of antibiotics, combined with knowledge of the importance of sanitation, saw a reduction of infant deaths to only 40 out of 1,000 by the 1940s. Continued advances in technology combined with better prenatal care have reduced the rate of infant deaths even more, to a current low of 6.4 out of 1,000 in the United States. Figure 6.1 compares rates of infant mortality in 1960 and 2011 among ten countries.

Despite the worldwide decline in infant mortality, birth complications persist; some of these complications appear to occur more frequently among teens and women over 35. Within all ethnic groups in the United States, rates of infant mortality are higher to women under the age of 20 than to women between the ages of 20 and 34. Aside from higher rates of infant mortality, babies born to teens are more likely to be premature and of low birth weight. For example, in 2011 in the United States, 11.7 percent of all babies were born prior to the thirty-seventh week of gestation and were considered premature. The rate for teens aged 15 to 19 was 13.5 percent, and for teens under the age of 15 the rate was 21.1 percent (Martin et al., 2013). Similar trends are evidenced for low birth weight, with 8.1 percent of all babies born in the United States weighing less than 2,500 grams (i.e., 5.5 pounds). Rates increase to 9.6 percent for teens aged 15 to 19 and to 11.7 percent for teens under the age of 15. In contrast to these negative outcomes, teens are less likely than older women to deliver by

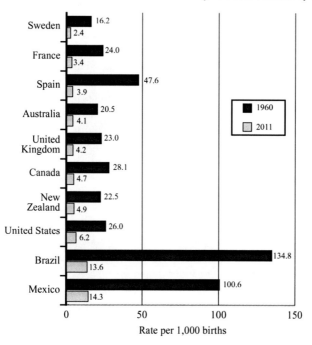

Figure 6.1 Rates of infant mortality in 1960 and 2011 for ten countries
Source: data.worldbank.org/indicator/SP.DYN.IMRT.IN

Caesarean section (Martin *et al.*, 2013). Teens are also less likely than women 20 or over to experience diabetes and hypertension (Osterman, Martin, Mathews, and Hamilton, 2011).

A cursory review of these statistics may be sufficient to infer that the cultural myth that teen pregnancies result in poor birth outcomes has a substantial basis in the reality of teen childbearing. However, these higher rates of infant mortality, prematurity, and low birth weight may be attributed to background socioeconomic and contextual factors that both predispose the women to an early pregnancy and increase the likelihood of adverse birth outcomes, rather than simply to the age of the mother at childbirth (Lawlor, Mortensen, and Andersen, 2011). As we first discussed in Chapter 2, this issue has been conceptualized as parsing *social influence effects* resulting from teen childbearing from *social selection effects* into teen childbearing. Social influence effects result *from* early childbearing and confer disadvantage to children of teen parents due to inadequacies in environments created by the teen parents, perhaps through harsh or insensitive parenting, parental irresponsibility, or immaturity. In contrast, social selection effects result from risk factors that exist *prior to* the pregnancy, which may lead to both increased likelihood of teen pregnancy and adverse child outcomes, making the age at childbirth irrelevant.

Risk factors associated with adverse birth outcomes include inadequate prenatal care (Vieira, Coeli, Pinheiro, Brandão, Camargo, and Aguiar, 2012), exposure to teratogens (Cornelius, Goldschmidt, De Genna, and Larkby, 2012; Mattson *et al.*, 2012), stress (Dunkel Schetter, 2011), abuse history (Gavin, Thompson, Rue, and Guo, 2012; Leeners, Stiller, Block, Görres, and Rath, 2010; Murphy, Schei, Myhr, and Du Mont, 2001), and having multiples (Branum, 2006) or short inter-pregnancy intervals (Kingston, Heaman, Fell, and Chalmers, 2012; Malabarey, Balayla, Klam, Shrim, and Abenhaim, 2012). These risk factors are concentrated among women living in poverty and tend to co-occur among pregnant teens (Markovitz, Cook, Flick, and Leet, 2005). Space limitations preclude further dis-cussion of these individual risk factors but the interested reader is encouraged to review the original sources cited.

Additional considerations, including shame and guilt, or perceived stigma, may lead some teens to hide their pregnancies (Hueston *et al.*, 2008) and create stressful conditions during gestation, which may precipitate adverse outcomes (Earnshaw *et al.*, 2013). Further, teens under the age of 15 may constitute a unique group and may experience more adverse outcomes due to biological immaturity (Kirchengast, 2009; Malabarey *et al.*, 2012). More specifically, there is some evi-dence that babies born to younger teen mothers (under the age of 15) may be small for gestational age (SGA) due to intrauterine growth restriction associated with incomplete pubertal maturation (Kirchengast, 2009). Collectively, these risk factors, rather than chronological age in and of itself, account for most of the differences in adverse birth outcomes between teen and adult women, and many can be mitigated by the provision of adequate prenatal care.

Inadequate prenatal care

Teen mothers are less likely than adult mothers to receive adequate prenatal care, thereby increasing the probability of prematurity, low birth weight, and other medical complications of pregnancy (Debiec, Paul, Mitchell, and Hitti, 2010; Okoroh, Coonrod, Chapple, and Drachman, 2012; Vieira *et al.*, 2012). In 2008, 7 percent of women of all ages in the United States reported initiating care dur-ing the third trimester of pregnancy or not at all. Pregnant teens were more likely than adults to report delayed or no care (12 percent). Rates of inadequate pre-natal care were even higher among younger teens; just under 16 percent of teens younger than 15 delayed prenatal care to the third trimester or had no prenatal care, but only 6 percent of teens over the age of 17 delayed care to the third tri-mester (Hueston *et al.*, 2008).

Lack of prenatal care has been linked to adverse birth outcomes. A study of teen pregnancies in Washington State found that young women without pre-natal care were over seven times more likely to have a preterm birth compared to teens who attended at least 75 percent of their recommended prenatal visits (Debiec *et al.*, 2010). Additionally, a study of over 40,000 birth records in Brazil found that rates of adverse birth outcomes for teens who received adequate pre-natal care did not differ from rates to adult mothers (Vieira *et al.*, 2012). Pregnant women with adequate prenatal care are encouraged to take prenatal vitamins, eat healthily, monitor weight gain, limit exposure to teratogens, and exercise. Other benefits of prenatal care include resolution of sexually transmitted and other infections, as well as general medical and dental care. In short, prenatal care is critical in preventing, monitoring, and correcting pregnancy problems that could lead to adverse outcomes.

Several studies have attempted to explain the relative lack of prenatal care among pregnant teens, particularly younger teens. Hueston *et al.* (2008) used data from birth certificates to analyze trends in prenatal care among 2.8 million teens who gave birth in the United States between 1978 and 2003. Trends over time indicated a dramatic increase in teens seeking prenatal care between 1988 and 1993, a time period that coincided with Medicaid expansion. The authors further suggested that younger teens may be more likely to attempt to hide their pregnancies and avoid prenatal care lest the pregnancies be discovered. Aside from cohort and age, being unmarried, having less education, and having a previous delivery were associated with an increased likelihood of delayed prenatal care.

Classifying teens by chronological age may not capture the most important differences affecting birth outcomes. While it is often assumed that those who are older are more mature, some younger teens may be more biologically and emotionally ready for childbearing than some older teens. Within a sample of 300 pregnant teens aged 12 to 19, those classified as emotionally not ready for childbearing had increased odds of inadequate prenatal care, symptoms of depression, and somewhat higher rates of smoking and drinking during pregnancy (Phipps and Nunes, 2012). Readiness to parent may need to be considered, along with chronological age, in predicting birth outcomes. Further reductions in infant mortality, preterm births, and low birth weights will require research that integrates multiple interacting risk factors into an interdisciplinary theoretical model (Dunkel Schetter, 2011).

A systems approach to birth outcomes

Dunkel Schetter (2011) describes an interdisciplinary model explaining processes and mechanisms during pregnancy, which may help explain the somewhat higher rates of adverse birth outcomes among teens. This model, which applies equally well to teen and adult pregnancies, is consistent with a systems approach, by proposing an interactive set of individual, interpersonal, sociocultural, and neighborhood characteristics (Madkour, Harville, and Xie, 2014) that collectively impact the likelihood of adverse birth outcomes. We describe this model in some detail using the case history of Amanda as an example. Consistent with current research, processes associated with preterm deliveries are somewhat distinct from processes associated with being small for gestational age (Dunkel Schetter and Lobel, 2012). Although the model by Dunkel Schetter (2011) specifically predicts preterm birth, she outlines a similar process model that predicts low birth weights, with symptoms of depression as the central focus instead of pregnancy anxiety (see also Grote *et al.*, 2010).

Pregnancy anxiety, a central construct in the model by Dunkel Schetter (2011), is specific to pregnancy and pregnancy outcomes, and has considerable evidence linking it to preterm births. Amanda, similar to most pregnant women, experienced some pregnancy anxiety and concerns about whether her baby would be born healthy, and felt some trepidation about the delivery process. Although a certain amount of pregnancy anxiety is to be expected, some women experience unhealthy levels (Dunkel Schetter, 2011). Excessively high pregnancy anxiety may be precipitated by major life events, including the death of a close friend or family, an anxiety disorder, or perceived risk of harm during the pregnancy. Although Amanda wasn't particularly anxious in general, she had started to worry since she had heard about other teens having problems with their pregnancies. Her health class had an invited speaker from the community, who talked to the students about the risks of teen pregnancy and the possible problems of children born to teen parents. After the talk, Amanda began to wonder if her body was capable of creating the right environment for her baby to grow in. Her concerns were reinforced when she went to the clinic for prenatal care and was lectured about the responsibility she had for making sure her unborn baby was healthy. She began to second-guess her meal choices, some days not eating much at all if she thought she was gaining too much weight, and then other days worrying that she wasn't eating enough. On top of everything else, her friends scared her by making her think about how the baby was going to get out of her body when the time came.

The amount of pregnancy anxiety Amanda and other women experience is hypothesized to be moderated by resilience resources that include self-esteem, optimism about the future, adequate support of family and romantic partners, coping skills, cultural values, spirituality, and biosocial factors that include physical health, socioeconomic status, and stature (Dunkel Schetter, 2011). Amanda was fortunate to have an abundance of resilience resources that served to buffer her pregnancy anxiety. For example, the support of her mother and her boyfriend enabled Amanda to remain optimistic and provided her with the resources, child care, and additional supports, so that she would be able to stay in school and achieve her goals. In addition, Amanda was in good health and had completed her pubertal growth process several years prior to the pregnancy. Although she grew up in a lower socioeconomic neighborhood, her mother made sure she always had enough to eat and that her major needs were met. The family relied on their faith to see them through when life got overwhelming. Since Amanda had relied on her faith in the past, she was confident that this same faith would see her through any pregnancy-related difficulties.

Pregnancy anxiety may cause babies to be born prematurely by three inter-related processes: neuroendocrine, inflammatory and immune, and behavioral (Dunkel Schetter, 2011; Wadhwa, Entringer, Buss, and Lu, 2011). High levels of pregnancy anxiety may trigger activation of a physical stress response that involves the hypothalamic–pituitary–adrenal (HPA) axis and release of cortisol, a stress hormone. Although a few studies with humans have linked excess cortisol production at key times during pregnancy to preterm births, the complexity of processes involved leaves evidence for a direct link to preterm births circumstantial.

Maternal health behaviors may also mediate the relationship between pregnancy anxiety and preterm birth by explaining how or why pregnancy anxiety may be related to an increased likelihood of prematurity. Some women may attempt to relieve their pregnancy-related anxiety through smoking cigarettes or marijuana, or turn to alcohol or other drugs to relieve the anxiety. Anxieties may also interfere with adequate sleep. These behaviors may interact with increased cortisol production to create changes in immune function and increase the likelihood of inflammation (Dunkel Schetter, 2011), consequently increasing the likelihood of premature birth.

Complexities regarding the interrelation of these three processes attenuate the ability to draw definitive conclusions about the role of inflammatory and immune processes on preterm births, although risks due to untreated urinary tract infections, sexually transmitted infections (STIs), and even periodontal disease, all examples of inflammatory or immune processes, have been well documented. Fortunately, Amanda neither smoked nor drank during her pregnancy. She began prenatal care in her fourth month, and was surprised when she was told she had an STI called trichomoniasis. She learned that "trich" could have caused the baby to be born early or to have other problems, so she was relieved when she and her boyfriend were treated and the infection was eradicated.

This theoretical model predicting preterm births fits teen and adult mothers alike. Differences in levels of pregnancy anxiety, as moderated by background characteristics and resilience resources, impact neurological, physiological, and behavioral responses to the life-changing event of pregnancy. Chronological age fades to insignificance once this set of interrelated elements is considered. Keith's healthy full-term birth was likely fully predictable by the factors described above, despite Amanda's young age of only 17 when she gave birth.

Summary and reframing

Comparisons of rates of birth complications – including preterm birth, low birth weight, and infant mortality – by maternal age provide only superficial support for the cultural myth that teen pregnancies result in poor birth outcomes. Reframing this myth to be consistent with evidence suggests that *most babies born to teen mothers who receive adequate prenatal care are born full-term and healthy*. The superficial support found, suggesting adverse outcomes for infants born to teen mothers, reinforces misperceptions and makes the cultural myth resistant to efforts to reframe in a more meaningful context, to provide the basis for effective prevention strategies, interventions, and policy decisions. Simplistic comparisons of rates between teens and adults fail to capture background characteristics associated with both early pregnancy and adverse birth outcomes which need to be considered when programs and policies are implemented. For example, simple postponement of childbearing from age 17 to age 20 does little to build resilience resources or address background cultural or neighborhood issues associated with heightened levels of pregnancy anxiety. Dunkel Schetter (2011) cautions against blaming mothers for less than optimal birth outcomes and instead suggests the blame should be placed on societies that inadequately support the health and well-being of women during pregnancy. She passes on the wisdom, "societies that nourish resilience in mothers and their families are surely likely to see maternal optimality" (p. 549).

Cultural myth: children of teen parents will experience cognitive delay, adjustment problems, and will themselves become teen parents

A second common belief is that the age of the mother at childbirth will place her children at risk for a multitude of problems including cognitive and academic delays, behavior and psychosocial problems, early pregnancy, attenuated economic prospects, and increased likelihood of arrest and incarceration. As we rethink this common belief we review evidence that attempts to determine the extent to which these problematic outcomes are causally related to the age of the mother at childbirth rather than to background characteristics that both place the mother at risk for an early pregnancy and contribute to adverse outcomes for her children. We begin with another fictionalized example from the Notre Dame Adolescent Parenting Project that highlights this dilemma:

Christine was only 14 years old when she found out that she was pregnant. She had been having sex for a while with a boy who was a senior in high school. She was only a freshman and was so flattered by his attention that she consented to his requests for unprotected sex. Christine felt lost and alone during her pregnancy. She was scared to talk to her mom, who had also been a teen parent and had warned Christine many times that she would be upset if Christine followed in her footsteps. She hid her pregnancy until it became undeniable, which was when she was seven months along. Her family didn't have good health insurance, but brought home just enough income that they didn't qualify for Medicaid, so even after Christine sought prenatal care she often missed appointments because she was worried about not being able to pay for her medical expenses. Because she was experiencing so much stress about her pregnancy, Christine stopped going to school and eventually dropped out after her son, Dominic, was born. Although Christine continued to live with her mother, their relationship was tense and Christine did not receive support from her mother or from the child's father, who broke up with her and refused to claim paternity after finding out that she was pregnant. By the time Dominic entered kindergarten, he was substantially delayed in terms of cognitive ability and social adjustment. Christine was unaware of how to advocate for intensive support services through the school, and although the school provided Dominic with minimal supports he still lagged behind his peers throughout childhood and into adolescence. At his 18-year assessment, Dominic met criteria for moderate intellectual disability, had dropped out of school, and was unable to secure employment that would allow him to be self-sufficient. In addition, a young woman in his neighborhood claimed that Dominic was the father of the child she was carrying. At the same visit, Christine reported that she had five more children after having Dominic, with her second oldest child being born shortly after Dominic turned one year old.

As we reviewed the stark contrast between Keith and Dominic's outcomes, we began to wonder about the extent to which Dominic's social and academic problems in school, his lack of employment, and his alleged teen fatherhood were a result of Christine's teen pregnancy (a social influence effect) versus factors in Christine's early life that both led to her early pregnancy and simultaneously continued to negatively impact the development of Dominic (a social selection effect). Numerous studies have been conducted over the past decades comparing developmental outcomes for children born to teen parents to children born to parents who delayed childbearing until at least age 20. Early studies, limited by technological constraints and simplistic analytical models, focused on simple between-group comparisons without consideration of background characteristics of the teen mothers. As computational models became more sophisticated, analyses began to account for these background characteristic in increasingly elegant designs. Many of the early studies reported meaningful differences in outcomes of children born to teen versus adult mothers, leading to misperceptions that still resonate today. As results of more sophisticated analyses began to be published, however, it became clear to us and others in this field that many of the differences between children born to teen and adult parents were due to background characteristics (a social selection effect) rather than age per se (a social influence effect).

We review some of this research below, organized by domain: cognitive and academic outcomes, behavioral adjustment and risky behaviors, teen pregnancy, unemployment, and criminal activity. We rely on the widely cited work of Hoffman and Maynard from the book *Kids Having Kids* (2008), and similar analyses conducted in the UK (Francesconi, 2008; Hawkes and Joshi, 2012), Australia (Bradbury, 2011; Harden *et al.*, 2007), New Zealand (Jaffee, Caspi, Moffitt, Belsky, and Silva, 2001), the Netherlands (Kalmijn and Kraaykamp, 2005), Sweden (Coyne, Långström, Rickert, Lichtenstein, and D'Onofrio, 2013), and Canada (Dahinten, Shapka, and Willms, 2007). Lack of consistency between findings from these studies, even those using the same data sets, makes it difficult to disentangle misperceptions from realities. However, careful perusal of the findings presented in these sections will provide ample evidence that maternal age, in and of itself, is less of a predictor of children's development than the multiple interacting risk factors that were often present in the lives of teen parents long before their pregnancies.

Cognitive and academic outcomes

Compared to children of adult moms, kindergarten-aged children born to teen mothers who participated in the Early Childhood Longitudinal Study (ECLS-B, Wave IV; see Appendix) scored lower on assessments of early reading, math, and general knowledge (Manlove, Terry-Humen, Mincieli, and Moore, 2008). Similar conclusions were reached by Hawkes and Joshi (2012) in a sample of children from the UK Millennium Cohort Study (MCS, see Appendix), with modest differences between young children born to teen and adult parents remaining even after accounting for background characteristics. A sample of Australian children born to teen mothers showed that these children were also less proficient in school at ages four and five than children born to older parents, but in this case the differences were accounted for primarily by their mothers' own educational attainment (Household Income and Labour Dynamics in Australia & Longitudinal Study of Australian Children, see Appendix; Bradbury, 2011) rather than age at childbirth.

Adolescent children born to teen mothers (NLSY97) continued to lag behind peers born to adult mothers on assessments of reading, general knowledge, and high-school graduation. However, after taking into account a variety of background characteristics including sex, race, the marital status of their mothers when they were born, maternal education, and educational levels of the grandparents, differences in cognitive and academic outcomes no longer differed significantly between children born to teen and adult parents (Manlove *et al.*, 2008).

In addition, young adult children born to younger teen parents (17 or less) were somewhat less likely to graduate from high school (Hoffman and Scher, 2008). These conclusions are similar to those reached by Jaffee and her colleagues (2001) in the Dunedin Multidisciplinary Health and Development Study (see Appendix). Although children born to teen mothers were 2.61 times as likely to leave school early, this difference was completely accounted for by parental characteristics that included mothers' IQ and educational attainment, and fathers' conviction histories, as well as family circumstances that included SES and number of caregiver changes before age 14. Using Australian data from the HILDA survey, Bradbury (2011) reached similar conclusions that the difference between educational attainment and educational performance of Australian children born to teen mothers and their cousins with adult mothers was eliminated when relevant background factors were controlled.

Behavioral and psychosocial outcomes

Manlove *et al.* (2008) also compared the behavioral adjustment of offspring born to teen versus adult mothers from the ECLS-K and NLSY97 studies. Children's behavioral outcomes, relationship quality and skills, and physical health and well-being were no different between the group of children born to teen mothers versus those born to mothers in their early twenties. In fact, the quality of the home environment was actually found to be significantly better for the children who were born to the youngest teens after controlling for confounds, potentially because the younger teens were more likely to reside with their parents. Few between-group differences were found even before taking into account background factors. No meaningful differences were found on use of alcohol, cigarettes, marijuana, or symptoms of depression. Slight differences in delinquency were explained by background characteristics associated with the age of the mother, rather than her age itself.

Risks attributed to children of adolescent mothers also include psychopathology and problems with substance use (De Genna, Larkby, and Cornelius, 2013; Harden *et al.*, 2007). A children-of-twins design was used to explain how and why age at motherhood was associated with psychopathology in an Australian sample of adolescents and young adults (Harden *et al.*, 2007). This strategy controls for background, family and genetic factors that may be correlated with the outcome variable by using children of twins who delayed childbearing as a comparison sample. Factor scores were derived for three types of psychopathology: behavior problems, substance use problems, and internalizing problems. Analyses suggested that becoming a mother as a teen was associated with increased behavioral problems, even after controlling for genetic influences and other family factors that were shared by children born to twin sisters who delayed motherhood. Causal effects were also reported for the impact of teenage motherhood on internalizing problems and, to a lesser extent, substance use problems. Although the innovative methodology of this study provides strong controls for many background factors, the role of fathers was unable to be quantified. The authors suggested that some of the problematic outcomes for children born to teen mothers may be attributed to genetic factors passed on by fathers.

Early pregnancy and parenthood

Adolescents and young adult women born to teen mothers are more likely than those born to adult mothers to have a teen birth by age 18, providing partial support for the cultural myth (Hoffman and Scher, 2008; Manlove *et al.*, 2008). Although some studies have concluded that differential rates of teen parenting dissipate when controls for background characteristics are considered (Jaffee *et al.*, 2001), other studies support a social influence effect in which age at childbirth remains significant even after including controls for background characteristics (Manlove *et al.*, 2008). Interestingly, aside from a teen birth, other relationship outcomes (including interpersonal skills, conflict and closeness with romantic partners, and the quality of the relationship with mothers), use of birth control, and health factors such as obesity, did not differ for children born to teen versus adult mothers, even before accounting for background characteristics. A significant exception was that the adolescent children born to teen mothers were more likely to have married or cohabited by age 20 than children born to adult mothers. While delaying the timing of a first birth is part of the story, postponing a first birth without improving the educational and social circumstances of teens prior to a first pregnancy may confer little advantage upon children's outcomes (Jaffee *et al.*, 2001, p. 394).

Employment, nonproductive activity, and earnings

Differences between the unemployment of young adults born to teen versus adult parents from the Dunedin sample were fully explained by parental characteristics, including fathers' arrest histories and SES (Jaffee *et al.*, 2001). Others agree that much of the association between attenuated financial outcomes and children born to teen mothers may be attributed to lower educational attainment rather than age at first birth (MCS Hansen, Hawkes, and Joshi, 2009; Hawkes and Joshi, 2012). In contrast, British children born to teen mothers were found to spend less time in productive activity and had lower levels of earnings than children of their mothers' siblings (i.e., their cousins) who delayed childbearing (BHPS, see Appendix; Francesconi, 2008). Discrepancies between outcomes of these studies suggest the need for further research that more fully explains how and why children born to teen parents may be at risk for economic adversities.

Arrests and incarcerations

Although differences between children born to teen versus adult parents in many domains are largely explained by factors other than maternal age at childbirth, more substantial differences were found on rates of incarceration among sons born to teen mothers using data from the NLSY79 (Grogger, 1997; Hoffman and Scher, 2008). By the time they were in their late thirties and early forties, 13.92 percent of sons born to mothers under the age of 18 had been incarcerated at least once, and had spent almost twice as much time incarcerated as sons born to women aged 18 to 22 (Hoffman and Scher, 2008). The size of the impact was reduced when background factors were considered, but age of mother at birth remained a meaningful predictor. Similar conclusions were reached by Jaffee *et al.* (2001), who reported that SES explained much of the difference in violent offending between children of teen and adult mothers, but that a significant and unexplained difference remained.

Important considerations

Despite the quality of the analyses described above, three constraints limit the validity of their findings: reliance on averages, how the questions were framed, and variability in controlling for background characteristics. Comparisons between children born to teen versus adult mothers typically rely upon average scores. For example, Manlove *et al.* (2008) reported that the average general knowledge score of kindergarteners born to teens under the age of 18 was 21.15, a significant difference from the 24.10 score of children born to women between the ages of 25 and 29. The average, 21.15, was a compilation of scores of 525 children born to mothers aged 17 and under. If 50 percent of the children scored higher than average, while 50 percent of children born to women 25 through 29 scored lower than average, then considerable overlap may exist between these distributions, with some children born to younger mothers performing as well as or better than many children born to adult mothers. Questions framed to identify characteristics of children born to younger mothers who are academically successful despite the youth of their mothers would provide direction for efforts to enhance these characteristics in young mothers and their children.

A second consideration is that results are limited by how the questions were framed. Comparisons between teen and adult mothers introduce maternal age as the most important characteristic in interpreting the results. Although age is typically associated with both biological and social maturity, individuals vary tremendously in biological and social maturity during the adolescent years. For instance, some youth may have completed puberty by age 10 or 11, while others may be just entering puberty at age 13. The timing of puberty is a better marker of physiological readiness to reproduce than chronological age. Physiological readiness, combined with measures of psychosocial maturity, is even better. Framing comparisons by chronological age implies that delaying childbearing by several years will improve outcomes. In contrast, framing questions in terms of physiological and psychosocial maturity implies that waiting to begin childbearing until bodies are ready and women have acquired sufficient perspectives on life is the goal of intervention. For some, this readiness could happen during the teen years, but others may need several years into their twenties before they acquire the level of maturity needed.

Reframing questions based on actual biological or psychosocial maturity does not eliminate the problem with how questions are framed. Comparing outcomes for children born to teen versus adult mothers assumes that the fathers' age and developmental maturity are irrelevant to child outcomes. This assumption is contrary to a considerable body of research suggesting that fathers' contributions begin even before conception (Crijns, Bos, Knol, Straus, and de Jong-van den Berg, 2012; Frey, Navarro, Kotelchuck, and Lu, 2008). Conclusions that adult men born to teen mothers are more likely to be incarcerated ignore the potential impact of genetic or epigenetic links to the fathers (Jaffee *et al.*, 2001).

Fathers are likely to contribute directly and indirectly to their children's antisocial behavior. One indirect route is through the process of *assortative mating* (Boutwell, Beaver, and Barnes, 2012). Assortative mating occurs when sexual partners are selected based on similarity in geographic location, peer group affiliation, and other characteristics and traits considered desirable. Similarity between sexual partners extends to antisocial and aggressive personality traits. For example, one study of over 10,000 couples from the Early Childhood Longitudinal Study (ECLS-B; see Appendix; Boutwell *et al.*, 2012) found that mothers' antisocial behaviors correlated highly with fathers' antisocial behaviors ($r = 0.51$). The correlations between parents' substance use was even higher ($r = 0.71$). Similarity between couples decreased somewhat with the length of time in the relationship, supporting arguments that the relationship was established based on similarity rather than partners becoming similar the longer they have been involved (Boutwell *et al.*, 2012). Assortative mating also accounted for arrest and incarceration history in youths from the Add Health study (Beaver, 2012). Although the quality of the relationships between youths and mothers was also significant, the effect size was over four times higher for links between paternal criminal history and children's criminal behavior.

A more direct route by which fathers contribute to their children's antisocial behavior is through the intergenerational transmission of criminal behavior. Analyses using data from the Pittsburgh Youth Study (see Appendix) revealed that the arrest histories of the fathers were strong predictors of their sons' arrests, even after controlling for other predictors including socioeconomic background, achievement, and parental supervision. Although boys with mothers under the age of 18 at their birth were more likely to admit to delinquent behavior, maternal age at childbirth was not an independent predictor of either arrest history or confirmed delinquent behavior (Farrington, Jolliffe, Loeber, Stouthamer-Loeber, and Kalb, 2001). Similar results were obtained using data from twins born in England and Wales (Twins Early Development Study, see Appendix; Jaffee, Moffitt, Caspi, and Taylor, 2003). The authors of this study concluded that "children born to highly antisocial men experience a double whammy of risk when their father resides with the family" (p. 120). The first aspect of the double whammy involves direct transmission of genetic risk for antisocial behavior. The second aspect involves the negative impact of fathers' behaviors on the rearing environment provided to the children (Jaffee *et al.*, 2003).

In addition to how the questions were framed, conclusions are limited by the information available in the data sets. Although most samples were large and nationally representative, they were typically not designed to test hypotheses about teen parenting. Data used to control for background differences between teen and adult mothers were limited to what was available in the data sets. Manlove *et al.* (2008) acknowledged this constraint as they discussed the significance of the cognitive and academic differences found between teen versus adult mothers. They suggested that some of the differences may have been due to unmeasured intellectual differences between the teen and adult mothers, which could have explained the results better than the attributions to maternal age at the time of childbirth. Studies that have included controls for maternal intelligence have typically found that this explains much of the difference in cognitive and academic outcomes between children born to teen versus adult parents (Jaffee *et al.*, 2001).

A few recent studies have addressed issues related to controlling for background characteristics by using more sophisticated analytic techniques (e.g., propensity matching, miscarriages as natural experiments, sibling comparisons). Comparisons of findings from different analytic techniques using the same NLSY data led Levine, Emery, and Pollack (2007) to conclude that characteristics in the lives of young women who become teen mothers, rather than early childbearing per se, were largely responsible for their children's outcomes in academics, aggression, and substance use. In contrast, the likelihood of grade retention, truancy, and early initiation of sexual activity were found to be more strongly predicted by teen motherhood status.

Despite the elegance of these methodologies, they are all variable-centered approaches that seek to identify associations between variables, rather than person-centered approaches that seek to identify patterns among people. A person-centered approach would assume considerable heterogeneity within a sample of children born to teenage mothers. Identification of subgroups of young adult children born to teenage mothers would provide valuable information for more tailored and streamlined intervention programs, as well as establishment of more focused policy efforts.

A person-centered approach

Evidence from our Notre Dame Adolescent Parenting Project (NDAPP; Whitman *et al.*, 2001) revealed high levels of resilience among 18- to 21-year-olds who had been born to teen mothers, with the majority of these youths graduating from high school, demonstrating a positive self-concept, and displaying low rates of developmental disabilities, criminal behavior, and psychopathology (Weed and Noria, 2011). In this analysis, we used latent class analysis (LCA) to classify emerging adults from a heterogeneous population into smaller, relatively homogeneous subgroups with different patterns of strengths and vulnerabilities. We used eight indicators in the domains of academics, substance use, health, risky behaviors, and psychological functioning to classify 113 emerging adults who were born to a sample of adolescent mothers and who have been followed longitudinally since the prenatal period (see Chapter 4).

The majority of children born to teenage mothers were classified as typical. As emerging adults they were engaged in productive activity, had good physical and mental health, and demonstrated few behavior problems. The relatively positive outcomes for these typical youths challenge the cultural myth that children of teen parents will experience cognitive delay, adjustment problems, and will themselves become teen parents, and suggest that the average penalty for being born to a teen mom does not apply universally to all families. Positive outcomes were concentrated among Black youths, with approximately two-thirds of children born to Black mothers classified as typical in every domain. In contrast, over 60 percent of children born to White teen mothers had problems in one or more domains, with 35 percent being classified as delinquent. Differential patterns of outcomes associated with race are consistent with different fertility-timing norms proposed by Geronimus (2003). Children who grow up in cultures where teenage parenthood is accepted as normative may fare better than those whose status is less accepted as normative (Béhague, Gonçalves, Gigante, and Kirkwood, 2012; Marie *et al.*, 2011).

Summary and reframing

The evidence reviewed above provides mixed support for the cultural myth that children of teen parents will experience cognitive delay, adjustment problems, and will themselves become teen parents. Limitations associated with how research questions have been framed and analyzed constrain our ability to draw robust conclusions. Studies that have looked for adverse consequences of teen parenting have sometimes found them and sometimes not. In general, alternative explanations (e.g., father characteristics) for adverse outcomes have not been adequately investigated. Despite these limitations, evidence suggests that *the majority of children born to teen parents do not have serious problems and do not become teen parents*. Although cognitive, psychological, and academic differences may be observed during early childhood, by adolescence these differences often dissipate (Farris, Nicholson, Borkowski, and Whitman, 2011; Manlove *et al.*, 2008; Weed and

Noria, 2011). Evidence for generalized adjustment problems is also weak, with most pointing to no meaningful differences for children born to teen versus adult parents once background differences are considered.

Two important qualifications to our general finding of few differences between children born to teen and adult mothers are in the areas of incarceration (Grogger, 2008; Jaffee *et al.*, 2001; Hoffman and Scher, 2008) and teen parenthood (Jaffee *et al.*, 2001; Manlove *et al.*, 2008). Although some evidence does suggest that children born to teen mothers are at increased risk for these outcomes, it is also true that most children born to teen mothers do not experience incarceration or teen births. To understand the association between maternal age at childbirth and adverse outcomes, more attention needs to be placed on the processes or mechanisms that lead to antisocial outcomes for some children born to teen mothers. The role of fathers and other contextual factors may be crucial in these processes. Further research also needs to integrate biological processes and consider how genetic or epigenetic processes may mediate or moderate associations between maternal age at childbirth and adverse outcomes (Miller *et al.*, 2010).

We propose a more nuanced view, which posits that children born to teen mothers are a diverse group, with some being resilient to the risks to which they are exposed whereas others will experience adverse outcomes at some point, or throughout, their development. In an effort to move away from this cultural myth, as well as the prior myth that children of teen mothers will certainly experience birth complications, we return to the systems perspective.

Understanding children's development from a systems perspective

Recall from Chapter 1 that a systems perspective involves multiple, interacting elements that combine synergistically to accomplish a specified function. Functions we have discussed in this chapter include the birth of a healthy baby as well as cognitive and academic achievement, psychosocial functioning, and reproductive behavior of children born to teen mothers. Each of these functions can be explained as a result of multiple, interacting influences. Bronfenbrenner's bioecological systems theory provides one way to conceptualize important elements that together impact birth outcomes and the ongoing development of children born to teen parents.

Applying Bronfenbrenner's model to the development of children born to teen parents begins with a focus on biological aspects of the newborn. Perinatal complications, congenital malformations, prematurity, low birth weight, and perhaps of even greater concern, being small for gestational age, confer a disadvantage right from the beginning that can be overcome only with strong supports within and between the surrounding systems; if not adequately addressed, these biological vulnerabilities may predict ongoing cognitive, behavioral, and psychosocial difficulties (Werner and Smith, 1992).

Families are an important component of the microsystem, along with day care, schools, neighborhoods, peers, and playgrounds. These are the settings where infants, children, and teens spend the majority of their time. The structure of the family may not be as important as how well it functions to socialize children. Two biological parents may do this as well or as poorly as a young mother living with her own mother, or as an older teen mother who lives alone with her child but relies on a new boyfriend to provide needed emotional and material supports. What is most important is how well the needs of the child are being met, rather than who is meeting these needs. Analyses by Manlove *et al.* (2008) found few differences in the home environments of children born to teen versus adult parents. However, children who experienced more instability in primary caregivers through age 15 had less successful outcomes in several domains; this sort of instability was found to occur more often in homes headed by teen parents and partially accounted for differences in outcomes found for children born to teen and adult parents (Jaffee *et al.*, 2001).

High-quality child care is important for all children, regardless of the age of their parents at childbirth (Pluess and Belsky, 2010; Pungello *et al.*, 2010). However, many child care settings that are affordable for teen parents lack the quality necessary to support the optimal development of children. In fact, poor quality child care settings could mediate the impact of SES on differences in outcomes between children of teen versus adult mothers. School-aged mothers' programs can be an important microsystem component that provides high-quality child care while simultaneously teaching and encouraging good parenting practices. Few studies have included the quality of child care as an explanatory variable; this clearly needs further investigation as one of the many factors that can affect the development of children born to teen mothers (Pungello *et al.*, 2010).

Three additional points relate to how individual factors interact with microsystem settings. First, the needs of infants born with complications due to prematurity, SGA, or other problems may be more difficult for families to handle. Teen parents, both mothers and fathers, may have limited experience with, or knowledge of, the additional challenges entailed in caring for an infant who doesn't conform to their expectations of what a healthy infant should be. Second, the role of fathers of children born to teen mothers has often been overlooked (Lu *et al.*, 2010). Understanding outcomes of children born to teen mothers requires attention to the role of fathers as well. A third consideration, only recently brought to light by scientific research, is that some infants and children may be impacted more by the quality of the home environment and parenting than others. Specifically, small genetic differences between infants may allow some children to thrive despite their family's inability to fully meet their needs, whereas a slight genetic variation in other infants may lead to greater sensitivity, and resulting distress, when their needs are not met (Ellis and Boyce, 2011; Pluess and Belsky, 2010).

The exosystem of children born to teen parents often includes health care settings, perhaps a state-run health department or private pediatrician, alternative child care providers, extended family, and parents' school or work settings. The importance of exosystem influences can be seen in the continuing account of Christine, as she tries to support her son, Dominic, now in 1st grade:

Christine had worked full-time in a local factory to make ends meet for her and her son, Dusty. Her own mother cared for Dominic, along with several of his cousins, during the day while Christine worked. Dominic began 1st grade less prepared than some of the other children in the class, so the teacher called Christine in for a conference. Christine requested time off from her job to attend the conference and was granted a half-day off, but without pay. Although Christine needed every penny to make ends meet, she also believed it was important to meet with Dominic's teacher, so she went to the conference. During the conference Christine felt that the teacher was judging her for being a teen mom and causing Dominic to have trouble learning to read. Christine tried to stay respectful to the teacher, but was both angry and frustrated when she left to return to work. Her supervisor even yelled at her a couple of times that afternoon for being inattentive. Only a week or two later, Dominic started bringing home notes from the teacher informing Christine that he was being disruptive in class. Christine needed to again request time off work for a conference. This time her supervisor denied her request and let her know that if she didn't show up for work she would lose her job. Christine was facing a dilemma with no good solution. If she skipped the teacher conference, Dominic would continue to have troubles in school, but if she went, she would lose her job and no longer be able to provide for his basic needs. Her youth and inexperience made her feel intimidated by both her supervisor and Dominic's teacher. She opted to keep her job and missed the conference with Dominic's teacher, probably reinforcing the teacher's judgmental attitudes about teen parents.

Christine's dilemma highlights the influential role of parental work environments in relationship to children's outcomes. This is yet another area relatively unintegrated in studies that compare outcomes of children born to teen versus adult mothers.

The outermost ring of Bronfenbrenner's bioecological model is the macrosystem that includes government ideology and policy, social and gender norms, cultural values and traditions, and economic trends. Macrosystem philosophies have a direct impact on exosystem settings, which, in turn, have tremendous potential to alter the trajectories of children born to teen parents. Although child care and parental work have direct, exosystem-level effects on children's development, these factors are influenced by macrosystem factors such as government assistance for child care and family leave policies. Family leave policies vary considerably among countries as do government-sponsored child care options (Braun and Glöckner-Rist, 2011). The restrictive policy in the United States triggers frequent conflicts, similar to Christine's, requiring parents to make choices between family and income, and leaving few options aside from neglecting some components of the system to attend to others. These policies may magnify, rather than reduce, initial differences between birth outcomes of infants of teen versus adult parents, as well as the ongoing development of the children.

General summary and reframing

In this chapter we have reviewed evidence from scientific studies to rethink two related cultural myths about children born to teen parents. Despite simple comparisons that show infants born to teen mothers have higher rates of infant mortality, prematurity, and low birth weight when compared directly with rates evidenced among children born to adult mothers, most babies born to teen mothers who receive adequate prenatal care are born full-term and healthy. However, perceived stigma, embarrassment, or shame may cause some teens to hide their pregnancies and delay care. Macro- and exo-system changes that facilitate early entry into prenatal care may reduce the likelihood of adverse outcomes for infants born to teen parents.

Just as most babies born to teen mothers are healthy, most will grow up without serious problems and will not repeat the cycle of becoming teen parents. However, the evidence we reviewed does suggest that some children born to teen parents will experience significant developmental problems, with an increased likelihood of early childbearing and criminal offences. Attempts to explain these adverse outcomes as selection effects have not been substantiated, suggesting that maternal age at childbirth may play an important predictive role. However, further process-oriented attempts to explain why maternal age at childbirth is associated with these adverse outcomes have not yielded robust explanations, perhaps due to limitations in the way that research questions have been framed or failure to account for the correct contextual factors.

Continued misperceptions about outcomes for children born to teen mothers may create a feedback or looping mechanism that may inadvertently promote more adverse outcomes. Pregnant teens who have been admonished to avoid pregnancy, lest their children have medical complications and behavioral problems, may experience more pregnancy anxiety, increasing the likelihood of premature birth. Replacing an exclusive focus on children of teen parents with the message that broader systems make a major contribution to the health and development of babies born to parents of all ages may be a good place to begin to change misperceptions.

7 Myths and misperceptions related to public policy

Why, then, is there such a yawning gulf between policy assumptions and the experiences of its subjects?

(Duncan, 2007, p. 320)

The goals of public policy overlap substantially with goals of scientific research. Both policy-makers and researchers strive to improve the lives of individuals within society and of society more generally. The research process does this by attempting to illuminate important truths whereas policy is based on the application of these truths. In Chapter 2 we focused attention on constraints inherent in scientific research that make it challenging for results to provide a valid representation of teens' lives and experiences. In this current chapter we turn our attention to theoretical and empirical constraints intrinsic to developing policy that reflects the diverse experiences of pregnant and parenting teens.

We begin with the story of a pregnant teen as a reminder that, in order to be most effective, policy needs to follow from the experiences of its constituents. *Cynthia was in her best friend's bathroom, staring down at a pregnancy test that confirmed her fears – she would be having a baby sometime in the summer before her senior year. She was worried how her parents and teachers would react – they had always told her to wait until marriage to have sex, and she had let them down. She thought about her boyfriend, Dave, and worried what this would do to their relationship. They had been together off and on since middle school. He was a great guy, but would he be able to help her? She would need money from him and help with child care if she was going to be able to finish high school. Her thoughts then turned to her mother. She knew her mother was going to flip out when she found out that Cynthia was no longer a virgin. They had been arguing a lot lately, ever since her parents announced they would be getting a divorce – this would only add fuel to the fire. Cynthia didn't want to be lectured by her mother on how to behave responsibly. She felt that her mother wasn't being very responsible herself, and Cynthia suspected that she was the one who asked for the divorce. Now that her parents lived apart, could she handle living alone with her mother once the baby came? With the financial strain of the divorce, would her parents be able to help her with the cost of diapers? Cynthia was scared. How would her parents react to this news? Could she count on Dave and her parents to help her with the baby? How would she finish up school and pay for what the baby needs? What would this do to her future? What would people think of her? There were more questions than answers. The only thing Cynthia was sure of was that she needed help.*

This chapter focuses on the empirical and theoretical basis for *prevention* and *intervention* efforts for teen pregnancy and parenting as reflected in policy. If Cynthia's pregnancy could have been prevented, her challenges and worries associated with being a teen mother would have been avoided. Further, once Cynthia became pregnant, effective policies would have ensured that she had the help she needed to promote both her own and her child's well-being. The dual focus on prevention and intervention has the potential to benefit not only teen parents and their children, but extends to society more generally.

The goal of this chapter is to propose that acceptance of cultural myths may lead to the development of policy that overlooks the actual experiences of the teens, families, and societies the policies are designed to benefit. The cultural myth that *abstinence education is the best way to prevent teen pregnancy* is one example of how common beliefs may impact pregnancy prevention policy. Relatedly, the cultural myths that *better outcomes are achieved when teen mothers live with their own mothers* and *it is better for teens and their babies if biological parents marry* illustrate how common beliefs impact policy designed to ensure more positive outcomes for teen parents and their children. The discussion of each of these myths begins with a brief review of the historical background of the relevant policy development, followed by an analysis of supporting empirical evidence and theoretical justification. Each section concludes with a reframing of the cultural myths, to better account for the actual experiences of pregnant and parenting teens. Overall, our examination suggests that each of the prevailing policies reviewed in the chapter may be effective for a subset of teen parents, but that this subset does not reflect the experiences of most teen parents. The mandates, which apply to all teens but are based on what works only for some, squander taxpayers' money and fail to provide the services and supports most needed.

Cultural myth: abstinence education is the best way to prevent teen pregnancy

Abstinence education was the US government's main approach to pregnancy prevention between 1982 and 2007; funding for abstinence-centered programs initially was estimated at $4 million per year; funding jumped to $59 million in 1998 with another jump to $102 million in 2002. Over $170 million dollars was allocated to abstinence education during 2005 to 2007 (Howell and Keefe, 2007). During this time, programs promoted abstinence until marriage, prohibited public schools from providing education regarding alternatives to abstinence, restricted dissemination of contraceptives, and made few allowances for discussion of safe-sex practices. This approach to teen pregnancy prevention focused almost exclusively on the sexual decision-making of young women and men, and ignored the role that contextual or societal factors played in adolescent sexual behaviors. In short, an exclusive focus on abstinence was promoted as a morally appropriate strategy to prevent teen pregnancy.

The abstinence-centered approach to teen pregnancy prevention in the United States began with the implementation of the Adolescent Family Life Act (AFLA) in 1981. Although the AFLA was written with a primary aim of support-ing pregnant and parenting teens, a secondary section of the act was dedicated to preventing teen pregnancy. In its first 15 years of existence the AFLA made some strides towards providing support for pregnant and parenting teens, as intended. The prevention section, however, found resurgence following a 1996 report sug-gesting that the societal cost of teen pregnancy was in the range of billions of dollars (Maynard, 1996).

A subsequent policy shift required the prevention section of the act to con-form to guidelines for abstinence education, where abstinence was defined as not engaging in premarital sex, and programs that received federal funding were required to comply with eight specific criteria listed in Section 510 of the 1996 Social Security Act (Table 7.1; Santelli *et al.*, 2006). When the abstinence-centered approach was initiated in the mid-1990s there was little empirical evi-dence supporting its effectiveness; rather, the policy was implemented with the assumption that research would confirm its utility (McClelland and Fine, 2008). In fact, most research providing any justification for abstinence-centered pro-grams was published after the policy was already broadly implemented (see Clark *et al.*, 2005; Denny and Young, 2006; Jemmott, Jemmott, and Fong, 1998, 2010; Lerner, 2005; Weed, Ericksen, and Birch, 2005; Weed, Ericksen, Lewis, Grant, and Wibberly, 2008).

A clear shift towards evidence-based policy decisions has been seen in recent US legislation. This shift is reflected in the remarks made by US Department of Health and Human Services Secretary Kathleen Sebelius: "Teen pregnancy is a serious national problem and we need to use the best science of what works to address it. This investment will help bring evidence-based initiatives to more communities across the country" (US DHHS, 2010). In 2010, a new Office of Adolescent Health (OAH) was established within the Department of Health and Human Services to coordinate programs related to adolescent health, com-pile empirical evidence to support such programs, and disseminate its findings to practitioners and the general public (Solomon-Fears, 2013).

Consequently, the AFLA program was supplanted by three new programs beginning in 2010 (Solomon-Fears, 2013). The Teen Pregnancy Prevention (TPP) program provides funding for "medically accurate and age-appropriate" prevention programs as well as their evaluation. The TPP was charged to pro-vide funding only for rigorously designed and tested programs. The Personal Responsibility Education Program (PREP) provides funds to educate teens on both abstinence and contraception, in addition to more general preparation for adulthood including education on healthy relationships, financial liter-acy, communication, and life skills. The third program, Title V Abstinence Education Block Grant, continues to provide funding for abstinence-centered education programs that have been deemed rigorously tested in a randomized-controlled trial.

Table 7.1 Federal definition of abstinence-only education

Under Section 510(b) of the 1996 Social Security Act, abstinence education is defined as an educational or motivational program that:

(A)	Has as its exclusive purpose, teaching the social, psychological, and health gains to be realized by abstaining from sexual activity
(B)	Teaches abstinence from sexual activity outside marriage as the expected standard for all school-age children
(C)	Teaches that abstinence from sexual activity is the only certain way to avoid out-of-wedlock pregnancy, sexually transmitted diseases, and other associated health problems
(D)	Teaches that a mutually faithful monogamous relationship in the context of marriage is the expected standard of human sexual activity
(E)	Teaches that sexual activity outside of the context of marriage is likely to have harmful psychological and physical effects
(F)	Teaches that bearing children out-of-wedlock is likely to have harmful consequences for the child, the child's parents, and society
(G)	Teaches young people how to reject sexual advances and how alcohol and drug use increases vulnerability to sexual advances
(H)	Teaches the importance of attaining self-sufficiency before engaging in sexual activity

Source: Title V, Section 510 (b)(2)(A–H) of the Social Security Act (P.L. 104–193)

Controversy surrounding the emphasis on abstinence education in programs designed to prevent teen pregnancy has polarized advocates into two camps. Advocates who support abstinence-centered education assert that teens cannot cognitively handle the mixed message that they should abstain from being sexually active, but use contraception if abstinence fails (Weed *et al.*, 2008). The opposing perspective (Kirby, 2002) suggests that abstinence-centered education withholds important information needed by teens as they develop knowledge, attitudes, values, and behaviors about sex and sexuality (i.e., sexual socialization). The polarization between the two camps has led to publications that appear more focused on discounting evidence provided by the opposing camp than on finding solutions that address substantiated needs of young people. Perhaps due to the philosophical differences, results of program evaluations have been inconclusive and, at times, contradictory. Both sides have criticized the other for poor methodology in study design, and both have overextrapolated their results. To best dissect the evidence for the cultural myth that abstinence education is the best approach to preventing teen pregnancy, we will present empirical evidence provided by both sides and a theoretical evaluation of abstinence approaches.

Empirical evaluations

A comprehensive review of abstinence programs presented by The Heritage Foundation, a conservative research think tank, took the stance that alternative approaches to abstinence-centered sex education condone sexual activity in youths (Kim and Rector, 2010). The report concluded that 17 of the 22 abstinence-centered studies evaluated demonstrated effectiveness in at least one outcome; therefore, abstinence education was determined to be effective and preferred over comprehensive sex education. Across 17 studies, there was evidence that abstinence education reduced the frequency of sexual activity, number of sexual partners, and teen pregnancies, with results documented between five weeks and 24 months after the program. A range of factors impacted effectiveness, including the age of the youths (i.e., middle school versus high school) and whether or not they had already engaged in sexual activity prior to the program.

The Heritage Foundation report included a review of six studies, based on data from the Add Health study, on the effectiveness of virginity pledges (Bearman and Brückner, 2001; Brückner and Bearman, 2005; Rector and Johnson, 2005a, 2005b; Rector, Pardue, and Martin, 2004; Resnick *et al.*, 1997). Teens responded to whether they had "ever taken a public or written pledge to remain a virgin until marriage" during the early waves of the study; their responses were matched with later sexual and reproductive behavior during the high-school years (Wave II) and in early adulthood (Wave III). In lieu of random assignment of teens to pledge or no pledge conditions, variables related to differential motivation and attitudes that may have predisposed some to endorse the pledge were controlled for in analyses (i.e., family structure, religiosity, age, gender, and ethnicity). Results revealed that teens who took virginity pledges were more likely to refrain from sex for almost a year and a half longer than teens who did not pledge abstinence, were less likely to engage in risky sexual behavior, and were less likely to have a teen or nonmarital birth.

Results from these virginity pledge studies were not uniformly positive, however. Although all studies used the same sample, analytic strategies differed. Two studies concluded that teens who reported that they endorsed virginity pledges were also less likely to use condoms if they had sex, and were more likely to engage in risky sexual behaviors (Bearman and Brückner, 2001; Brückner and Bearman, 2005). Bias seems likely due to which outcomes were reported and which were ignored, how data was analyzed, and how nonsignificant outcomes were interpreted. In addition to these problems, since studies relied on regression techniques to control for selection effects rather than random assignment to conditions, drawing conclusions about the role of virginity pledges in causing delayed sexual initiation should be interpreted cautiously (see Santelli *et al.*, 2006).

In summary, although The Heritage Foundation review provides some evidence that abstinence can be effective for some outcomes (Kim and Rector, 2010), conclusions were overextrapolated from the data reviewed, and it therefore represents a biased perspective. For example, the review provided no evidence of programs that compared abstinence-centered education to a more comprehensive sexual education program, yet made interpretations that abstinence programs were better than comprehensive ones. The generalizability of the studies must also be considered. For example, one study demonstrated effectiveness of the "Sex Can Wait" curriculum, but further examination of the primary article revealed that only teens who completed the 18-month follow-up were included in the analysis. Because the authors did not report whether or not there was a baseline difference in those who completed the study and those who dropped out, and whether more individuals from the intervention or the control group completed the study, it is unclear whether results may have been biased (Denny and Young, 2006). Finally, individual differences were evident suggesting that some teens might benefit more from abstinence approaches than others, yet this was not adequately emphasized in analyses or study conclusions. Teens who are already sexually active, for instance, may benefit less from an abstinence-based approach, yet some programs only examined the effectiveness of their program for those who reported being sexually inactive at baseline (Weed, Ericksen, and Birch, 2005). The effectiveness of abstinence programs, evaluated and described in this manner, cannot be generalized to all and should not provide a foundation for policy decisions.

A comprehensive review of pregnancy prevention programs by Kirby (2007) concluded that there was insufficient evidence to support the widespread dissemination of abstinence-based sex education as a means of teen pregnancy prevention. Abstinence programs often demonstrate short-term effectiveness on delay of intercourse, but limited outcome data is available for pregnancy prevention. Although delay in sexual initiation has been demonstrated, and would be expected to reduce the potential for pregnancy, if teens who participate in abstinence-centered programs are less likely to use birth control when they do become sexually active (Bearman and Brückner, 2001; Dailard, 2002), program participation may actually be associated with increased rates of teen pregnancy. Thus, Kirby called for the implementation of more comprehensive programs that target both *sexual* and *nonsexual antecedents* of pregnancy. Sexual antecedents include knowledge of reproduction, sexually transmitted infections (STIs), contraception, and interpersonal skills to avoid unplanned pregnancy (Kirby, 2002, 2007). Nonsexual antecedents of pregnancy include social skills, self-esteem, and a positive future orientation that may trickle down to impact sexual health and decisions about sexual behaviors.

Kirby argued against the common belief that providing education on contraception use may undermine the message of the importance of delaying sexual intercourse. He presented evidence that programs using a more *comprehensive* approach do not appear to confuse teens, show no evidence that the programming results in teens having sex more often or earlier, and have demonstrated a variety of positive behavioral effects (Kirby, 2002; Kirby, Laris, and Rolleri, 2007). In contrast to The Heritage Foundation review, Kirby's summary of the literature suggested that research conveys only limited evidence that encouraging abstinence alone adequately impacts sexual or nonsexual antecedents of teen pregnancy. In fact, abstinence-centered programs and policy do little to substantially delay sexual intercourse, prevent pregnancy, or improve self-efficacy, self-esteem, or perceived self-control (Kirby, 2007; Scher, Maynard, and Stagner, 2006; Trenholm, Devaney, Fortson, Clark, Quay, and Wheeler, 2008). More comprehensive programs, on the other hand, have shown ample evidence of delaying sexual initiation, reducing frequency of sexual intercourse, and reducing the number of partners (Kirby, 2007).

Advocates from both sides of the abstinence debate are quick to pigeonhole the other into an extreme position, instead of allowing recognition of how their missions may have common groundings. For example, abstinence researchers have referred to comprehensive studies as "condom studies" (Weed, Ericksen, and Birch, 2005); comprehensive researchers narrow the approach of abstinence studies as being "abstinence-only" programs and reject the other camp's title of "abstinence-centered." Comprehensive programs cannot be whittled down to just condoms, and abstinence programs are not just preaching abstinence. In fact, two-thirds of the comprehensive programs in Kirby's review included an abstinence component along with sexual antecedent messages such as contraception use. Ideally, both camps would work towards building stronger teens who can make important sexual decisions in light of contextual factors and avoid adverse outcomes such as unwanted pregnancies and STIs.

Not surprisingly, both sides of the debate surrounding abstinence education are quick to point out methodological flaws for the counterevidence, and less likely to be up front on limitations of studies supporting their own views. Important considerations for both sides of the divide include:

- The necessity of not overextrapolating results. Support for one type of program does not imply that other types of programs are ineffective.
- Conclusions that program participation was responsible for causing changes in sexual or reproductive behaviors need to be based on rigorous methodology. Statistical controls for background characteristics (found in many virginity pledge studies) are not as rigorous as random assignment. Conclusions that one type of program causes more effective outcomes than another should only be drawn from research that randomly assigned youths to program conditions.
- More attention needs to be placed on the process of change. Theoretical models of change are needed to guide program development. Factors that mediate change (e.g., nonsexual antecedents including self-esteem, locus of control, resistance skills, and parent communication) need to be identified, evaluated, and included in future programs (Trenholm *et al.*, 2008).

Theoretical foundations

The theory of reasoned action and its extension, the theory of planned behavior (Ajzen, 1991; Montano and Kasprzyk, 2008), provide the theoretical foundation for several abstinence-based prevention programs as well as many comprehensive sex education programs. The theory of planned behavior was designed to predict human behavior in specific contexts (e.g., substance abuse, volunteering, reproductive behaviors). The model explains behavior as intentional; intentions to act are proposed to be caused by attitudes about the behavior, subjective norms, and perception of control over actions. Related to teen pregnancy prevention, the theory of planned behavior attempts to explain which teens will become pregnant based on their attitudes about pregnancy, perceived norms, and perceptions of control. Changing behavior, therefore, most directly requires changing intentions – an important component of virginity pledge programs. Most programs also target attitudes about sexual and reproductive activity within the context of normative beliefs. Finally, similar to Bandura's concept of self-efficacy, perceived behavioral control would reflect the confidence with which teens believe they will be able to effectively abstain from sexual activity or to protect themselves from unwanted side effects, such as STIs or pregnancy, should they have sex.

Several shortcomings of this theoretical approach to pregnancy prevention are evident. First, research has demonstrated that changing attitudes about sexual and reproductive behavior does not always lead to behavioral change (Trenholm *et al.*, 2008). This disconnect could be a result of how attitudes interact with subjective norms and perceived control. Second, although curricula may effectively change attitudes and improve skills needed to maintain control over sexual and reproductive behaviors, impacting subjective norms by targeting individuals is a bit more complicated. For example, fertility-timing norms are established by groups outside of the programs' purviews. Changing subjective norms without a corresponding focus on the reality of these norms will likely be ineffective. Finally, enhancing perceptions of control may be less effective in contexts where teens' intentions to remain abstinent are thwarted by sexual coercion, abuse, or rape. Intentions reflect a motivation component provided the action is under voluntary control.

Although the theory of planned behavior (Ajzen, 1991; Montano and Kasprzyk, 2008) provides a somewhat reasonable explanation for teen sexual and reproductive behaviors, its basic assumptions are inconsistent with general systems theory. The theory of planned behavior suggests that attitudes, subjective norms, and perceived behavioral control each exert independent impacts that can be combined in a linear manner to predict intentions. In contrast to this reductionist approach, the more holistic systems approach acknowledges that although attitudes, subjective norms, and perceived behavioral control may be important, in reality they interact synergistically with intentions to predict behavior. In addition, the theory of planned behavior places ultimate responsibility for behavioral decisions on the individual. Although social and cultural factors are considered, their relevance is always filtered through individual perceptions. For example, social pressures towards virginity or sexual experience aren't measured directly, but rather as perceived subjective norms. Programs that target individuals will have an exceptional challenge overcoming subjective norms if the objective norms and social pressures are omitted from intervention efforts. Consequently, by reinforcing assumptions of rational choice, the theory of planned behavior may contribute to the "yawning gulf" that Duncan (2007) identified between policy and constituent experiences.

In contrast to many prevention programs that target individual change, a systems approach to intervention may identify multiple targets and the interaction of these targets. Most pregnancy prevention programs discussed so far have targeted individual teens directly, thereby limiting the amount of change possible.

Targeting parents of teens may also be beneficial, as has been done with the "Start the Conversation" strategy through The National Campaign to Prevent Teen and Unplanned Pregnancy; this strategy encourages communities to reach out to parents, to teach skills and improve parents' confidence in talking with their children about sexual and reproductive behaviors.

Even if the individual or familial intervention is successful in the short term, if the environment in which the teens live does not change, the program's long-term effectiveness may be less likely (Trenholm *et al.*, 2008). Thus, a systems perspective would also necessitate intervention at the school and community levels, and consideration of how the effectiveness of any program is relative to the different populations and settings that are targeted (Scher *et al.*, 2006). A systems approach suggests that teen pregnancy prevention programs that target multiple systems will be more effective than programs that focus exclusively on teens' attitudes and behaviors on abstaining from sex. Why, then, have policy-makers continued to invest funds in programs that are not supported by theory and research? For example, funding for abstinence-centered education is still earmarked at approximately $50 million per year; consequently, from fiscal year 2010–2014, $250 million will be allocated to abstinence-centered programs, despite a lack of strong theory or evidence, supporting the utility of these programs (Solomon-Fears, 2013).

As described in the quote that opened this chapter, Duncan (2007) acknowledged the role of both research and cultural beliefs in widening the gulf between policy and constituent experiences, and described a potential culprit for this disconnect as a *rationality mistake*. In essence, policy-makers commit a rationality mistake by assuming that teens' reproductive decisions should be based on the same educational and economic ramifications seen by the policy-makers. If policy is based upon this erroneous premise, then it likely discounts the experiences of some teens who make reproductive decisions that are rational for their unique contextual circumstances. Further, the rationality mistake places responsibility for teen pregnancy and parenting on the decision-making skills of the teens themselves, while minimizing contributions of societal constraints (Duncan, 2007).

Policies that avoid this rationality mistake will be more responsive to the actual experiences of people. It can be challenging to form these responsive policies, however, because they require valid knowledge of what the people's experiences are. Thus, policy decisions need input from empirical evidence that provides accurate and relevant information about the needs of pregnant and parenting teens, the challenges they and their children face, and the strengths and opportunities they possess. Furthermore, ongoing evaluation of the extent to which programs are meeting needs is imperative. Policy decisions are all too often disconnected from this empirical foundation. Abstinence policy is just one example of government-funded programs fueled by political agendas instead of previously established empirical evidence and supportive theory. In order to truly meet the goals of bettering the lives of individuals and society, policy-makers need to base their decisions on empirical evidence from studies that are appropriately designed, analyzed, and interpreted.

Summary and reframing

In sum, there is not a one-size-fits-all approach to the prevention of teen pregnancy; although some teens may respond well to abstinence-centered programs,
others need a more comprehensive approach. Returning to the example of
Cynthia allows for consideration of how individual differences might impact program effectiveness: *Cynthia was embarrassed to go to class today. She knew they were
starting their final year with a program called "My Choice, My Future!" in her health
class. She had just run across the packets she used in her 8th and 9th grade years. She
looked at their titles, "Reasonable Reasons to Wait: The Keys to Character" and "Art of
Loving Well: A Character Education Curriculum for Today's Teenagers." She felt sick
thinking about what she would say. Both years her teachers had used different ways to
explain the reasons to wait until marriage to have sex. She remembered last year reading
short stories, poetry, and even fairy tales on what to look for in healthy relationships. As
she sat down, her belly barely fitting in the desk any longer, she knew her teachers would
be disappointed that she had failed them.*

Cynthia's shame and embarrassment over her pregnancy, and her willingness
to take responsibility for it, are all consistent with the rationality assumption
(Duncan, 2007). Although she felt as though she had failed those who taught her
and cared for her, in reality the well-meaning adults in her environment should
share the blame for her pregnancy for implementing curricula that lacked robust
evidence of effectiveness. "My Choice, My Future!" was one of four abstinence-
centered programs experimentally evaluated with random assignment of youths
to program and control conditions (Trenholm et al., 2008). No significant differences in sexual activity, number of sexual partners, contraceptive use, pregnancy, or STIs were found between youths who participated in any of the four
abstinence-centered programs compared to control youths.

Successful programs are those that maintain a focus on positive youth development while simultaneously addressing specific issues related to sexual and
reproductive behaviors. The consensus from evaluation studies is that the most
effective programs are those that focus on positive youth development through
nonsexual antecedents (e.g., improving social skills, self-esteem, and relationship
expectations) as well as sexual antecedents related to teen pregnancy (Gavin,
Catalano, David-Ferdon, Gloppen, and Markham, 2010; Mawer, 1999). These
types of program goals may best explain why and how various curricula work (i.e.,
by explaining processes such as mediators of intervention efficacy).

Targeting nonsexual antecedents goes beyond telling teens not to engage in
sex, by providing them reasons *why* this choice is in their best interests (e.g., they
have goals to achieve, a promising future, a need to be self-sufficient), so they can
come to the decision not to engage in sex until they are prepared for its potential
consequences. In a similar manner, teaching about contraception does not ensure
that teens will use it consistently or properly. There is building evidence, both
quantitative and qualitative, that teens' misunderstanding of how to use contraception is not solely to blame for teen pregnancy (Arai, 2003; DiCenso, Guyatt,
Willan, and Griffith, 2002; Duncan, 2007; Graham and McDermott, 2006).

Nonsexual antecedents may need to be strengthened to ensure teens actually apply their contraceptive knowledge.

In conclusion, preventing teen pregnancy requires an ongoing understanding of the challenges, strengths, and opportunities of youth. Public sex education based on an abstinence-centered message lacks both a basis in scientific evidence and a strong theoretical grounding. Fortunately, the current approach to adolescent health in the United States is shifting to becoming more evidence-based. Collectively the evidence we have examined provides a convincing rationale to refute the cultural myth that abstinence education is the best way to prevent teen pregnancy. Reframing this common belief requires attention to the actual experiences of today's youth. Choices made by youths related to sexual initiation, use of contraception, and pregnancy are partially determined by a thought process that takes into consideration both current and future life options, but are also influenced by factors not directly under their control (e.g., fertility-timing norms).

Acknowledging that abstinence remains the only 100 percent effective way to prevent pregnancy, we propose that *abstinence education is only one important component of a multifaceted strategy that targets not only teens, but also families, communities, and broader social values and beliefs.* Programs should have multiple, clear, programmatic goals that may include sexual health, reducing sexual risk-taking, abstinence, relationship skills, and more general life skills, in addition to a focus on preventing unwanted or mistimed pregnancies. In most cases these goals are complementary and have the potential to make a positive impact in several areas.

Cultural myth: better outcomes are achieved when teen mothers live with their own mothers

Concerns about high rates of teen pregnancy and parenting were addressed in US policy changes as part of the 1996 welfare reform (Acs and Koball, 2003). Two stipulations had to be met in order for teen parents to receive federal funds. First, minor parents (those under the age of 18) were required to live with a responsible adult, generally regarded as the teen mother's mother (i.e., the child's grandmother). Second, minor parents had to return to school or training programs with direct job consequences within 12 weeks of giving birth (Duffy and Levin-Epstein, 2002). Teen parents who did not comply would lose welfare benefits; exceptions were allowed if a parent or other adult relative was unable to be located, or if a state agency determined that the home would be unsafe or not in the teen mother's best interests. In addition to reducing rates of teen pregnancy and parenting, these policy changes were expected to decrease nonmarital births, encourage stable families, and provide teens with financial support and self-sufficiency skills (Levin-Epstein and Schwartz, 2005). For this section, we will focus primarily on the aspect of the policy that is driven by the cultural myth that better outcomes are achieved when teen mothers live with their own mothers.

The current policy that requires teen mothers to live with their own mothers in order to receive governmental assistance has historical roots reflecting societal shifts in social norms (Blank and Blum, 1997). This *minor mandate* stemmed from a program originally developed in 1935 to provide support for widows, the Social Security Act in the United States providing Aid to Dependent Children (ADC). The targeted group soon expanded to support poor single mothers. However, despite the reflection of social norms that mothers should stay at home to raise children, concerns were immediately raised that the provision of support was encouraging nonmarital births (Blank and Blum, 1997). In response, several States enacted legislation to block support to children born to unmarried mothers. After World War II, social and demographic changes in the United States resulted in tremendous expansion of the population served by ADC. Consequently, a new emphasis was placed on families in 1962, accompanied by a name change to Aid to Families with Dependent Children (AFDC). It wasn't until the late 1960s that provisions were added to require welfare recipients to "make good-faith efforts to become economically self-sufficient" (Blank and Blum, 1997). This reflected changing social norms that mothers were no longer expected to stay at home, but to assist the family financially by working outside the home. These provisions became known as "Welfare-to-Work."

The Personal Responsibility and Work Opportunity Reconciliation Act of 1996 (PRWORA) replaced AFDC with the Temporary Assistance for Needy Families (TANF) program. The major goals of TANF are to provide for families, so children can be cared for in their own homes, reduce financial dependence of needy families by enhancing employability, prevent pregnancies outside of marriage, and encourage the formation of two-parent families and sustained marital relationships (Levin-Epstein and Schwartz, 2005). PRWORA subsumed ideals embodied in Welfare-to-Work provisions and was established with the assumption that young people would adjust their sexual behaviors if they understood that there would be economic constraints that prohibited reliance on the government for assistance if children were born outside of marriage (Hao, Astone, and Cherlin, 2007).

The impact of these policies is illustrated by returning to the case of Cynthia at the point when her son, Jayden, is two months old. *Cynthia looked at the monthly TANF check she held in her hand. She was so grateful for the help to pay for Jayden's diapers and formula. Dave was working hard to save up so they could live on their own when she turned 18. He had another year of saving and she couldn't wait for that day. She had to live with her mother until then to keep receiving these checks. She knew she also had to continue going to school. That wasn't the hard part – she wanted to finish up high school as soon as possible so she could start dental hygiene school, become self-sufficient, and no longer need TANF. The hard part was enduring the fights with her mom and the constant nagging over how to take care of Jayden. Her mom was stressed out now that the divorce was final. Cynthia tried to keep that in mind – plus the fact that she knew her mom was just doing what she thought was best. Sometimes it was just too much though. She was ready to be on her own. Just one more year!*

Requiring teen mothers like Cynthia to live with their parents was based, much like abstinence policy, more on assumptions than on research evidence. The policy assumed that living with the grandmother would result in better child outcomes, help the mother complete her education, and reduce the likelihood of repeat pregnancies. The policy also assumed that stipulations put in place would deter teens from becoming pregnant in the first place. Little evidence has been found to support these assumptions, and some evidence has demonstrated opposite effects. For example, one study, published prior to policy implementation, observed that teen mothers who resided with their parents immediately after the baby was born were more likely to stay in school, but the benefits were completely reversed in the two-year follow-up. By that time, teens who still lived with their parents were actually less likely to achieve economic security (Furstenberg *et al.*, 1987). Other studies have found similar negative consequences of teen mothers living with their own parents (e.g., Horvath-Rose and Peters, 2001).

Evaluation of the success of the minor mandate in decreasing nonmarital births, encouraging stable families, and providing teens with financial support and self-sufficiency skills has been hampered by unreliable data. Implementation of the policy occurred at the State level, but States were not required to report data (Offner, 2003). One evaluation conducted by the Center for Law and Social Policy (CLASP) concluded that teen parents were "undercounted, untracked, oversanctioned, and underserved" (Duffy and Levin-Epstein, 2002). Although these concerns were largely based on frustrations over validity of reports from State agencies, the data that were available indicated that teens were overrepresented among families who received sanctions. The limitations of State reports prevented the authors of this evaluation from drawing definitive conclusions about the impact of policy stipulations.

In lieu of reliable State data to evaluate the effectiveness of policy decisions, a handful of researchers have attempted to compare outcomes for teens prior to policy changes with outcomes that occurred following the policy changes, using data from national data sets (e.g., NLSY; Acs and Koball, 2003; Hao *et al.*, 2007; Kaestner, Korenman, and O'Neill, 2003; Offner, 2003). Overall, conclusions from these studies found no direct impact of the minor mandate on preventing nonmarital childbearing or school dropout. The study by Hao and colleagues (2007) provided the most detailed analysis and was consistent with a systems perspective in that the authors examined reciprocal relationships between policies requiring teen mothers to stay in school and to live with their parents to receive welfare benefits, and State policies aimed at paternal child support. General conclusions from these analyses were that changes in welfare policy were unrelated to teens' reproductive behaviors. Teen mothers who lived with their own mothers were no more or less likely than other teen mothers to stay in school or to have subsequent children while unmarried. However, the authors interpreted their results as marginal support for an indirect effect of child support policy on reducing rates of teen pregnancies, suggesting that men are somewhat less likely to cause a pregnancy in States that have tougher child support policies (Hao *et al.*, 2007).

The assumption that living with the grandmother will provide greater support is simplistic and fails to take into account the quality of the relationship, any social strain that might exist between the mother and daughter, and how the mother's relationship with the baby's father might impact the need for support from the grandmother. Mothers with low support from the grandmothers have demonstrated better parenting outcomes if they were living on their own (Spieker and Bensley, 1994). Grandmothers can also infringe upon teen mothers' ability to be independent parents (Rosman and Yoshikawa, 2001), and living with them may even cause distress (Kalil, Ariel, Spencer, Spieker, and Gilchrist, 1998). The transition of teens into parenthood inherently brings stress that can be compounded if teens are unable to gain support (McLaughlin and Micklin, 1983), but social support is multifaceted (Thompson, Flood, and Goodvin, 2006) and can cover emotional, informational, tangible, social, and practical needs. Functional provision of social support needs to be matched with the specific stressors the mothers are facing (Toomey, Umaña-Taylor, Jahromi, and Updegraff, 2013); simple co-residence with a member of the social support network, such as living with the grandmother, does not mean that teens are receiving the help they need to become independent adults. In contrast, parenting supports that are meaningful and accessible can have substantial effects on the development of young mothers and their children (cf. Bert, Farris, and Borkowski, 2008; Farris, Bert, Nicholson, Glass, and Borkowski, 2013).

Lack of consistency in evaluation findings may be partially attributed to heterogeneity inherent in any sample of teen mothers. The Three Generation Study (see Appendix) has studied relationships between teen mothers and grandmothers as they have unfolded over time, and has identified two specific types of support relationships: *Parental Supplement* and *Supported Primary Parent* (Krishnakumar and Black, 2003). The most typical model, describing about two-thirds of the dyads, was the Parental Supplement model in which the teen mother and grandmother shared caregiving responsibilities. The other one-third of the dyads was consistent with a Supported Primary Parent model in which the teen mother was the primary caregiver, with only occasional assistance from the grandmother (Oberlander, Black, and Starr, 2007). Greater *maternal* caregiving over the first two years of a child's life, consistent with a Supported Primary Parent model, predicted more positive outcomes for children. The authors suggested that the teen's adoption of the role of parent may lead to more positive long-term outcomes for children of teen mothers (Oberlander and Black, 2011). These results are generally consistent with findings from the Family Life Project (FLP, see Appendix; Barnett, Mills-Koonce, Gustafsson, and Cox, 2012), suggesting that greater conflicts in relationships between mothers and grandmothers were related to children's behavior problems. More problematic outcomes, therefore, are observed when grandmother support allows teen mothers to relegate the primary responsibility of parenthood to others or when teen mothers are stuck in a conflictual relationship with their mothers. Taking this heterogeneity into account, requiring all teen mothers to live with their own mothers might not allow for teens to gain primary responsibility in cases when either the grandmothers are overbearing or the teens are not proactive.

Stipulations that require teen parents to live with family members may be most detrimental for more vulnerable teens (Duffy and Levin-Epstein, 2002). For example, one study found that, of over 500 girls who became pregnant as teens, two-thirds reported sexual abuse, with close to one-half of the perpetrators identified as family members (Boyer and Fine, 1992). Forcing teen mothers who may have experienced sexual abuse by a family member to live in the same household not only puts the teens at risk for continued abuse but also endangers their children.

A growing number of studies suggest the need for more flexible policies supporting teen parents and their children (Levin-Epstein and Schwartz, 2005; Shapiro and Marcy, 2002). For example, a study by Shapiro and Marcy (2002) found that up to 46 percent of teens who applied for TANF were turned away without being given the chance to apply. The authors attributed the denial of services to insufficiently trained case workers and to the lack of a transition period to give teens a chance to comply with stipulations. A transitional period would also allow time for State agencies to investigate housing options before requiring teen parents to return to abusive, or otherwise inappropriate, home situations. Reports have indicated a number of unmet service needs of teen parents who received aid (Duffy & Levin-Epstein, 2002). Only a couple of States had made significant progress in supporting the needs of teen parents regarding education and training, although most endorsed this as an important area of continued emphasis. In contrast, few alternative housing options (e.g., Second Chance homes) were available for teen mothers who were unable to reside with their own parents. Consequently, teen parents most in need of support may be denied the support they need (Duffy and Levin-Epstein, 2002). Duffy and Levin-Epstein (2002) surmised that "much of the Congressional impetus for the mandates may have been intuitive ... However, the imposition of the mandates may keep particularly vulnerable teen parents and their children away from needed assistance with schooling and living arrangements" (p. 4).

Summary and reframing

In summary, there is little evidence to support the belief that *better outcomes are achieved when teen mothers are required to live with their own mothers*. Co-residence stipulations in TANF regulations undoubtedly benefit some teen mothers. Both teen mothers and their children may benefit from temporary residence with grandparents who provide a safe environment, encourage continued education, and allow the teen mothers to assume primary parent roles but provide supports as needed. These grandmothers may encourage autonomy and independence, while maintaining a close connection with their daughters and their children.

In contrast, not all homes provided by grandparents share these characteristics. Requiring parenting teens to co-reside with parents who abuse alcohol or other drugs, or who have failed to protect teen mothers from abuse, is obviously counterproductive. Although not as obvious, grandparents who adopt a primary caretaking role and allow the teen parents to resume their lives as adolescents may also be counterproductive in the long run (Oberlander and Black, 2011). Although TANF policy acknowledges that co-residence is not always the best option, alternatives for teen mothers are lacking. Second Chance homes are infrequently available (Andrews and Moore, 2011), and few foster homes are willing to accept a teen parent with a child. The optimal situation for some teens may be to move into independent households while retaining access to high levels of support from their mothers and from well-trained case workers (Chase-Lansdale, Brooks-Gunn, and Zamsky, 1994; Spieker and Bensley, 1994).

Reframing the cultural myth to more closely match the challenges, strengths, and opportunities of parenting teens needs to consider the diversity in response to becoming a parent. Current policy is an example of an uneasy compromise between beliefs that teen mothers need support and that simultaneously limit this support. The belief that *better outcomes are achieved when teens are provided resources to support their transition to parenthood* may be closer to the actual experiences of youth. Supportive resources for teen parents are similar to resources beneficial for parents of any age and include affordable high-quality child care, including school-based care, provision of emergency sick-child care, support for age-appropriate parenting practices, and safe, affordable living situations.

Cultural myth: it is better for teens and their babies if biological parents marry

Historically, teen pregnancy and parenting were problems only because they were an observable consequence of sexual activity outside of marriage. As a consequence, marriage between young couples was promoted to avoid illegitimate births. However, as illustrated in the story of Claire and Jeremy from Chapter 1, many of these early marriages were unsuccessful. This section rethinks the myth that it is better for teens and their babies if biological parents marry. We begin with a brief overview of policy in the United States that promotes marriage, followed by a comparison of the stability of teen marriages to marriages that occur between adults. We subsequently examine evidence that has evaluated the benefits of marriage for women and children. Little research is available that focuses exclusively on teens, but some studies have included low-income and young mothers more generally. Our examination highlights the difficulty of definitively attributing differences between married and unmarried parents to marriage per se, since people who choose to marry may be different from those who remain single. The many different types of family structures also make it difficult to find an appropriate comparison group for married parents. We end by reframing the cultural myth to be more consistent with the evidence.

Welfare legislation in the United States includes policy designed to promote healthy marriages. This *marriage initiative* (Healthy Marriage and Responsible Fatherhood Program, administered by the Administration for Children and Families of the US Department of Health and Human Services; Brotherson and Duncan, 2004) is based on the assumption that children are better off if raised by two biological parents who are married (McLanahan, 2007). This policy was implemented, in part, by concerns over high rates of divorce, combined with steep rises in rates of nonmarital births. The policy encourages the formation of healthy marriages by providing incentives to seek premarital counseling (e.g., reduced cost of marriage license), by providing tax or economic assistance for low-income couples, and by providing relationship education to teens (Brotherson and Duncan, 2004).

Despite changes in national policy, each State has the authority to design how the marriage initiative is implemented. A 2006 review suggested that policy implementation in many States actually provided a disincentive to marry, especially if the intended spouse was also father of some or all of the children (Moffitt, Reville, Winkler, and Burstain, 2009). The marriage disincentive was primarily attributed to inclusion of the man's income in welfare eligibility determination, which could lead to denial of benefits. A preliminary study to determine whether policy changes actually changed marriage decision-making suggested that there were few effects (Moffitt et al., 2009). Evidence from other countries, however, has suggested that government policy may be effective in promoting marriage.

Researchers in Austria took advantage of a natural experiment to evaluate the impact of policies promoting marriage on the stability of unions (Frimmel, Halla, and Winter-Ebmer, 2012). The natural experiment was based on an abrupt policy change in Austria: whereas marriage had been encouraged among Austrian couples with the provision of a cash benefit, this benefit was suddenly discontinued. An ensuing marriage spike occurred during the short period between the announcement of the policy change and when the change actually took place. Many of these marriages were considered "marginal marriages" because of the presumption that they only occurred to receive the cash benefit. However, when the stability of these marginal marriages was compared to average marriages, no differences in divorce rates were found. These results suggested that marriage-promoting policies may actually create stable marriages. However, this study did not report comparisons specifically for teen mothers.

Among recent cohorts, marriage is becoming increasingly dissociated with childbearing (Teen Births, 2013). More women of all ages are choosing to become mothers outside of a marital relationship. Until recently in the United States, teens who became pregnant often were forced into early marriages to avoid the shame and embarrassment of an illegitimate birth (Cherlin, Cross-Barnet, Burton, and Garrett-Peters, 2008). However, nonmarital births have more recently become increasingly common. For example, in 2011, 89 percent of births to teens in the United States between ages 15 and 19 were to unmarried mothers, up from 51 percent in 1982 (Teen Births, 2013).

Marriages to women under the age of 20 are less stable than marriages to women over 20 (Copen, Daniels, Vespa, and Mosher, 2012). Approximately 54 percent of marriages to women under the age of 20 were intact after ten years of marriage, compared to 69 percent of those to women between the ages of 20 and 24, and 78 percent of those to women over the age of 25. However, educational level at the time of marriage was a better predictor of instability than chronological age, suggesting that much of the instability may be due to an *immaturity effect* (NSFG; Lehrer and Chen, 2011). The immaturity effect emphasizes mistaken expectations based on inadequate self-knowledge and uncertainty about their own and their partners' potential trajectories. In addition, premarital cohabitation remains a risk for relationship disruption, as does having a child from a previous union.

Despite postponement in the normative age of marriage, most teens report positive attitudes towards marriage and see prior cohabitation as a means to ensure they are making good choices in partners (Wood, Avellar, and Goesling, 2008). However, attitudes towards marriage and cohabitation vary by both sex and by race. Compared to women, fewer men opt to both marry and to cohabit during their early twenties. Marriage and cohabitation during emerging adulthood are also less likely among Blacks compared to Whites or Latinas (Wood *et al.*, 2008). Racial differences in the rates of marriage may suggest a difference in the value placed on marriage. However, Oberlander and her colleagues (2010) challenge this interpretation with the suggestion that some Black mothers hold marriage "in such high esteem that it is difficult to find a suitable partner" (p. 32).

Consistent with the other cultural myths we have discussed in this chapter, the marriage initiative has generated considerable debate and disagreement among policy analysts and researchers. One side of the debate emphasizes the benefits attributed to children who grow up in homes with two biological parents who are married (Amato, 2007). The other side of the debate argues that there is insufficient evidence that marriage confers the same benefits to all families, especially those with lower incomes, and that forcing couples who would not have chosen marriage into marriage in order to receive benefits is not beneficial for any (Furstenberg, 2007).

Several publications have relied on data collected from the Fragile Families and Child Wellbeing Study to investigate the impact of fathers in the lives of young mothers and their children (Cooper, McLanahan, Meadows, and Brooks-Gunn, 2009; Liu and Heiland, 2012). Few benefits of marriage were observed in one study with this sample (Liu and Heiland, 2012). Although the study revealed that children of married parents tended to be healthier, had fewer behavior problems, and scored higher on vocabulary development, these differences were attributed to a selection effect as opposed to an influence of marriage itself. In other words, older, more educated people with better jobs were more likely to marry than younger people with less education. The supposed benefit of marriage was actually attributed to these confounding factors. Differences in children's outcomes were associated with these preexisting differences between couples who married compared to those who remained single.

The study by Liu and Heiland (2012) did find a small, but significant, impact of marriage on children's vocabulary scores at three years of age. However, some of the difference in scores between children from the two groups was attributed to the inclusion of cohabiting couples in the nonmarried group. The authors suggested several reasons that the vocabulary scores of children living with cohabiting parents would be lower, including stigma and less paternal investment in the children. Conclusions imply that much of the benefit attributed to marriage among young, low-income families is really the result of a selection effect, and when controls are included for this selection effect, the benefit of marriage dissipates (Liu and Heiland, 2012).

Studies using other data sets (e.g., The National Survey of Families and Households: Choi and Marks, 2013) concurred that relationships between marriage and outcomes differed for people based on socioeconomic status (SES). Specifically, marital happiness was more associated with positive health outcomes for those with higher SES, while marital conflict was more associated with negative health outcomes for those with lower SES. In other words, people from higher SES benefitted more from good marriages, and those from lower SES suffered more from bad marriages.

An analysis conducted by the Center for Law and Social Policy specifically focused on the potential impact of marriage for pregnant teens (Seiler, 2002). Marriage typically improves the economic status of women, but divorcing puts women at higher risks of poverty than never marrying. The economic benefit for a teen mother may be less than for women in their twenties if the father of the baby is also still a teen who has few economic resources to contribute. Marriage also increases the likelihood of a closely spaced second birth, which has been linked to worse economic and educational outcomes for both young mothers and their children. With or without this second birth, teens who marry are significantly less likely to return to school following childbirth than those who don't marry. One specific study that explored relationships among poverty, early teen marriage, and dropping out of high school concluded that there was a strong relationship between early teen marriage and later poverty (Dahl, 2005). In addition to economic and educational consequences of teen marriage, Seiler (2002) expressed concern about the high rates of violence observed in young relationships. In sum, Seiler concluded that "the instability of teen marriage and the risks it can pose should give pause to any policymaker who is eager to encourage pregnant adolescents to walk down the aisle" (p. 10).

Not only may marriage be detrimental to the pregnant teens, but the presumed benefits of growing up in a two-parent home may not always accrue for their children. Characteristics of the fathers may play a large role in determining whether children will benefit or not from the marriages. One interesting study took into account the likelihood of incarceration of potential mates based on the premise of *assortative mating* that occurs when sexual partners are selected based on similarity of important characteristics and traits considered desirable (Finlay and Neumark, 2010). Basically, findings suggested that finding good fathers and good spouses may not be easy for some young women with low education. Within a limited selection of quality partners, marriage may result in partners with undesirable characteristics including violence, aggression, or criminal tendencies. Instead of benefitting children, these characteristics may actually be detrimental (see also Jaffee *et al.*, 2003).

Summary and reframing

To summarize, current policies are often based on the assumption that it is better for teens and their babies if biological parents marry. The relationship between marriage and positive outcomes, however, appears to be primarily due to a selection effect. Marriage itself may have less of an impact than the characteristics of couples who choose marriage. These couples tend to be older, more educated, and have better jobs. Unstable relationships create stress, and high levels of marital conflict are associated with negative outcomes for parents and children (Cummings, Davies, and Campbell, 2000). Relationships that have high conflict and are not meeting the needs of the mothers or children do not get better simply because the couples get married. Young couples should be discouraged from forming unions with little chance of success, but rather should be supported in recognizing, developing, and maintaining quality relationships. Reframing this cultural myth based on empirical evidence suggests that *marriage is good for some teens and their babies, but not for all*. Marriage may be especially appropriate for older teen mothers who have finished high school, and who have the maturity and support to manage an intimate relationship.

Difficulty with policy development for prevention and intervention

Closing the gap between policy assumptions and the actual experiences of youth (Duncan, 2007) requires three overlapping strategies. First, cultural myths based on misperceptions need to be eradicated and replaced with insights that more closely approximate actual challenges, strengths, and opportunities. Second, policy-makers need to rely on research studies that have been appropriately designed, rigorously examined, and properly interpreted. Finally, the assumption that pregnancies result solely from irrational choices made by teens needs to be replaced with a systems perspective that acknowledges the contributions of families, communities, and broader society to rates of teen pregnancies and teen births. Policies that are informed by cultural myths rather than scholarly evidence often derail progress and hinder outcomes. Closing the gap between policy and the experiences of teen parents requires insight into meaningful differences between teen mothers.

To examine how these overlapping strategies could help create meaningful policy, we will examine the UK's approach to teen pregnancy with a comprehensive, research-based initiative consistent with a systems perspective during the time period when the United States enacted an abstinence-centered curriculum. Both approaches received controversial reviews and should be considered in light of prevalent cultural myths during their implementation. We previously reviewed the historical and political basis for the United States to specifically target the cultural myth on abstinence, but will now present a short synopsis of the approach taken by the UK, as part of their approach was aimed at questioning how a predominant societal belief may impact how teen mothers are treated, and consequently, how well they fare.

In 1999, the Social Exclusion Unit (SEU) in the UK established a Teenage Pregnancy Unit (TPU) that was charged with crafting policy to prevent teen pregnancy, reduce abortions among teens, and improve the quality of life for teens who did become young parents. The TPU was established at a time when other countries in Western Europe were seeing a decline in teen pregnancies that had yet to reach the UK (Botting, Rosato, and Wood, 1998). The very name of the Social *Exclusion* Unit conveys an awareness by policy-makers of the difficulty that many young parents face. The UK's perspective on the origin of the high teen parenting rate was clearly outlined in a report by the SEU that went against some commonly held beliefs (SEU, 1999). For example, the report questioned a cultural belief that pregnant teens had failed society, and replaced this belief with a viewpoint that somehow society had failed these teens and put them at greater risk for social exclusion. The policy strived to take into account the perspective of the teens themselves, and not just society's perspective (Graham and McDermott, 2006).

The report summarized research portraying that teen parents and their children were not doomed to a downward spiral of substandard living and poor outcomes, but that they were at greater risk for challenges such as poverty, single parenting, lower educational attainment, and unemployment (SEU, 1999). The SEU's plan was founded in research documenting that the high rate of teen pregnancy was likely not due to teen mothers wanting to gain from the welfare system, but more from the teens' pessimistic views of other options that would be available to them if they postponed motherhood. Young mothers conveyed low expectations of employment, ignorance of how to access resources, and poor education on sexual health and contraception (SEU, 1999). By questioning and reframing common beliefs, the UK was taking responsibility for how its culture and society could contribute to and help to remedy the high rate of teen pregnancy, instead of placing the majority of blame on the teen mothers themselves.

These reframed cultural myths were then integrated into policy designed to accomplish the goals of the SEU relevant to youth and teen mothers. One aspect of the approach taken by the UK was to improve teen mothers' social support and connectedness to resources through the Sure Start Plus program, which connects young mothers with case workers, or personal advisors. These advisors were educated females who could help young mothers avoid and overcome challenges related to poor outcomes (e.g., poverty, lower education, unemployment). Sure Start personal advisors were intended to improve teens' self-esteem and confidence, counteract any negative feedback from society or their families, and provide resources to ensure their educational and financial situations were trending towards independence and self-reliance (Wiggins, Oakley, Sawtell, Austerberry, Clemens, and Elbourne, 2005). While not specific to teen mothers, reviews of the Sure Start Plus program, and the effectiveness of the personal advisors, have revealed a modest economic benefit and small but significant effect sizes in terms of less harsh discipline, family chaos, and better home environments (Meadows, 2010). A long-term analysis of the effectiveness of the program that includes a specific focus on teen mothers, will be telling if this comprehensive approach to supporting underprivileged mothers is effective.

Ten years following the implementation of strategies suggested by the TPU, the UK boasted a reduction in teen pregnancy, to less than 40 conceptions per 1,000 young women between 15 and 17 years of age (Dickins, Johns, and Chipman, 2012). Although this reduction was far from the original goal of less than 20 pregnancies per 1,000 teens, the UK's approach provides an example of how the issue of using science to inform policy can be utilized, but also highlights the difficulties in obtaining large effects even when policy is based on good empirical and theoretical foundations. Inspection of Figure 4.1 from Chapter 4 reveals a consistent pattern in the declining trajectories of teen births since the UK policy was implemented. The difficulty with implementing policy that benefits the development of individuals and of society more generally can be inferred from examination of the decline in birth rates to women aged 15 to 19 in the UK and the United States. The striking declines in both countries over the past 20 years have occurred despite very different approaches to teen pregnancy prevention. The UK attempted a progressive approach that questioned common beliefs about teen mothers (SEU, 1999); the United States implemented abstinence policy based on the assumption that pregnancies result mainly from irrational choices made by teens (Duncan, 2007). Even with these vastly different approaches, year-to-year fluctuations in rates of birth to teens in both countries eventually stabilized on a declining trajectory that appears remarkably resistant to the implementation of sweeping policy changes. For example, short-term declines between the years 2001 and 2005 were offset by increases from 2006 through 2009, but the overall general trajectory remained unchanged.

General summary and reframing

The acknowledgement that abstinence from sexual intercourse is the only 100 percent effective way to prevent teen pregnancy is an important message to disseminate to young people. Concurrently, teens need to be provided valid and convincing reasons to postpone sexual activity or parenthood. Many programs that have received past funding, however, have lacked both solid theoretical foundations and empirical evidence of effectiveness. In contrast, comprehensive approaches that also target nonsexual, psychosocial antecedents associated with the likelihood of pregnancy have received more empirical support. Based on this, we have reframed the cultural myth to state that abstinence education is only one important component of a multifaceted strategy that targets not only teens, but also families, communities, and broader social values and beliefs.

Policy established to improve social support to teen mothers by requiring them to live with their own mothers or to marry their babies' fathers can have unintended effects. Although many young mothers benefit from a supportive relationship with their own mothers and a stable romantic relationship, grandmothers and fathers can create difficulty for teen mothers and their children if the relationships are strained or they do not appropriately support the mothers' needs. Consequently, we have reframed this myth as, better outcomes are achieved when teens are provided resources to support their transition to parenthood and marriage is good for some teens and their babies, but not for all.

Although we believe that replacing unsubstantiated cultural myths with beliefs reframed to better reflect the actual experiences of teen parents and their children will provide more effective social policy, we have already provided evidence that even the best developed policies can be slow to create change. Until these reframed beliefs are largely integrated into societal beliefs at the macro-level, meaningful changes are not likely to occur. As an example of how reframing cultural myths may lead to more effective policy, consider the different policy implications of the current cultural myth that all teen pregnancies are unintended and unwanted compared to the reframed version that many teen pregnancies occur to youths who have conflicting feelings and attitudes about becoming parents. Providing knowledge of and access to contraception is a magic bullet to pregnancy prevention if pregnancies are unintended and unwanted. However, knowledge of and access to contraception will have limited effectiveness if many teens are actually ambivalent about becoming pregnant (see Chapter 4). Beliefs at the macro-level that allow for teens' daily fluctuations in emotions and feelings in swaying the decision-making process would trickle down to programming focused at the exo- and microsystems, thereby resulting in positive changes for individuals and society at multiple levels.

A systems perspective targeting overarching beliefs applies equally well to conceptualizing the multiple, interactive elements involved in prevention, intervention, and subsequent policy formation. This book could be broadly summarized as an attempt to target macro-level influences on teen pregnancy and parenting by trying to clarify societal beliefs based on empirical and theoretical justification, and not misperceptions and stereotypes. While we have focused on three cultural myths in this chapter, reframing cultural myths based on appropriate research and theory for all ten of the myths we have covered in the book would narrow the gulf between policy assumptions and constituent experiences.

8   Rethinking cultural myths

> The progress this country has made in reducing teen pregnancy resulted in public
> sector savings of $12 billion in 2010 alone. Therefore, funding proven efforts to
> reduce teen pregnancy is important, timely, and should be a high priority.
>
> (Public Cost: FAQs, n.d.)

Continuing economic downturns have resulted in cuts to social programs that
target the prevention of teen pregnancy and interventions for adolescent parents. Cutbacks in program funding make it imperative that policies and programs are based on actual experiences of pregnant and parenting teens rather
than on cultural myths or long-held misperceptions. Ill-informed policies and
programs drain economic resources, diverting funds from vulnerable populations. Alternatively, policies and programs based on rigorous evaluation have
the potential to save substantial money by preventing costly consequences of
teen parenting for youths who are unprepared for parenthood or who lack appropriate supports.

The cultural myth that *teen pregnancy costs taxpayers lots of money* has been a
driving force in policy development (Maynard and Hoffman, 2008; Solomon-
Fears, 2013). Strategies to reduce associated costs have taken three directions.
First, predicated on the belief that young women were becoming pregnant to
gain government benefits, and had little incentive to become independent and
self-sufficient, welfare reform in the United States in 1996 was partially designed
to curtail childbearing as a means of securing additional financial support
(Dickins *et al.*, 2012). Second, sanctions to restrict welfare benefits if conditions
are not met (e.g., education and living arrangement) and set a lifetime limit for
the receipt of welfare dollars (Duffy and Levin-Epstein, 2002; Hao *et al.*, 2007)
are other strategies used to reduce costs attributed to teen childbearing. Third,
appeal to the high costs associated with teen pregnancy and parenting may be an
effective strategy to secure funding for programs that support pregnancy prevention and services to teen parents (Maynard and Hoffman, 2008). Provided these
programs work, costs associated with teen parenthood should decrease. In sum,
policy has been developed with the intent to reduce taxpayer costs, to motivate

teens towards independence, and to a lesser extent, provide supports that comes with strings attached.

In this concluding chapter, we rethink the common belief that teen pregnancy costs taxpayers money. Adherence to this cultural myth has created a paradox that may well undermine the good intentions associated with its widespread dissemination. Although appeal to the cost savings associated with implementation of pregnancy prevention programs may be used to leverage funding, it does so by perpetuating negative stereotypes of teen parents. Belief that teen pregnancy costs taxpayers money implies acceptance of many of the cultural myths we have reevaluated in prior chapters. For example, people may believe that costs are associated with derailed educational attainment of teen parents, with adverse perinatal outcomes of their children, or with increased likelihood of incarceration of these children as adults. Continued reinforcement of these negative stereotypes may exacerbate adverse outcomes and, in turn, inadvertently create barriers to more optimal outcomes. Our intent in this chapter is to suggest that replacing cultural myths based on misperception with understandings based on actual experience of pregnant and parenting teens is a critical component of a systems approach to improve outcomes for youths and their children.

We begin this chapter with a summary of evidence that has been used to support the high costs of teen childbearing. Our summary includes attention to both methodological and theoretical constraints that plague this evidence, and the challenges inherent in producing valid estimates of costs. Next, we return to the story of Claire and Jeremy, first introduced in Chapter 1 with continued development in Chapter 3, to highlight the actual experience of pregnant and parenting teens from a systems perspective. In this final chapter we explore how outcomes for the young couple and their child may have been different had appropriate beliefs, policies, and programs been in place. We conclude the chapter with a synthesis of recommendations based on the reframing of the ten cultural myths. As cultural myths and misperceptions are gradually replaced with more accurate understandings of the diversity of lives touched by teen pregnancy and parenting, not only will the lives of youths and their children improve, but also society more generally.

Cultural myth: teen childbearing costs taxpayers lots of money

The costs of teen childbearing have been disseminated in the book *Kids Having Kids* and through publicity sponsored by The National Campaign to Prevent Teen and Unplanned Pregnancy. The first edition of *Kids Having Kids* relied on data collected from the National Longitudinal Survey of Youth 1979 cohort (NLSY79), which followed a nationally representative sample of US teens from ages 14 to adulthood, the NLSY97 cohort that oversampled minority youths, and supplemental samples from the state of Illinois (Maynard, 1997). Analyses were revised and extended for the 2008 publication, to take into account long-term outcomes and comparisons between cohorts (Maynard and Hoffman, 2008). We have reviewed these studies in prior chapters; studies that focused on outcomes for teen mothers and teen fathers were reviewed in Chapter 5 and studies that focused on children born to teen mothers were reviewed in Chapter 6.

Analyses attempted to move beyond simple comparisons of teen and adult parents by controlling for selection effects (e.g., education level or poverty) that would independently account for less optimal outcomes. Regression analyses were most typically used to explain the incremental variance attributed to teen parenting over and above variance explained by the background factors. Other analyses relied on more sophisticated techniques by creating miscarriage or cousin comparison groups. Researchers calculated the size of the effect explained only by the age of the mother at childbirth (i.e., social influence effect). Effect sizes, regardless of significance level, were used to compute the cost in actual dollars, based on the assumption that even a small, nonsignificant effect may be meaningful if spread out over a large number of families headed by teen parents (Maynard and Hoffman, 2008).

The annual cost of teen childbearing in the United States in 2010 was estimated at $9.4 billion (Counting it Up, 2013). The 2013 report further estimated that the average annual societal cost per child born to a teen mother during each year from birth to age 15 was $1,682, resulting in a total cost of $25,230 per child. The bulk of the costs were associated with health care, child welfare, and incarceration. These costs accrue when Medicaid is relied on rather than private insurance, for investigations of child abuse and neglect, for foster care or other out-of-home placements, and for continued incarcerations due to criminal offenses. Earlier estimates by Hoffman (2006) suggested that costs were not distributed equally and that teen mothers aged 17 or younger accounted for approximately $8.6 billion of the $9.1 billion incurred, or 94.5 percent of all costs. Our intent is not to dispute the cost estimates resulting from these analyses, but rather to question the assumptions on which they were based and to suggest that the results perpetuate negative stereotypes of pregnant and parenting teens and reinforce cultural myths. We turn first to methodological considerations that may constrain the usefulness of these cost estimates.

Methodological constraints

A challenge inherent in social science research is ensuring that the true experiences of individuals are adequately represented. Duncan expanded on this challenge: "evidence about the actual experience and outcomes of teenage parenting is ignored, discounted, or re-interpreted in line with the expected, 'common sense', view. Sometimes researchers do this themselves" (Duncan, 2007, p. 321). In Chapter 2 we focused on the specific difficulties social scientists face in their attempts to generate valid knowledge. In the next section we review several of the points we made in Chapter 2 and apply them specifically to research designed to estimate the costs of teen pregnancy. Five important methodological constraints that may affect the interpretation of results are: (1) reliance on averages, (2) confusion between significant and meaningful findings, (3) the file-drawer problem, (4) how questions are framed, and (5) determinism.

Reliance on averages

Despite the elegance of methodologies used in many of the studies to estimate costs attributed to teen childbearing, almost all have been variable-centered approaches that sought to identify associations between variables. When relationships were found they were described in terms of *average* effect sizes. For example, men who fathered the children born to teen mothers were reported to have lifetime earnings that were, on average, $1,548 less compared to men who fathered children of women aged 20 to 21 (Maynard and Hoffman, 2008). This approach fails to account for the diversity of responses of young men to becoming fathers; some young men respond by intensification of achievement efforts sparked by perceived responsibility of their new role (Tuffin *et al.*, 2010). Inclusion of all teen fathers in cost estimates, despite the diversity of responses, reinforces stereotypes that all teen fathers share characteristics that do not apply to most.

In contrast to these variable-centered methodologies, person-centered approaches can provide important insights into the diversity of responses to a common experience (i.e., teen parenthood). Person-centered approaches seek to identify patterns among people, and allow for categorization of people into different typologies or subgroups. For example, although Jaffee *et al.* (2001) reported that being born to a teen mother was a risk factor for violent offending, the study also concluded that approximately one-half of all children born to teen mothers stayed in school, were employed, postponed parenthood until adulthood, and were not violent offenders. Focusing only on a statistically significant association between two variables (i.e., having a teen parent and becoming a violent offender) would have masked the more important conclusion indicating that most children did not experience adverse outcomes. The incidence of incarceration observed by some studies needs to be interpreted with caution, and can be better understood by supplementing the findings with qualitative studies. Averaging costs over the entire population of children born to teen parents obscures the reality that few, if any, costs are associated with close to one-half of these children, while many others may incur minor financial obligations, and just a small percent account for the majority of the costs of incarceration. Identification of meaningful subgroups provides valuable information for more tailored and streamlined intervention programs, as well as the establishment of more focused policy efforts.

Confusion between significant and meaningful findings

In contrast to quantitative studies, qualitative studies can detail unique and complex experiences of teen parents, allowing for the identification of individual differences in how teens respond to challenges provoked by early childbearing. However, qualitative studies that rely on small samples to provide in-depth insight into the strengths and challenges of teen pregnancy and parenting may not have enough statistical power to produce significant results. Although findings from these studies may be meaningful, due to nonsignificance they lack conviction that other teens would respond similarly. Many large quantitative studies have the opposite problem: a small, but statistically significant effect of teen parenting is generalized as a negative effect for all teen parents. This small average impact may be obtained in a number of ways, including many slightly positive or neutral outcomes offset by a small percentage of extremely negative outcomes.

Conclusions drawn from qualitative studies often suggest that the consequences of teen parenthood are more complicated and multidirectional than conclusions drawn from quantitative studies (Clemmens, 2003; Duncan, 2007; Graham and McDermott, 2006; Phoenix, 1991). In other words, becoming a parent is often experienced as a life-changing event, and some of these changes may actually be positive. Estimates of the costs of teen childbearing based solely on quantitative research may be missing the bigger picture that includes both positive and negative impacts depending on the contexts of the early childbearing (Graham and McDermott, 2006; Pettigrew, Whitehead, Macintyre, Graham, and Egan, 2004).

The file-drawer problem

The file-drawer problem occurs when research that fails to find significant differences between groups is stored in office files rather than disseminated through a publication process. Research reviews or syntheses may be biased to the extent that they are based on only research that supports hypotheses of group differences. Conclusions that would refute the hypotheses remain hidden in file drawers. The file-drawer problem is essentially an issue of how well the research used to draw conclusions represents the population under investigation.

Application of the file-drawer problem to cost estimates of teen childbearing focuses attention on the samples used to generate these costs. Our review of outcomes for teen parents in Chapter 5 and for children of teen parents in Chapter 6 revealed considerable inconsistencies between studies. Many studies found few differences in outcomes that could be attributed to teen parenthood status per se, independent of selection effects. However, conclusions drawn from other samples tended to find stronger influences of teen childbearing. We urged caution in drawing conclusions from any one study. Cost estimates have been based largely on data collected in the NLSY79 (Maynard and Hoffman, 2008), although other studies were used when data was unavailable in the NLSY79 data set. Although the NLSY79 is a well-designed study with a nationally representative sample, relying on one source to compute cost estimates carries the bias that may exist in that one study through to the conclusions. Cost estimates derived from several independent samples should yield more valid cost estimates.

Framing of questions

Framing questions based on the age of the mother at childbirth focuses attention on the agency of young women and diverts attention from the role of fathers and other important systemic influences. The vast majority of births to teen mothers overlap with births to unwed mothers. One analysis concluded that "family fragmentation costs US taxpayers at least \$112 billion each year, or over \$1 trillion dollars per decade" (Scafidi, 2008, p. 5). These costs are close to 12 times the costs associated with teen childbearing. Perhaps the majority of the costs attributed to teen childbearing could actually be attributed to nonmarital childbearing.

Another review estimated costs associated with unintended pregnancies, which also overlap substantially with teen pregnancy. Conclusions from this analysis revealed that \$11.1 billion in government expenditure was attributed to unintended pregnancies in 2006 (Sonfield, Kost, Gold, and Finer, 2011). Aside from the alternative framing of questions based on marital status or intendedness, costs attributed to births to teen fathers may also overlap considerably with costs attributed to teen mothers. Although marital status, intendedness, and father characteristics were controlled in some analyses that estimated costs associated with maternal age at childbirth, few studies controlled for all these factors simultaneously. Framing questions in terms of costs attributable to teen mothers as opposed to unwed mothers, unintended pregnancies, or teen fathers continues to reinforce stereotypes of teen mothers and perpetuate unsubstantiated cultural myths.

In fact, the focus on age differences by Maynard and Hoffman (2008) went as far to suggest an actual cost savings to society by delaying childbearing by several years. Translating these results into policy would suggest that pregnancy prevention efforts should focus on convincing all teens to delay childbearing. Campaigns based on this philosophy have included the "Not Me, Not Now" slogan (Doniger, Riley, Utter, and Adams, 2001). However, as reviewed by Scher in *Kids Having Kids* (2008), evaluations have not supported the utility of this strategy. The weak findings of these evaluative studies should not be surprising, as we have argued that multiple systems interact synergistically to lead to teen pregnancy. Intervention and prevention need to be approached with an understanding that many factors, not just age, are influential.

Further, framing questions based on differences between groups, whatever these groups may be, does little to explain the process leading to more or less optimal outcomes. For example, establishing a significant relationship between maternal age at childbearing and child incarcerations does little to explain why this relationship exists. Conceptual and theoretical models need to guide research questions that will address the processes leading to more or less optimal outcomes. For example, the model proposed by Dunkel Schetter (2011) explains a process, consistent with systems theory, leading to premature births, and provides a context for understanding how age of the mother may impact this more general process. Reframing questions to identify processes leading to more optimal outcomes in other areas will yield more meaningful results than simply comparing outcomes between groups.

Determinism

The studies used in Maynard and Hoffman's (2008) analyses of cost estimates were not designed to test hypotheses about teen childbearing. Rather the

aims of these studies were to provide descriptive information about significant life events, with a focus on labor market activities of several groups of
men and women. Testing hypotheses about the causal influence of maternal
age at childbearing requires careful measurement of background factors that
may predispose some young women to both teen childbearing and also lead to
more negative outcomes. Although most data sets contain demographic information related to these background characteristics, often critical variables are
missing. Manlove *et al.* (2008) acknowledged this constraint, as they discussed
the significance of the cognitive and academic differences found between teen
and adult mothers. They suggested that some of the differences may have been
due to unmeasured intellectual differences between the teen and adult mothers, which could have explained the results better than the attributions to the
mothers' age at the time of childbirth. Studies that have included controls for
maternal IQ have typically found that this explains much of the difference in
cognitive and academic outcomes between children born to teen and adult
parents (Jaffee *et al.*, 2001).

Omission of important variables in regression models may overestimate the
effect size associated with maternal age at childbirth. Implications that postponing childbearing until the mid-twenties would reduce negative outcomes, and
thus lower costs, may be exaggerated to the extent that differences were actually
based on unobserved selection characteristics. Studies that have moved beyond
regression approaches, or *third-generation designs*, have attempted to overcome
limitations due to unobserved factors, by reliance on comparisons groups formed
to reduce selection effects. Cost estimates based on third-generation designs are
typically less than those from regression approaches and may more closely approximate actual values. However, even third-generation designs may not adequately
account for all individual differences in response to teen parenthood.

Summary and reframing

Evidence for the cultural myth that *teen pregnancy costs taxpayers lots of money* is
mixed. Several well-designed studies with different samples and using different
analytic techniques have documented some negative outcomes and resulting
societal costs that may be attributed to maternal age at childbearing. On the
other hand, methodological constraints preclude unconditional acceptance of
the conclusions. Confirmation from studies designed to test a priori hypotheses about these associations are needed. These confirmatory studies need to
be based on measures that are selected in advance to assess critical constructs
rather than relying on proxy variables available in a data set. Confirmation
studies also need to include both quantitative and qualitative data that test
process models, to answer questions of how and why teen parenting may cause
more adverse outcomes for the teens and their children. Finally, studies need
to compare alternative framing of questions to allow outcomes to be attributed
to marital status, intendedness, or paternal characteristics rather than maternal
age at childbirth. In consideration of these constraints we suggest reframing the

cultural myth as *costs attributed to teen pregnancy may be limited to a subset of teen parents and their children*.

Rethinking costs from a systems perspective

Theoretical models that explain teen pregnancy and parenting based on reductionist perspectives may also constrain the types of programs and policies developed. Consistent with the cultural myth that teen childbearing costs taxpayers lots of money, a reductionist perspective suggests implementing programs that persuade young people to postpone childbearing until age 20 or older. In other words, once a statistical link between variables has been observed (e.g., between teen motherhood and child incarceration), a reductionist perspective suggests that intervention aimed at changing the link will have direct implications on the outcome. In contrast, a systems perspective is at odds with reductionist thinking, and suggests that changing only one link will result in adaptations in other parts of the system that will counter the change to produce homeostasis, leaving the important outcomes unchanged. Effective policies and programs, therefore, need to be based on an understanding of system properties, not just statistical relationships between variables (Midgley, 2006).

Rethinking teen pregnancy and parenting from a systems perspective focuses attention on the ultimate goals of programs and policies (Bird, 2011; Chilman, 1990; Fine and McClelland 2006; Harden, Brunton, Fletcher, Oakley, Burchett, and Backhans, 2006; SmithBattle, 2012). One way to look at goals is from the standpoint that all teens should have access to knowledge and resources that will prepare them for productive societal roles and relationships (Tolman and McClelland, 2011) and that all babies should be born to parents prepared to provide sufficient nurturing to allow for optimal development. Framed this way, parental age at childbirth becomes less important than the parents' capacity to provide for their children. Prevention programs targeting teens then become the comprehensive, multicomponent programs that we advocated for in Chapter 7. Interventions to improve infant outcomes need to include not only teens, but expectant mothers and fathers more generally. Misperceptions that age alone instills the capacity for nurturant parenting lead to a focus on programs for pregnant teens, while many adult parents also lack cognitive readiness to parent (Whitman *et al.*, 2001).

The explicit stated goals of policies and programs may sometimes mask an underlying implicit agenda. This implicit agenda may be based on one or more of the regulatory functions described in Chapter 1. For example, pregnancy prevention programs may be used to further a moral agenda intended to curtail expressions of teen sexuality. Consistent with this supposition, the review of abstinence education, by Kim and Rector (2010), opens with the observation that "sexual activity during teenage years poses serious health risks for youths and has long-term implications" (p. 1). Pregnancy prevention, in this manner, is not the actual goal, but rather used as a means to promote abstinence. Abstinence until marriage may be perceived as an important goal in its own right by parents and by some religious organizations, but policies and programs to promote abstinence differ from those aimed at preventing teen pregnancy. Within the context of pregnancy prevention programs, abstinence may be encouraged as the only sure way to prevent pregnancy, but should be taught as a means to an end, not the end itself.

Thoughtful reflection on the ultimate goals of programs and policy also needs to disentangle them from goals based on myths and misperceptions. Knowledge of contraception may also be perceived as an important goal of pregnancy prevention efforts. However, this goal may be based on the myth that all teen pregnancies are unintended and unwanted. If this myth were true then teens who had better knowledge of and access to birth control would use contraception to prevent the unwanted pregnancies. However, we have reviewed evidence that many teens may have ambivalent attitudes towards pregnancy and childbearing that lead to ineffective and inconsistent use of birth control. Programs and policies that are clear that the goal is to reduce teen pregnancies are more likely to acknowledge the sometimes contradictory and inconsistent feelings and intentions of teens, and provide strategies to deal with the feelings in addition to information about contraception.

Myths and misperceptions about the types of teens who become pregnant may also obscure program goals. Goals may become focused on perceived lack of morals, character, or judgment of teen parents. Acknowledgement that most teen parents do not have behavior problems would allow programs to build on the enthusiasm and motivation that most teens have to become good parents and provide effectively for their children, thereby minimizing the risk that children of teen parents will have adjustment problems.

Goals to improve outcomes for teen parents and their children may also become entangled with goals to save taxpayers money. Improving outcomes may save money, but focusing on the dollars (or euros) and cents as opposed to the ultimate goals is often counterproductive. Campaigns that attribute costs to teen pregnancy and parenting reinforce negative perceptions of teen parents that may actually create additional challenges and hurdles for young parents. These campaigns may indirectly, therefore, perpetuate the negative outcomes they are intended to prevent.

In addition to careful attention to goals, a systems approach to prevention and intervention requires the collaboration of relevant stakeholders (Midgley, 2006). Stakeholders need to agree on programmatic goals and strategies before they can achieve them. Evidence reviewed throughout this book reveals little collaboration among stakeholders. Policy is often implemented by legislators without consideration of findings from empirical research. Advocacy groups have reinforced some ill-informed cultural myths in attempts to garner funding and other resources. Even researchers have framed research questions based on prevailing beliefs about differences between teen and adult mothers. Public health initiatives address important needs of pregnancy and parenting teens, but are often uncoordinated with other services. Often the voices of teen parents and their families have been discounted. Integration and collaboration from these diverse stakeholders is a daunting and challenging, but imperative, task. In the United States, The National Campaign to Prevent Teen and Unplanned Pregnancies has sometimes taken the lead to convene diverse stakeholders to address important program and policy issues. Recent policy in the UK puts more responsibility on local councils to draft policy to impact teen pregnancy and parenting (Local Government Association, 2013). Further efforts along these lines are encouraged, with the recommendation that groups implement a systems perspective as they aim to influence policy and practice.

Practical challenges

An understanding of systems dynamics reveals that established systems are difficult to change. Feedback loops serve to maintain *homeostasis* despite changes in any one component. Homeostasis refers to a process that returns systems to a prior stable level following disruption. This dynamic stability may be beneficial in some instances; for example, trends over time in both the United States and the UK show declines in the birth rate to teen mothers (see Figure 4.1). These trends in both countries are ideal examples of homeostasis. Despite year-to-year fluctuations, teen birth rates continue to decline at a consistent rate that has varied little over the past 20 years. More specifically, both countries experienced stronger declines in the teen birth rate followed by mirrored increases. For the UK decreases were seen in 1994 and 1995 followed by increases in 1998 and 1999. In the United States, similar declines were seen a few years later around 2002 and 2003 followed by mirrored increases in 2006 and 2007. Year-to-year fluctuations eventually stabilized, with a return to a declining rate predicted by trends beginning in 1991. Attempts to explain US declines based on changes in sexual activity among teens, or to changing welfare policies, were only able to account for 12 percent of the observed decline (Kearney and Levine, 2012), leading to the conclusion that:

> Most targeted policies had no effect on teen birth rates. The two policy changes that do seem to matter some, expanded family planning services through Medicaid and reduced welfare benefits can only combine to explain 12 percent of the decline in teen childbearing between 1991 and 2008.
>
> (p. 164)

Transformational change (i.e., the type of change required to actually produce a steeper declining trajectory) requires a more systemic approach that focuses not only on the teens themselves, but also on broader social and cultural systems that may be more stable influences on teen births (SmithBattle, 2012).

Reframing cultural myths

Despite the wealth of research on teen pregnancy and parenting, cultural myths remain pervasive. The central tenet of this book is that although cultural myths

Table 8.1 Cultural myths reframed

Chapter	Cultural myth	Myth reframed	Evidence	Recommendations for policy and programming
3	Providing media visibility of pregnant or parenting teens will encourage others to become pregnant.	Providing media visibility that emphasizes sexual risks, and responsibilities and the challenges resulting from teen parenting can help prevent teen pregnancy.	Youth with characteristics that place them at risk for early pregnancy may be drawn to media focused on pregnant and parenting teens. The impact of media visibility is dependent on both the context of the viewing and the viewers' characteristics. Viewers who perceive the content as realistic and identify with the characters are more likely to absorb content. Communications about sexuality and pregnancy during childhood may create cognitive filters for how media content is perceived by youth.	Foundations with missions to prevent teen pregnancy should provide support for TV programs that highlight sexual risks and responsibilities in addition to the realistic challenges of teen pregnancy. Parents need to be aware of the importance of communicating with their children regarding sexual content of media, and provided supports to do this effectively. Popular culture has the potential to counter negative stereotypes of pregnant and parenting teens. However, portrayals should be careful to avoid placing full responsibility on the teens, and must consider the role of broader social and cultural forces.

Table 8.1 (cont.)

Chapter	Cultural myth	Myth reframed	Evidence	Recommendations for policy and programming
4	Most pregnant teens have behavior problems.	The majority of teen pregnancies occur to, or are caused by, young women and men without a history of behavior problems.	Although teens with behavior or substance abuse problems may be more likely to experience early pregnancy, these account for only a small percentage of the total number of pregnant teens. Many pregnant teens have a history of sexual abuse.	Universal sexual health programs need to be implemented for all teens, not just those perceived to be at risk. Application of a systems approach to sexual abuse, which targets influences at the levels of the individual, interpersonal relationship, community, and society more generally, is needed. Provide targeted teen pregnancy prevention programs or services for youths who have experienced sexual abuse. Apply conceptual models that integrate externalizing problems, including substance abuse and aggression, in explanations for unplanned and unwanted pregnancies at any age.

All teen pregnancies are unintended and unwanted.

Many teen pregnancies occur to youths who have conflicting feelings and attitudes about becoming parents.

A biologically based desire to have children is felt by many youths.

Some teens may misrepresent their true pregnancy intentions due to perceived social censure.

Consistency of contraceptive use may be affected by fluctuations in desire for children.

Younger teens may have a more difficult time resolving conflicting feelings about pregnancy and childbearing.

Childbearing decisions may represent a trade-off between the immediate rewards of having children versus waiting for more long-term rewards associated with educational and career investments.

Educational programs for youth need to acknowledge that the desire for children may be both strong and socially adaptive, but at the same time, help youths develop strategies to cope with these feelings until a more appropriate time in their lives.

Increase educational and occupational opportunities for youths at risk for early pregnancy, to provide greater incentive for postponing childbearing.

Changing fertility-timing norms may require campaigns that include education for parents and grandparents, not just the youths themselves.

Explanations for teen pregnancies need to be integrated with conceptual models that clarify the timing of fertility decisions for men and women of all ages.

Table 8.1 (cont.)

Chapter	Cultural myth	Myth reframed	Evidence	Recommendations for policy and programming
5	Parenthood derails the trajectories of the teens' lives.	Becoming a parent has the potential to transform lives for men and women of all ages.	Growing up with few economic advantages sets a course that leads to both early parenthood as well as a continuation of the original low economic trajectory. Whether the transformation triggered by parenthood is positive, negative, or neutral depends on a variety of past and present contextual factors including socioeconomic status, culture, motivation, and relationship status.	Support programs during the prenatal period, for both men and women, can help prospective parents prepare for challenges of parenthood. Programs that target first-time parents of all ages may reduce the stigma of teen parenthood and reinforce the understanding that parenthood entails challenges even for adult parents. Improved family-friendly school and work policies for teen parents can help them stay in school and maintain employment. More affordable child care options for teens, especially those with parent support and education components, can help teen parents stay in school and receive guidance to be successful in their new parenting roles. Explanations for the impact of parenthood during the teen years need to be integrated with conceptual models that clarify how parenthood impacts lives of men and women of all ages.

6	Teen pregnancies result in poor birth outcomes.	Most babies born to teen mothers who receive adequate prenatal care are born full-term and healthy.	The lack of adequate prenatal care is associated with poor birth outcomes for children of teen mothers. Children born to young teen mothers who have not completed puberty may experience some growth restriction and associated complications. Anxieties about the pregnancy and delivery may increase the likelihood of premature births.	Evidence-based, teen-friendly prenatal care should be provided in ways that can be coordinated with teens' school schedules. Schools should provide consideration for absences due to prenatal medical care. Comprehensive youth development programs that build resilience resources – including optimism about the future, relationship skills, and healthy behaviors – should be encouraged.
9	Children of teen parents will experience cognitive delay, adjustment problems, and will themselves become teen parents.	The majority of children born to teen parents do not have serious problems and do not become teen parents.	Most children born to teen parents will graduate from secondary school, will not become dependent on substances, and will be psychologically and emotionally well-adjusted. Although children born to teen parents are more likely to also become teen parents, most children born to teen parents postpone childbearing until age 20 or beyond. Fathers of children born to teen mothers play a role in determining the well-being of their children. Teen mothers and teen fathers are often similar on antisocial behaviors; this similarity may lead to an increased likelihood of adult arrest and incarceration for children born to teen mothers.	School-based mental health services for all children, not just those born to teen parents, can provide a safe, confidential, and therapeutic environment for children to share information about and gain support for difficult home situations. These programs should be preventative in nature, but also provide individualized referrals for youths who report maltreatment or have symptoms of serious problems. Government policies related to child-support enforcement, family leave, and affordable child care are needed. Provide research funding to understand the processes by which birth to teen parents leads to adverse outcomes for some children.

Table 8.1 (cont.)

Chapter	Cultural myth	Myth reframed	Evidence	Recommendations for policy and programming
7	Abstinence education is the best way to prevent teen pregnancy.	Abstinence education is only one important component of a multifaceted strategy that targets not only teens, but also families, communities, and broader social values and beliefs.	Sexual health education must encompass a comprehensive curriculum that, while recommending abstinence as the best approach, addresses sexual antecedents of pregnancy, such as information on contraception, and nonsexual antecedents, such as building personal skills, interpersonal relationships, and future-oriented goals.	Public funding should only be provided to programs that take a comprehensive, empirically supported approach to sexual health education and pregnancy prevention. Prevention efforts focused on changing teens' attitudes and behaviors will have little impact without simultaneous efforts that address broader social and cultural factors that contribute to the high teen pregnancy rate.
7	Better outcomes are achieved when teen mothers live with their own mothers.	Better outcomes are achieved when teens are provided resources to support their transition to parenthood.	Teens who live with mothers who are supportive yet allow the teens to assume the role of primary caregiver achieve the best outcomes. Over-involvement from the grandmother or conflictual relationships may undermine maternal caregiving. Requiring teens to live with their own mothers when the household is dysfunctional may be detrimental to all involved.	Programming should focus on the grandmother's role in helping the teen mother succeed as an emerging adult and as a parent; conflict-resolution skills should be an essential part of the program. Social services personnel need to be sensitive to diverse living arrangements and be willing to propose options for pregnant teens. Alternatives, such as Second Chance homes, need to be supported, to provide options for teen mothers from dysfunctional homes. States need to collect at least minimal data to support the continued effectiveness of this mandate.

7	It is better for teens and their babies if biological parents marry.	Marriage is good for some teens and their babies, but not for all.	Programs should be developed to target and support teen fathers' early involvement in the babies' lives, to encourage sustained and positive relationships with the mothers and children.
		More optimal outcomes of children raised by two parents are primarily attributed to characteristics of people who marry compared to those who remain single.	Programs should be available to counsel teen parents on their relationship. Programs should not emphasize marriage as the end goal, but rather focus on co-parenting skills regardless of the relationship status of the parents.
		Teen marriages are associated with subsequent teen births, dropping out of school, and later poverty for women.	Couples with high levels of conflict should seek support to resolve their differences before deciding whether to marry.
		Teen marriage may result in partners with undesirable characteristics including violence, aggression, or criminal tendencies.	

Table 8.1 (cont.)

Chapter	Cultural myth	Myth reframed	Evidence	Recommendations for policy and programming
8	Teen pregnancy costs taxpayers lots of money.	Costs attributed to teen pregnancy may be limited to a subset of teen parents and their children.	Cost estimates are based on an "average" effect size that is unlikely to apply equally to all teen parents or their children. Estimations of cost savings due to society from this average effect size are inappropriate. Teen pregnancy can be adaptive for some young people, and therefore should not be prevented across the board. Rather, the emphasis should be on preventing pregnancy among people who are not ready to become parents regardless of their specific ages. Campaigns that highlight costs may inadvertently perpetuate negative stereotypes and stigma, and may actually contribute to less optimal outcomes and increased costs.	Prevention of unintended or unwanted pregnancies among women of all ages is warranted to reduce society's costs related to providing services to mothers who otherwise would have been able to provide for themselves. Sexual health programs should incorporate education on cognitive models of parenting to prepare people to be successful parents whenever they have children. Costs should be attributed to social and cultural factors, rather than to teen mothers themselves, to eradicate negative stereotypes that may contribute to additional societal costs.

may hold a kernel of truth, many are irrelevant (and potentially harmful) when overgeneralized to all pregnant or parenting teens. Through a broad and comprehensive review of the literature, we carefully evaluated ten common beliefs and have reframed them to more closely approximate reality. Each of the reframed myths is summarized in Table 8.1 to provide a concise summary. The table lists each cultural myth according to the chapter in which it was reviewed, reframes the myth based on evidence, summarizes key points from the evidence, and offers specific recommendations for policy and programming.

We maintain that it is essential to create a dialogue about the more nuanced reality underlying each cultural myth; doing so will afford an opportunity for researchers, practitioners, policy-makers, and laypersons to optimize the development and delivery of programs aimed at preventing teen pregnancy or helping teen parents and their children. We have offered a set of solutions, framed as recommendations for policy and programming. We envision these recommendations as guidelines to use in the design and implementation of policies and programs. We illustrate some ways in which our recommendations could be utilized by returning to the example of Claire and Jeremy.

An applied example: Claire and Jeremy

Recall that Claire and Jeremy were a young couple who faced parenthood at the ages of 14 and 15. Forced into an early marriage by parents who were embarrassed by their children's behavior, the newlyweds and their baby moved in with Jeremy's family. When Claire turned 18, she divorced Jeremy and moved out on her own with their young child. We now revisit this young couple with the goal of highlighting some things that could have been done to optimize outcomes for Claire, Jeremy, and their child in consideration of the reframed myths presented in Table 8.1. In doing so, we utilize Bronfenbrenner's systems perspective to demonstrate how the refinement of cultural myths is relevant at various systems levels. The sections below provide examples from the micro-, exo-, and macrosystems.

Our exclusive focus on these three system levels is not intended to convey the unimportance of the mesosystem. However, we have emphasized the importance of connections between the systems (i.e., the mesosystem) throughout this book and trust that we have made our points sufficiently clear. Although our hypothetical example considers independent changes that may have had the potential to positively impact outcomes, as we have emphasized throughout this book, individual changes interact synergistically, often with unanticipated results. Changes at all levels simultaneously should have an exponentially greater impact. In other words, any one change is valuable, but changing the entire system is critical to bringing about the most optimal outcomes for the individuals, their families, and society.

Microsystem factors

The microsystem includes daily settings and the roles and relationships encountered in these settings. Cultural myths infiltrate how roles and responsibilities are understood and thus impact microsystem functioning. Claire's parents believed that teen pregnancies would only occur to youths who were delinquent or substance abusers, and that abstinence education would be effective in preventing teen pregnancy. These beliefs led them to avoid speaking with Claire about sex, lest they put ideas into her head. They assumed she would avoid sexual activity, since she was neither delinquent not substance abusing. Their belief that teen pregnancies were unintentional and unwanted reinforced their sense of security, since they felt Claire typically made good decisions and wouldn't do anything that would jeopardize her future (Elliott, 2010).

Claire's microsystem may have functioned more effectively had her parents endorsed our reframed versions of cultural myths. Armed with the understanding that most pregnant teens are not problem children may have allowed them to realize the need to ensure that their daughter participate in a comprehensive sexual health program. Realizing that many teens may actually have ambivalent feelings about childbearing may have led them to incorporate youth sessions at church that focused on awareness of the ambivalent feelings and ensured youths had strategies to deal with them.

Once Claire's pregnancy became known, instead of revising their long-held beliefs, her parents changed their perceptions of their daughter. Since they endorsed the cultural myth that only delinquent or otherwise problem children became pregnant, then they figured that Claire must actually be a problem child who made an impulsive, irrational decision, which resulted in a pregnancy that she did not want and that would derail her future opportunities. Their reaction – spurred by embarrassment, shame, and misperceptions – was anger at Claire and Jeremy, leading to the stipulation that she move out until she was able to get her act together.

Rather than withdrawing support because they felt that her life was irrevocably derailed, Claire's parents could have helped the situation by providing supports that allowed her to embrace her off-timed transition to parenthood. Enrolling Claire in a prenatal support program, helping ensure that she stay in high school, and helping her find child care could have gone a long way towards providing a more optimal microsystem for Claire and her child. Perhaps even more importantly, Claire's parents needed to continue to maintain their pre-pregnancy beliefs about Claire's character rather than be swayed by cultural myths that she must be troubled or delinquent.

In contrast to Claire, Jeremy engaged in some problem behavior prior to the pregnancy. He had experimented alcohol and other drugs, and had skipped school on occasion when he had the opportunity to do more exciting things with his brother who was in college. After the birth of his child, Jeremy quit these activities, focusing on his education and picking up an after-school job to help with Claire's expenses. Jeremy provides a good example of how teens who are initially struggling can step up to the responsibilities of teen parenting. Although the role of teen fathers has often been ignored, recent evidence suggests they contribute importantly to both the well-being of their partners and their children. Thus, teen fathers need familial and social supports to be able to help their partners emotionally and financially, and to be constructively involved in their children's lives.

Like Claire's parents, Jeremy's mother was also influenced by cultural myths that may have contributed to less than optimal outcomes for the young couple. Her belief that teen pregnancies result in poor birth outcomes led her to vigilant oversight of Claire's diet and behavior. The concern expressed by Jeremy's mother that the baby was going to have problems, since Claire was too young and too small to have a healthy baby, began to increase Claire's own anxiety about the pregnancy and upcoming birth. Since Claire was only 14, some of these concerns may have been valid; however, Jeremy's mother was unaware that most babies born to teen mothers who receive adequate prenatal care are born full-term and healthy. Just like for adult mothers, adverse pregnancy-related events are avoided, prevented, or quickly responded to if teens receive early and consistent prenatal care. Whereas increased anxiety associated with cultural myths of impending pregnancy-related complications may actually precipitate these complications, reassurance of healthy births contingent on following recommendations of her OB/GYN may have alleviated much of Claire's anxiety.

In addition, both families believed that everything would turn out better if Claire and Jeremy married. Claire and Jeremy were pressured into a shotgun wedding based on the firmly held conviction that children need two biological parents to be successful in life. Despite the early marriage, however, Jeremy's mother was skeptical of Claire's ability to provide the quality of parenting a newborn would need. She believed that it would be better for Claire to live with her own mother, who would assume much of the early caregiving responsibilities. However, since Claire's own mother had refused to accept this responsibility, Jeremy's mother felt obligated to step in and allow the young family to live with them, seeing herself as somewhat of a surrogate parent to Claire and the baby.

The grandmother's overcompensation caused strife with Claire, and also prevented Claire from fully taking on the parenting responsibilities and decision-making necessary to feel confident as a mother. Due to the influence of these cultural myths, the grandmother's actions pushed Claire away, while simultaneously not providing her the chance to learn the proper skills to be an independent parent. Endorsement of the reframed versions of the cultural myths may have enabled the microsystem of the young couple to function more adequately. Jeremy's mother could have been more helpful by aiding Claire in obtaining high-quality prenatal care, working with the school to excuse Claire for prenatal care appointments, and preparing both teens for their parenting responsibilities. In addition, the early marriage, with a high probability of divorce, may have been avoided.

Other microsystem components in the lives of both Claire and Jeremy included their peers, school, extracurricular activities, and church. Their school and church were largely influenced by the cultural myth that abstinence education is the best way to prevent teen pregnancy. Religious institutions are important sources of values and messages about sexuality for many youths, including Claire and Jeremy. Somewhat surprisingly, teen births are more common in geographic areas that more strongly endorse conservative religious beliefs (Strayhorn and Strayhorn, 2009); this association may be attributed to lower rates of contraceptive use and, to a lesser extent, lower rates of abortion should pregnancy occur. In addition, some religious groups stress obedience to authority, which may make it difficult for some young women to resist pressure to become sexually active. Although churches may hold strong beliefs about sexual activity of youths, they also may be in unique positions to help develop skills in youths, which would enhance motivations to resist sexual activity and risks of pregnancy.

Many prevention and intervention programs are school based. However, as we have reviewed in Chapter 7, the type of abstinence-centered programs that were permitted in schools have largely been shown to be ineffective. If Claire and Jeremy had been provided with a more comprehensive sex education program that focused on skill- and goal-building, even if grounded in abstinence promotion, they may have made different choices in their sexual decision-making. Although pregnancy prevention efforts are important at the microsystem level, without corresponding efforts at both the levels of the exosystem and macrosystem, microsystem prevention efforts may be insufficient.

Exosystem factors

Cultural myths also permeate how social structures beyond the immediate day-to-day settings perceive and respond to pregnant and parenting teens. School boards, health departments, recreational centers, and extended social networks are all embedded in the exosystem and play a role in preventing pregnancy and supporting teen parents. Negative stereotypes about teen parents conveyed by members of these institutions discouraged Claire and Jeremy from seeking help and support due to perceived stigma. The isolation and exclusion created by the stigma likely contributed to the eventual dissolution of the young family (Breheny and Stephens, 2007a; SmithBattle, 2013).

Exosystem structures may also reinforce existing cultural myths. For example, the media can inform cultural myths related to the perception of teen pregnancy and parenting, by perpetuating beliefs that are unsubstantiated but provide a dramatic and engaging entertainment format (e.g., *16 and Pregnant*, *Teen Mom*), or by conveying important messages to society (e.g., PR campaigns). Many people believe that providing media visibility of pregnant or parenting teens will encourage others to become pregnant. Although this is not true in and of itself, it is possible that oversimplified portrayals that do not present the true depth of the consequences associated with teen pregnancy and parenting may be a contributing factor to teens' sexual and reproductive decision-making.

Claire and Jeremy's time spent watching popular shows about teen pregnancy on MTV, applying their own interpretations without input from parents, may have contributed to their early childbearing. While *16 and Pregnant* conveys a somewhat realistic depiction of the challenges of teen pregnancy, the series *Teen Mom* provides a more sensationalized portrayal. Networks such as MTV that broadcast shows about teen pregnancy and parenting should recognize that youths at risk for early pregnancy may be drawn to these types of shows, and that viewers who perceive the content as realistic and identify with the characters are more likely to be affected by the shows. In turn, producers should ensure that portrayals on their shows highlight sexual risks and responsibilities in addition to the realistic challenges of teen parenthood. Moreover, portrayals should avoid placing full responsibility for pregnancy on the teens themselves, by acknowledging the role of broader social and cultural forces that have contributed to the situations depicted on the shows.

Macrosystem factors

The macrosystem contains the blueprints for how a society should function. These blueprints may take the form of informal and implicit cultural myths or as more explicit laws, regulations, and rules (Bronfenbrenner, 1977). An important theme throughout this book is that explicit laws, regulations, and rules are often based more on implicit cultural myths than on the actual experiences of constituents. For example, welfare policies that impact pregnant and parenting teens are based largely on cultural myths that better outcomes are achieved when teen mothers live with their own mothers, that it is better if biological parents marry, and that teen pregnancy costs taxpayers lots of money.

Replacing these cultural myths that are based on misperceptions with a reframed understanding derived from the actual experiences of pregnant and parenting teens would enable the macrosystem to more effectively support teens like Claire and Jeremy. Acknowledgement of the reality of individual circumstances surrounding teens would insert more flexibility in the rules and regulations. Whereas some teens may be better off living with their own mothers, or married to the babies' fathers, other teens may best thrive when provided with supports that enable them to live independently. More flexible governmental supports for Claire and Jeremy may have allowed them to develop a plan that would have encouraged both parents to continue their education, to develop parenting and co-parenting skills, and to work towards productive careers that would allow them to eventually become self-sufficient contributors to society.

Macro-level changes in how schools respond to pregnant and parenting teens may also have benefitted Claire and Jeremy. Some school districts require pregnant teens to seek alternative educational experiences (e.g., home schooling, alternative schools), perhaps due to an implicit belief that visibility of pregnant teens will encourage other teens to become pregnant. As a consequence, the educational rigor or perceived status of these alternative programs may be diminished, making it difficult for graduates to qualify for college entrance. In contrast, policies that enable pregnant and parenting teens to remain in a regular school setting, with allowances for medical appointments, and perhaps additional instruction in relationship development and parenting, would reinforce the value of continued education following high school.

Perhaps the most influential cultural myth for the macrosystem is the belief that teen pregnancy costs taxpayers lots of money. This belief directly impacted elements of the exosystem, and indirectly impacted elements of the microsystem, in ways that influenced people's reactions to Claire and Jeremy as they navigated teen pregnancy and parenthood. Widespread acceptance of this myth may also have affected the development of Claire and Jeremy's child, as service providers including caregivers, educators, and medical professionals may have consciously or subconsciously treated the child differently if they felt that he was a burden on society. Instead, if people began to accept the reality that costs should be attributed to social and cultural factors, rather than to teen mothers themselves, individuals and society could begin to eradicate the negative stereotypes that may contribute to negative outcomes and additional societal costs. This macrosystem shift would, in turn, trickle down to the exo- and microsystems, and to the individual teen parents themselves, with the long-term result being a more accurate dialogue about teen pregnancy and parenting that could lead to lower rates of teen pregnancy as well as more optimal outcomes for teens who do become pregnant and their children.

Summary

Evaluation of the cultural myth that teen childbearing costs taxpayers lots of money highlights several misperceptions about pregnant and parenting teens. In contrast to headlines implying that costs are equally distributed among all teen parents, our review suggests that costs are primarily associated with a subset of children born to teens under the age of 18. Explanations that account for the increased health and welfare costs of this subset of children remain elusive. Further prospective research that tests specific hypotheses aimed at disentangling maternal age at childbirth from paternal age at childbirth, relationship status, intentionality, prenatal care, and psychosocial and physiological maturation (e.g., timing of puberty), is needed to further advance our understanding of the processes by which teen childbearing may lead to either adaptive or dysfunctional outcomes. Process-oriented explanations will be enhanced by supplementing quantitative research with related qualitative studies.

Consistent with a systems perspective, process-oriented models need to move beyond theories focused solely on individual behavior (e.g., theory of planned behavior) and consider system dynamics. Clearly articulated goals devoid of hidden agendas are an important first step (e.g., achieving reductions in unintended pregnancies to teens rather than using teen pregnancy prevention to advance moral agendas). A coordinated approach that targets multiple levels of the system, from the individual to the macrosystem level, will be more transformative than efforts focused on the teens themselves. Collaboration among diverse stakeholders, including pregnant and parenting teens, is required to achieve this coordinated approach.

In essence, a primary goal of this book has been to expose cultural myths based on misperceptions of pregnant and parenting teens. Shifting long-held beliefs closer to actual experience of youths, as they confront challenges and opportunities associated with early childbearing, alters the macrosystem in important ways. This shift or alteration in the informal blueprint for society has the potential to trickle down through the exo- and microsystem levels, ultimately leading to more effective societal responses to teen pregnancy and parenting. The provision of more optimal policies, programs, and individual supports has the potential to enhance outcomes for teens in general, as well as for teen parents and their children.

Effective policy development requires attention to the diversity of responses to teen parenthood. Our reframed versions of the cultural myths presented in Table 8.1 emphasize this diversity. Our intent is that our recommendations will be used by researchers, policy-makers, and practitioners as a general guideline, with the realization that they may need to further refine reality for the particular teens or group of teens with whom they are working. Moreover, it is essential not to discard our recommendations simply because policy-makers or program providers have seen a few situations that reinforce the cultural myths. We have acknowledged that all of the myths contain some kernel of reality. However, we have conducted an extensive review of decades' worth of evidence in order to summarize a reality that does not reflect our own personal biases but rather brings together and contextualizes data from a variety of countries, cultures, and perspectives.

Optimizing development for all teens, some of whom may be parents, will also benefit society more generally. Achieving this goal requires attention to implicit beliefs that may take the form of cultural myths. Policies and programs built on myths as opposed to the actual experiences of teens' lives will have little chance of success. Rethinking cultural myths within a framework of systems theory, as we have done throughout this book, provides a direction for more effective policies and programs. This direction suggests macrosystem forces, including stigma, educational disadvantage, and poverty, need to be a focus of intervention efforts in addition to individual decision-making of teens. If overarching beliefs are not reframed to bring cultural myths closer to reality, individual changes at the micro- or exosystem levels will have minimal impact.

Appendix: Select studies used to investigate teen pregnancy and parenting

United States samples

The National Longitudinal Study of Adolescent Health (Add Health)

Add Health is an ongoing longitudinal study of a nationally representative sample of over 15,000 teens who were in grades 7–12 during the 1994–1995 school year. Four waves of data were collected, with the most recent in 2008 when the sample was aged 24 to 34. The primary means of data collection was self-report, with teens responding to computerized surveys designed to enhance the validity of sensitive information about risky health behaviors. This self-report data was supplemented with contextual information about neighborhoods, schools, and the broader community. In addition, biological data was collected on the young adult sample during the fourth wave of data collection. Principal funding came from the Eunice Kennedy Shriver National Institute of Child Health and Human Development with 23 other federal agencies and foundations providing additional funding (Harris et al., 2009).

Research utilizing the Add Health sample makes a major contribution to our rethinking of myths presented in Chapters 4 through 7. For instance, data from this sample was used by several investigators including Brückner et al. (2004) to investigate predictors of pregnancy during the teen years. Fletcher (2012) and Fletcher and Wolfe (2009) also used data from the Add Health study to investigate the impact of early parenthood for both young women and young men, using teens who miscarried as a comparison group. Relationships between childhood SES, childhood maltreatment, and low birth weight babies were also investigated with this sample (Gavin, Thompson, Rue, and Guo, 2012). Finally, since teens responded to questions about sexual and reproductive behaviors as well as intentions to avoid sexual activity, data was used by several investigators to evaluate the effectiveness of virginity pledging.

Annenberg Sex and Media Study (ASAMS)

The ASAMS was a five-year longitudinal study began in 2005 with a sample of 547 male and female youths aged 14 to 16 from the Philadelphia area (Hennessy,

Table A.1 Table of major studies

Studies from the United States of America

Abbreviation	Full name and website (if available)	Design	Waves (if longitudinal)	Year study began	Sample at initial interview	Sample size at initial interview
Add Health	The National Longitudinal Study of Adolescent Health www.cpc.unc.edu/projects/addhealth	Longitudinal	**Wave I:** 7th–12th grade **Wave II:** 8th–12th grade **Wave III:** 18–28 years old **Wave IV:** 24–34 years old	1994	Male and female teens from 7th–12th grade	20,745
ASAMS	Annenberg Sex and Media Study (Hennessy, Bleakley, Fishbein, and Jordan, 2009)	Longitudinal	**Wave I:** age 14–16 **Wave II:** age 15–17 **Wave III:** age 16–18	2005	Male and female teens aged 14 to 16	547
Baltimore Study	Baltimore Study of Unplanned Teen Parenthood www.socio.com/dap6366.php	Longitudinal	**Wave I:** 1966–1968, during pregnancy **Wave II:** 1968–1970, 1 year after delivery **Wave III:** 1970, 3 years after delivery **Wave IV:** 1972, 5 years after delivery	1966	Teen mothers under age 18	404
ECLS-B	The Early Childhood Longitudinal Study, Birth Cohort http://nces.ed.gov/ecls	Longitudinal	**Wave I:** 2001–2002, children ~9 months old **Wave II:** 2003–2004, ~2 years old **Wave III:** 2005–2006, ~4 years old/ preschool age **Wave IV:** 2006–2007, kindergarten or higher	2001	Children 9 months old	14,000

Table A.1 (cont.)

Abbreviation	Full name and website (if available)	Design	Waves (if longitudinal)	Year study began	Sample at initial interview	Sample size at initial interview
Family Life Project	Family Life Project http://flp.fpg.unc.edu	Longitudinal	**Wave I:** infant 2 months **Wave II:** infant 6 months **Wave III:** child 15 months **Wave IV:** child 2 years –annual through- **Wave IX:** child 2nd grade	2002	Newborns	1,292
Fog Zone	National Survey of Reproductive and Contraceptive Knowledge http://thenationalcampaign.org/resource/fog-zone-0	Survey	n/a		Men and women between 18 and 29 years of age	1,800
Fragile Families	Fragile Families and Child Wellbeing Study www.fragilefamilies.princeton.edu	Longitudinal	**Wave I:** time of child's birth **Wave II:** child 1 year **Wave III:** child 3 years **Wave IV:** child 5 years **Wave V:** child 9 years	1998	Children born in 1998–2000	4,700
MIDUS	Midlife in the United States http://midus.wisc.edu	Longitudinal	**Wave I:** 1995 **Wave II:** 2004 **Wave III:** 2013	1995	Adult men and women between 25 and 74	7,108
NDAPP	Notre Dame Adolescent Parenting Project http://ccf.nd.edu/research-projects/all-research-projects/adolescent-parenting/	Longitudinal	**Wave I:** prenatal **Wave II:** child 3 years **Wave III:** child 5 years **Wave IV:** child 8 years **Wave V:** child 10 years **Wave VI:** child 14 years **Wave VII:** child 18–21 years	1984	Pregnant teens and their firstborn children	281

Study	Name	Type	Waves	Year	Population	Sample size
NELS: 88	National Educational Longitudinal Study of 1988 http://nces.ed.gov/surveys/nels88/	Longitudinal	**Wave I:** 1988 **Wave II:** 1990 **Wave III:** 1992 **Wave IV:** 1994 **Wave V:** 2000	1988	Male and female teens in 8th grade	~25,000
New York Study	New York Study (Leadbeater and Way, 2001)	Longitudinal Qualitative	**Wave I:** 3–4-week-old infant **Wave II:** 6-month-old infant **Wave III:** child 1 year **Wave IV:** child 2 years **Wave V:** child 3 years **Wave VI:** child 6 years	1987	Teen mothers aged 14 to 19 and their children	126
NLSY79	National Longitudinal Survey of Youth 1979 www.bls.gov/nls/	Longitudinal	**Wave I:** 14 to 21 -annual through- **Wave XXI:** 35 to 42	1957–1964	Young men and women between ages 14 and 21	12,686
NLSY79C	Children of the NLSY79 www.bls.gov/nls/	Longitudinal	**Wave I:** birth to age 14 -biennial through- **Wave XX:** age 14	1986–2004	Newborns to age 14	3,000
NLSY79YA	Young Adult Children of the NLSY79 www.bls.gov/nls/	Longitudinal	**Wave I:** 1994, age 15 -biennial through- **Wave VI:** 2004	1994	Male and female teens at age 15	
NLSY97	National Longitudinal Survey of Youth 1997 www.bls.gov/nls/	Longitudinal	**Wave I:** 1997 -annual through- **Wave VIII:** 2004	1997	Male and female teens aged 12 to 16	Close to 9,000
NSFG	National Survey of Family Growth www.cdc.gov/nchs/nsfg.htm	Longitudinal	**Wave I:** 1973 **Wave II:** 1976 **Wave III:** 1982 **Wave IV:** 1988 **Wave V:** 1995 **Wave VI:** 2002 **Wave VII:** 2006–2010 **Wave VIII:** 2010–2015	1973	Adult men and women age 15–44 years	12,571

Table A.1 (cont.)

Abbreviation	Full name and website (if available)	Design	Waves (if longitudinal)	Year study began	Sample at initial interview	Sample size at initial interview
PYS	Pittsburgh Youth Study www.wpic.pitt.edu/research/famhist/index.shtml	Longitudinal	**Wave I:** 1987 -biannual or annual through- **Wave XVIII:** 2000	1987	3 cohorts: boys in 1st, 4th, and 7th grades	Close to 1,000 from each grade
SSDP	Seattle Social Development Project www.ssdp-tip.org/	Longitudinal	**Wave I:** 1981 **Wave II:** 1985 -annual through- **Wave XX:** 2011, age 33	1981	Children in 5th grade	808
Three Generation Project	Three Generation Project http://medschool.umaryland.edu/growth/3.asp	Longitudinal Intervention	**Wave I:** infant 3 weeks **Wave II:** infant 6 months **Wave III:** infant 13 months **Wave IV:** infant 24 months **Wave V:** child 7 years	1997–1999	Teen mothers under the age of 18	181
YDS	Youth Development Study www.icpsr.umich.edu/icpsrweb/ICPSR/studies/24881	Longitudinal	**Wave I:** 1988; 9th graders -annual through- **Wave XV:** 2004; ~age 31	1988	Adolescent males and females in 9th grade	1,139
Studies from the United Kingdom						
BCS	1970 British Cohort Study www.cls.ioe.ac.uk/page.aspx?&sitesectionid=795	Longitudinal	**Wave I:** 1970, birth **Wave II:** age 5 years **Wave III:** age 10 years **Wave IV:** age 16 years **Wave V:** age 26 years **Wave VI:** age 30 years **Wave VII:** age 34 years **Wave VIII:** age 38 years **Wave XI:** age 42 years	1970	Infants born in 1970	Over 17,000

	Study	Design	Waves	Participants	Year	Sample size
BHPS	British Household Panel Survey www.iser.essex.ac.uk/bhps	Longitudinal	**Wave I:** 1991 -annual through- **Wave 18:** 2009	Teens and adults age 16 and older	1991	5,500 households (10,300 participants)
MCS	Millennium Cohort Study www.cls.ioe.ac.uk/page.as px?&sitesectionid=851&s itesectiontitle=Welcome+ to+the+Millennium+Coh ort+Study	Longitudinal	**Wave I:** infant 9 months **Wave II:** child 3 years **Wave III:** child 5 years **Wave IV:** child 7 years **Wave V:** child 11 years	Children born in 2000–2001	2000	~19,000
TEDS	Twins Early Development Study www.teds.ac.uk	Longitudinal	**Annual waves from 1995 to 2013**	4 cohorts beginning with all twins born in 1994 and 1995		~15,000
Studies from the Commonwealth of Australia						
HILDA	Household, Income and Labour Dynamics in Australia Survey www.melbourneinstitute. com/hilda/	Longitudinal	**Wave I:** 2001 -annual through- **Wave 12:** 2013	Adult men and women	2001	7,682 households (19,914 participants)
LSAC	Growing Up in Australia: The Longitudinal Study of Australian Children www.growingupinaustralia. gov.au/	Cross-sequential	**Wave I:** 2004 **Wave II:** 2006 **Wave III:** 2008 **Wave IV:** 2010 **Wave V:** 2012	2 cohorts: infants, and children aged 4 to 5 years	2004	10,090
WACHS	1993 Western Australia Child Health Survey www.abs.gov.au/ausstats/ abs@.nsf/productsbyCatal ogue/9DA45E9B6C00CD 28CA25722E001A3723?	Survey	n/a	Children and youths from 4 to 16 years of age	1993	2,737

Table A.1 (cont.)

Abbreviation	Full name and website (if available)	Design	Waves (if longitudinal)	Year study began	Sample at initial interview	Sample size at initial interview
Studies from New Zealand						
CHDS	Christchurch Health and Development Study www.otago.ac.nz/christchurch/research/healthdevelopment/	Longitudinal	**Wave I**: infants in 1977 -biennial through- **Wave XX**: age 30	1977	Children born in 1977	1,265
DMHDS	Dunedin Multidisciplinary Health and Development Study http://dunedinstudy.otago.ac.nz/	Longitudinal	**Wave I**: birth **Wave II**: age 3 years **Wave III**: 5 years **Wave IV**: 7 years **Wave V**: 9 years **Wave VI**: 11 years **Wave VII**: 13 years **Wave VIII**: 15 years **Wave IX**: 18 years **Wave X**: 21 years **Wave XI**: 26 years **Wave XII**: 32 years **Wave XIII**: 38 years	1972	Children born in 1972	1,037
Cross-national studies						
FFS	Fertility and Family Surveys www.unece.org/pau/ffs/ffs.html	Retrospective	n/a	1988	Adult women	2,941–4,824 adult women for each of 23 countries

Bleakley, and Fishbein, 2012). Participants responded to a follow-up survey one year later (Wave II) and a year after that (Wave III). The final sample included 457 youths. Youths responded to online surveys with questions about where their knowledge of sex and sexual behaviors came from, and questions about their attitudes, perceived norms, and self-efficacy with respect to engaging in sexual intercourse. We rely on analyses of data from this sample in Chapter 3 to inform our evaluation of the extent to which media contributes to the sexual socialization of youth (Bleakley *et al.*, 2009; Hennessy *et al.*, 2009).

The Baltimore Study of Unplanned Teen Parenthood (Baltimore Study)

The Baltimore Study led the way in scientific investigation of teen parenting (Furstenberg, 1976). The study began as an evaluation of a prenatal program for teens at the Sinai Hospital. The sample included over 400 women who were under 18 and pregnant in 1966. The study continued through 1995 with four waves of data collected. Plans include research with the grandchildren born to the original sample of teen mothers. Recent funding has been provided by the William T. Grant Foundation. Data from the Baltimore Study have provided an unparalleled impetus for rethinking myths and misperceptions of teen pregnancy and parenting, as many of the families studied by Frank Furstenberg defied negative stereotypes and demonstrated success despite multiple contextual challenges. Data from this sample have informed policy development; we refer to data from this sample in our discussion of the policy requirement that teens reside with their own mothers in order to receive governmental assistance (Furstenberg *et al.*, 1987).

The Early Childhood Longitudinal Study (ECLS)

The ECLS is comprised of three studies: ECLS: Birth Cohort, and two cohorts of kindergarten children. The ECLS-K followed over 21,000 children from kindergarten in 1998 through to 8th grade. The ECLS-B followed a nationally representative cohort of 14,000 children born in 2001, from birth through the start of kindergarten. Children of Asian and Native American descent were oversampled, as were twins, and those with low and very low birth weight. Four waves of data were collected beginning at nine months of age and concluding in 2007 as children entered kindergarten. Information was collected from mothers and fathers as well as teachers and child care personnel. Children were also directly assessed by study personnel. Funding for the ECLS-B was provided by the United States Department of Education – National Center for Education Statistics. We rely on data from these samples in our evaluation of cultural myths surrounding children born to teen mothers in Chapter 6 (Manlove *et al.*, 2008). We also rely on information collected from parents of these children to support the important role of fathers in children's outcomes (Boutwell *et al.*, 2012).

Family Life Project (FLP)

The Family Life Project is a longitudinal study that followed children from birth in 2002 through 2013. The project represents a collaborative effort between researchers at the University of North Carolina Chapel Hill and Penn State University. It is funded by the National Institutes of Health and the Eunice Kennedy Shriver National Institute of Child Health and Human Development. As stated on their website "the overarching goal of the project is to develop an understanding of the unique ways community, employment, family economic resources, family contexts, parent–child relationships and individual differences influence development and competencies in children," with a focus on children and families who live in rural areas. Data has been collected on 1,100 families through in-home interviews and observations, phone calls with families, and questionnaires. Data from this sample informs our discussion in Chapter 7 of how relationships between teen mothers and their own mothers impact children's behavior problems (Barnett *et al.*, 2012).

The National Survey of Reproductive and Contraceptive Knowledge (Fog Zone)

This survey was funded by The National Campaign to Prevent Teen and Unplanned Pregnancy and conducted by the Guttmacher Institute. Approximately 1,800 men and women between the ages of 18 and 29 were surveyed by telephone about contraceptive knowledge, attitudes, and beliefs. We rely on data from this study to inform our review of attitudes towards pregnancy in Chapter 4 (Higgins *et al.*, 2012; Kaye *et al.*, 2009; Yoo *et al.*, 2012).

The Fragile Families and Child Wellbeing Study (Fragile Families)

Fragile Families, an ongoing longitudinal study that began in 1997 with approximately 3,600 married and 1,100 unmarried families, focused on the role of fathers in single-parent households. Initial interviews were conducted with parents in the hospital immediately following birth. Four additional waves of data were collected when children were one, three, five, and nine years of age, with a 15-year follow-up currently in progress. In-home assessments of child well-being were conducted at each follow-up, beginning at age three. Fragile Families was established by researchers at Princeton and Columbia universities, and has received funding from several government agencies, including the Eunice Kennedy Shriver National Institute of Child Health and Human Development and the National Science Foundation, and over 20 private foundations, including the Robert Wood Johnson Foundation. We rely on data from the Fragile Families study in Chapter 5 as we discuss relationship outcomes for teen mothers and teen fathers, and again in Chapter 7 as we evaluate pro-marriage policies (Cooper *et al.*, 2009; Liu and Heiland, 2012).

Midlife Development in the US (MIDUS)

MIDUS included a sample of over 7,000 men and women between ages 25 and 74. The study began in 1995 with funding from the John D. and Catherine T. MacArthur Foundation. Additional funding has been provided by the National Institute on Aging. Comprehensive data was collected from the sample, and their siblings, some of whom were twins. A second wave of data was gathered from the sample in 2002, coordinated by scientists at the University of Wisconsin-Madison, and a third wave is planned that will include an additional 2,600 participants. The maturity of this sample allows a retrospective examination of the long-term consequences of teen parenting. As we report in Chapter 5, Fletcher (2012) analyzed data collected from this study to draw conclusions about the potentially transformational nature of teen parenthood.

Notre Dame Adolescent Parenting Project (NDAPP)

The NDAPP began in 1984 with a sample of 281 pregnant teens between the ages of 13 and 19. The sample of teen mothers and their children were followed longitudinally for 18 years, with data collected over seven waves. The initial goals of the research focused on identifying predictors of cognitive and academic development of the children, but were later expanded to include socioemotional functioning of the children as well as maternal outcomes. The conceptual model that guided analyses is described more fully in Chapter 2. The project was coordinated by researchers at the University of Notre Dame and the University of South Carolina Aiken, and was funded by the National Institutes of Health and the Eunice Kennedy Shriver National Institute for Child Health and Development (Whitman *et al.*, 2001). We use data from this sample as we evaluate cultural myths in several chapters.

The National Educational Longitudinal Study of 1988 (NELS:88)

NELS:88 focused on close to 25,000 students from an eighth grade cohort in 1988, with four additional waves of data collection through the year 2000 (1990, 1992, 1994, 2000). Data included achievement testing of the sample, evaluation of high-school and postsecondary transcripts, surveys of parents, teachers, and school administrators, and extensive self-report questionnaires. NELS:88 was sponsored by the National Center for Education Statistics, US Department of Education's Institute of Education Sciences. Data from this study was used by Levine and Painter in 2003, and by Strange in 2011 to investigate educational outcomes of teen parents compared to a sample of teens with the same propensity to become pregnant, but who didn't (see Chapter 5).

New York Study

The sample for this six-year longitudinal study included 126 teen mothers between the ages of 14 and 19 and their children from the New York City area

(Leadbeater and Way, 2001). Six individual interviews were conducted with the mothers, beginning at 3–4 weeks postpartum and continuing until the children were between six and seven years of age. Measures included responses to in-depth interviews, observations of interactions between mothers and children, and standardized assessments. Funding came from the Smith Richardson, Spencer, and Spring Foundation, and other grants to the principal investigators. The study includes a unique blend of quantitative and qualitative methodologies that provide a rich description of the experiences of the teen mothers. Results are also somewhat unique in their emphasis on processes of resilience observed in the families, which we integrate in our discussion of resilient parenting in Chapter 5.

The National Longitudinal Surveys (NLS)

The NLS includes a set of eight studies. The NLSY79 sample included 12,686 youths aged 14 to 21, who were born between 1957 and 1964. This cohort was interviewed annually, with a total of 21 waves through 2004. The Children of the NLSY79 sample included children from birth to age 14, born to women who participated in the original NLSY79. Ten waves of biennial data have been collected from this cohort, which included over 3,000 participants between 1986 and 2004. Once children reached age 15, they transitioned into the NLSY79 Young Adult cohort. Six waves of data have been collected between 1994 and 2004.

A new, nationally representative cohort was added to the NLSY97 that included just under 9,000 teens aged 12 to 16, who were born in 1980 to 1984. Black and Hispanic teens were oversampled. Annual data collection began in 1997 and is ongoing, with eight waves of data collected through 2004 with a retention rate of 86 percent. Self-report survey data, using a computer-assisted personal interviewing system to promote reliability and validity, was supplemented with parental measures, high-school transcripts, cognitive testing, and contextual information about the educational environment. The additional four studies, which included two earlier cohorts of younger and older men and two earlier cohorts of older and younger women, are no longer active. The studies were sponsored and funded by the US Bureau of Labor Statistics with additional support from the Eunice Kennedy Shriver National Institute for Child Health and Human Development. The Ohio State University provided a home for the study with collaboration from the University of Chicago.

Several studies that are based on data collected from the NLSY cohorts are included in our rethinking of myths and misperceptions. For example, the intergenerational nature of the data allows conclusions to be drawn about intergenerational similarities in family size (Miller *et al.*, 2010), as we discuss in Chapter 4. We also rely on data from the NLSY to inform our review of earnings of both men and women, based on the timing of marriage and childbearing (Brien and Willis, 2008; Loughran and Zissimopoulos, 2007). Analyses of data from the three NLS data sets comprise the evidence used to explore differences in outcomes for children born to teen and adult mothers, as reviewed in Chapter 6. These data are also used to compute costs of teen pregnancy and childbearing (Hoffman and Maynard, 2008), as reported in the book *Kids Having Kids*, informing our rethinking of policy-related myths in Chapter 7 and Chapter 8.

The National Survey of Family Growth (NSFG)

The first five cycles, 1973 to 1995, of the NSFG were conducted with 15- to 44-year-old women, to acquire in-depth information about marriage, divorce, contraception, infertility, and the health of women and infants. Beginning in 2002, Cycle 6 included men, for a total sample of 12,571. Cycle 7 included data from over 10,000 men and 12,000 women, collected between 2006 and 2010. Cycle 8 is ongoing through 2015. Surveys are designed to provide data that will be used to inform policy-makers who craft reproductive health services and health education programs. The NSFG is sponsored by the Centers for Disease Control and Prevention's National Center for Health Statistics, with additional funding from various agencies within the US Department of Health and Human Services. Interviews have been coordinated by the University of Michigan's Survey Research Center, Institute for Social Research. We rely on studies utilizing data from the NSFG in Chapter 4 to investigate macro-level factors related to teen pregnancy. Data from this study was also used by Lehrer and Chen (2011) to investigate stability of marriage, a topic we consider in Chapter 7.

Pittsburgh Youth Study (PYS)

The focus of the PYS was on antisocial and delinquent behavior of inner-city boys. The longitudinal study included 1,517 boys initially from the 1st, 4th, and 7th grades in 1987. The boys were re-interviewed every six months at the beginning and then yearly. Measures included self-report and reports from parents and teachers. Funding was provided by the Office of Juvenile Justice and Delinquency Prevention (OJJDP), the National Institute of Mental Health, the National Institute on Drug Abuse, and the Pew Charitable Trusts. We rely on data from the PYS sample in Chapter 6 to inform our discussion of incarceration of boys born to teen mothers (Farrington *et al.*, 2001).

Seattle Social Development Project (SSDP)

The cohort for the SSDP included 808 5th-grade students from the Seattle, Washington, public schools. This longitudinal study began in 1981, and data has been collected annually since 1985, with the most recent wave at age 33. Risky health behaviors were a major focus on survey questions for youths and their parents, as was positive youth development. The study also included an intervention component focused on risk-reduction and social skill development (Hawkins, Kosterman, Catalano, Hill, and Abbott, 2005; Lonczak, Abbott, Hawkins, Kosterman, and Catalano, 2002). The study is based at the University of Washington's School of Social Work, and has received funding from the

National Institute on Drug Abuse, the Office of Juvenile Justice and Delinquency Prevention, the Robert Wood Johnson Foundation, and the Burlington Northern Foundation. The sample provides evidence of how role transitions during emerging adulthood are based on circumstances during late childhood and early adolescence, as we discuss in Chapter 5 (Oesterle *et al.*, 2010).

Three Generation Project

This longitudinal study began as a randomized control trial to evaluate the effectiveness of a home intervention study to support the parenting skills of teen mothers (Black *et al.*, 2006). The sample included 181 Black unmarried mothers who gave birth to their first children before the age of 18, and who lived with their own mothers. Five waves of data were collected beginning at birth, with the fifth wave at age seven, with 120 families. The study was located at the University of Maryland. We use publications from this sample to inform our evaluation of parenting skills of teen mothers in Chapter 5, and our evaluation of marriage policy in Chapter 7 (Krishnakumar and Black, 2003; Oberlander *et al.*, 2010).

Youth Development Study (YDS)

This longitudinal study began in 1988 with a sample of over 1,000 9th-grade students from the St. Paul, Minnesota, school district. Research questions focused on the costs and benefits of early youth involvement in the labor force. Comprehensive data was collected from the youths and their parents about multiple contexts and outcomes. By 2007, when participants were around age 35, 15 waves of annual data had been gathered. The YDS was co-funded by the National Institute of Mental Health and the Eunice Kennedy Shriver National Institute for Child Health and Human Development. Analyses of data from the YDS (Aronson, 2008) inform our discussion of normative trajectories of the transition from adolescence to emerging adulthood in Chapter 5.

United Kingdom samples

British Cohort Study (BCS)

All 17,000 infants born in England, Scotland, and Wales during a single week of 1970 were included in the cohort. Nine waves of data have been collected, beginning at birth and continuing through age 42 in 2012. The longitudinal study has been funded by the Economic and Social Research Council and managed by the Centre for Longitudinal Studies (CLS) at the University of London. We reference data from the BCS in our Chapter 5 comparisons of employment and financial outcomes for teen versus adult fathers (Sigle-Rushton, 2005).

British Household Panel Survey (BHPS)

This ongoing longitudinal study began in 1991 with a nationally representative sample of 5,500 households in England. Every member of the household aged 16 and over participated, with some information collected from children aged 11 to 15. Subsequent waves added households from Scotland, Wales, and Northern Ireland, with 18 waves of data collection completed by 2009. The study has been funded by the Economic and Social Research Council, and is overseen by a multidisciplinary Scientific Steering Committee. Data from the BHPS are used in Chapter 6 to compare employment and financial outcomes of children born to teen versus adult mothers using a children-of-siblings design (Francesconi, 2008).

Millennium Cohort Study (MCS)

A nationally representative sample of 19,517 children born in 2001 in the UK constitutes the Millennium Cohort. Children from minority ethnic backgrounds, from disadvantaged circumstances, and from Scotland, Wales, and Northern Ireland were oversampled. This is an ongoing longitudinal study with five waves of data collected to date, beginning when children were nine months of age, and the latest wave at age 11 (n = 13,287). The study is multidisciplinary in focus and collects extensive data about multiple contexts of the children's lives. The study is funded by the Economic and Social Research Council, along with several government departments. We rely on data from the MCS as we rethink myths surrounding outcomes of children born to teen parents in Chapter 6 (Hawkes and Joshi, 2012).

Twins Early Development Study (TEDS)

All twins born in 1994 and 1995 in England and Wales were invited to participate in this longitudinal study, with a 71 percent acceptance rate resulting in a sample of over 11,000. A smaller sample of 1,116 twins, representing those predicted to be at risk for adverse outcomes, was identified for inclusion in the E-Risk Study, with children born to teen mothers oversampled. Data was collected from in-home interviews and observations when children were five years of age. Father involvement and children's behavior problems were targeted areas of interest. Conclusions from this study inform our evaluation of cultural myths related to differential outcomes for children born to teen versus adult mothers in Chapter 6 (Jaffee *et al.*, 2003).

Australia samples

Household Income and Labour Dynamics in Australia (HILDA)

HILDA began in 2001 with a sample of 7,682 households in Australia. These households and individuals have been followed yearly for 12 years, with plans to continue.

Data is collected through interviews with each adult member of the household. Questions focus on economic and subjective well-being, work and careers, and family processes. HILDA is managed by the University of Melbourne Institute of Applied Economic and Social Research, with funding provided by the Australian Department of Families, Housing, Community Services and Indigenous Affairs.

Longitudinal Study of Australian Children (LSAC)

The overarching goal of this cross-sequential study was to investigate the impact of early experiences on later development, with the intent to use findings to inform policy and optimize the development of Australian children. Two cohorts of children were included; at Wave I over one half of the 10,090 children were under the age of two, and the other half were between four and five years of age. Measures were selected to include not only individual factors, but also social, economic, and cultural influences that might have long-term impacts on development. Data was collected from parents, other caregivers, teachers, and the children themselves. Fives waves of data have been collected through 2012, with plans to continue through 2018 when the children will be between ages 14 and 19. While many studies have been published using this data, in Chapter 6 we rely on analyses by Bradbury (2011) that compared outcomes for children born to teen versus adult mothers.

Western Australia Child Health Survey (WACHS)

This survey of Australian children and adolescents was conducted to provide program and policy-makers information about the physical and mental health, risky health behaviors, academic competence, utilization of health care and social services, and protective factors in the lives of school-aged youth. The survey was conducted in 1993 and included 2,737 youths from ages 4 to 16. Surveys were completed by the principal caregiver to the youths, their school principals and teachers, and the youths themselves if aged 12 or over. The study was initiated by the TVW Telethon Institute for Child Health Research, with funding provided by the Western Australian Health Promotion Foundation, the Health Department of Western Australia, and the State Statistics Committee (Zubrick *et al.*, 1997). We rely on data from the WACHS study in Chapter 4 to rethink myths associating teen pregnancy with problem behaviors (Gaudie *et al.*, 2010).

New Zealand samples

Christchurch Health and Development Study (CHDS)

The CHDS is a comprehensive ongoing longitudinal study of 1,265 children born in New Zealand during mid-1977. The sample was followed from infancy to age 30. Themes of the research include alcohol and other substance use, mental health and suicide, domestic violence, the transition to parenthood, and overall adjustment. The study has received funding from the Health Research Council of New Zealand, National Child Health Research Foundation, Canterbury Medical Research Foundation, and the NZ Lottery Grants Board. The study is housed at the University of Otago and overseen by faculty at the university. We review research using the Christchurch study in Chapter 4, suggesting that childhood behavior problems are a risk factor for teen pregnancy (Woodward, Fergusson, and Horwood, 2006), and to emphasize the importance of cultural differences in fertility-timing norms (Marie *et al.*, 2011).

Dunedin Multidisciplinary Health and Development Study

Children included in this sample were born in Dunedin between 1972 and 1973, and have been followed since birth. This is an ongoing longitudinal study with 13 waves of data collection through 2012 when the sample was 38 years of age. Offshoots of this study include research with the main sample's parents, and with children born to the sample. The study is housed at the University of Otago, and is multidisciplinary in nature. Funding has been provided by several agencies including the Health Research Council of New Zealand, the US National Institute for Mental Health, the Eunice Kennedy Shriver National Institute for Dental and Craniofacial Health, the US National Institute of Child Health and Human Development, the US National Institute on Aging, and the UK Medical Research Council. Analyses of data from the DMHDS are used as we rethink the myth in Chapter 6 that most children born to teen mothers will have adverse academic and psychosocial outcomes (Jaffee *et al.*, 2001).

Cross-national samples

Fertility and Family Surveys (FFS)

Surveys were completed by approximately 3,000 to 5,000 adult women in 23 of the member states of the United Nations Economic Commission for Europe (UNECE), between 1988 and 1999. Financing was provided by the Population Activities Unit of the United Nations Population Fund (UNFPA). The objectives were to gather comparative data across countries that could be used to examine contextual factors related to sexuality and reproduction (Festy and Prioux, 2002). This data was used by Kearney and Levine in 2012 to investigate social and economic factors associated with early childbearing, as we discuss in Chapter 4.

References

Acs, G., and Koball, H. (2003). *TANF and the status of teen mothers under age 18* (New federalism: Issues and options for States series A. No. A-62). Washington, DC: The Urban Institute.

Afable-Munsuz, A., Speizer, I., Magnus, J. H., and Kendall, C. (2006). A positive orientation toward early motherhood is associated with unintended pregnancy among New Orleans youth. *Maternal and Child Health Journal*, 10(3), 265–276.

Ajzen, I. (1991). The theory of planned behavior. *Organizational Behavior and Human Decision Processes*, 50(2), 179–211.

Albert, B. (2010, December). With one voice 2010 – America's adults and teens sound off about teen pregnancy. *The National Campaign to Prevent Teen Pregnancy and Unplanned Parenthood*, p. 5. Retrieved January 7, 2014, from http://thenationalcampaign.org/resource/one-voice-2010.

Amato, P. R. (2007). Strengthening marriage is an appropriate social policy goal. *Journal of Policy Analysis and Management*, 26(4), 952–955.

Amato, P. R., and Kane, J. B. (2011). Life-course pathways and the psychosocial adjustment of young adult women. *Journal of Marriage and Family*, 73, 279–295.

Andrew, M., Eggerling-Boeck, J., Sandefur, G. D., and Smith, B. (2006). The "inner side" of the transition to adulthood: How young adults see the process of becoming an adult. *Advances in Life Course Research*, 11, 225–251.

Andrews, K. M., and Moore, K. A. (2011). *Second Chance homes: A resource for teen mothers* (publication no. 2011–14). Washington, DC: Child Trends. Retrieved January 7, 2014, from www.childtrends.org/wp-content/uploads/2011/04/child_trends-2011_04_15_rb_2nd chancehomes.pdf.

Arai, L. (2003). Low expectations, sexual attitudes and knowledge: Explaining teenage pregnancy and fertility in English communities. Insights from qualitative research. *The Sociological Review*, 51(2), 199–217.

Arai, L. (2009a). *Teenage pregnancy: The making and unmaking of a problem*. Bristol: The Policy Press.

Arai, L. (2009b). What a difference a decade makes: Rethinking teenage pregnancy as a problem. *Social Policy and Society*, 8(2), 171–183.

Arnett, J. J. (2000). Emerging adulthood: A theory of development from the late teens through the twenties. *American Psychologist*, 55(5), 469–480.

Arnett, J. J. (2007). Emerging adulthood: What is it, and what is it good for? *Child Development Perspectives*, 1(2), 68–73.

Aronson, P. (2008). The markers and meanings of growing up: Contemporary young women's transition from adolescence to adulthood. *Gender and Society*, 22, 56–82.

Atwood, J. D., and Kasindorf, S. (1992). A multi-systemic approach to adolescent pregnancy. *The American Journal of Family Therapy*, 20, 341–360.

Aubrey, J. S., Harrison, K., Kramer, L., and Yellin, J. (2003). Variety versus timing: Gender differences in college students' sexual expectations as predicted by exposure to sexually oriented television. *Communication Research*, 30(4), 432–460.

Bales, S. N., and O'Neil, M. (2008). *Gaining support for teen families: Mapping the perceptual hurdles* (a report from the FrameWorks Institute to Healthy Teen Network). Washington, DC: FrameWorks Institute.

Bamji, Z., Eichelberger, J., Homick, J., and Loy, A. (2013, April). *Portrayals on teen parenting in the media: A quantitative analysis of MTV's* Teen Mom *series*. Presented at the Penn State Harrisburg Student Symposium.

Barnett, M. A., Mills-Koonce, W. R., Gustafsson, H., and Cox, M. (2012). Mother-grandmother conflict, negative parenting, and young children's social development in multigenerational families. *Family Relations*, 61(5), 864–877.

Basten, S. (2009). *The socioanthropology of human reproduction* (The Future of Human Reproduction Working Paper no. 1). University of Oxford. Retrieved January 7, 2014, from www.spi.ox.ac.uk/fileadmin/documents/PDF/WP_43_The_socioanthropology_of_human_reproductionx.pdf.

Bauer, K. (2011, June 10). What's being done to cut teen pregnancy rates in Louisville. *The Wave*. Retrieved January 7, 2014, from www.wave3.com/story/14673093/16-and-pregnant-whats-being-done-to-curb-teen-pregnancynumbers-in-louisville.

Baumrind, D. (1966). Effects of authoritative parental control on child behavior. *Child Development*, 37(4), 887–907.

Bearman, P. S., and Brückner, H. (2001). Promising the future: Virginity pledges and first intercourse. *American Journal of Sociology*, 106(4), 859–912.

Beaver, K. M. (2012). The familial concentration and transmission of crime. *Criminal Justice and Behavior*, 40(2), 139–155.

Béhague, D. P., Gonçalves, H. D., Gigante, D., and Kirkwood, B. R. (2012). Taming troubled teens: The social production of mental morbidity amongst young mothers in Pelotas, Brazil. *Social Science and Medicine*, 74(3), 434–443.

Belsky, J. (1984). The determinants of parenting: A process model. *Child Development*, 55(1), 83–96.

Benson, J. E., and Elder Jr., G. H. (2011). Young adult identities and their pathways: A developmental and life course model. *Developmental Psychology*, 47(6), 1646–1657.

Benson, J. E., Johnson, M. K., and Elder, G. H. (2012). The implications of adult identity for educational and work attainment in young adulthood. *Developmental Psychology*, 48(6), 1752–1758.

Bert, S. C., Farris, J. R., and Borkowski, J. G. (2008). Parent training: Implementation strategies for "Adventures in Parenting." *Journal of Primary Prevention*, 29, 243–261.

Biello, K. B., Sipsma, H. L., and Kershaw, T. (2010). Effect of teenage parenthood on mental health trajectories: Does sex matter? *American Journal of Epidemiology*, 172(3), 279–287.

Billari, F. C., and Liefbroer, A. C. (2010). Towards a new pattern of transition to adulthood? *Advances in Life Course Research*, 15(2), 59–75.

Billari, F. C., and Philipov, D. (2004). *Education and the transition to motherhood: A comparative analysis of Western Europe* (working paper). Vienna Institute of Demography, Austrian Academy of Sciences.

Bird, K. (2011). Against all odds: Community and policy solutions to address the American youth crisis. *University of Pennsylvania Journal of Law and Social Change*, 15, 232–250.

Black, M. M., Bentley, M. E., Papas, M. A., Oberlander, S., Teti, L. O., McNary, S., Le, K., and O'Connell, M. (2006). Delaying second births among adolescent mothers: A randomized, controlled trial of a home-based mentoring program. *Pediatrics*, 118(4), e1087–e1099.

Blank, S. W., and Blum, B. B. (1997). A brief history of work expectations for welfare mothers. *The Future of Children*, 7(1), 28–38.

Bleakley, A., Hennessy, M., Fishbein, M., Coles Jr., H. C., and Jordan, A. (2009). How sources of sexual information relate to adolescents' beliefs about sex. *American Journal of Health Behavior*, 33(1), 37–48.

Bleakley, A., Hennessy, M., Fishbein, M., and Jordan, A. (2008). It works both ways: The relationship between exposure to sexual content in the media and adolescent sexual behavior. *Media Psychology*, 11(4), 443–461.

Bleakley, A., Jamieson, P. E., and Romer, D. (2012). Trends of sexual and violent content by gender in top-grossing US films, 1950–2006. *Journal of Adolescent Health*, 51(1), 73–79.

Boden, J. M., Fergusson, D. M., and Horwood, L. J. (2008). Early motherhood and subsequent life outcomes. *Journal of Child Psychology and Psychiatry*, 49(2), 151–160.

Borkowski, J. G., Farris, J. R., Whitman, T. L., Carothers, S. S., Weed, K., and Keogh, D. A. (eds.) (2007). *Risk and resilience: Adolescent mothers and their children grow up*. Mahwah, NJ: Lawrence Erlbaum Associates.

Borkowski, J. G., and Weaver, C. M. (eds.) (2006). *Prevention: The science and art of promoting healthy child and adolescent development*. Baltimore: Paul H. Brookes Pub. Co.

Botting, B., Rosato, M., and Wood, R. (1998). Teenage mothers and the health of their children. *Population Trends*, 93, 19–29.

Boutwell, B. B., Beaver, K. M., and Barnes, J. C. (2012). More alike than different: Assortative mating and antisocial propensity in adulthood. *Criminal Justice and Behavior*, 39, 1240–1254.

Boyd, H. (2011, July 30). Sex and television: How America went from "I Love Lucy" to "Playboy Club." *Deseret News*. Retrieved January 7, 2014, from www.deseretnews.com/article/700167256/Sex-and-Television-How-America-went-from-I-Love-Lucy-to-Playboy-Club.html?pg=all.

Boyer, D., and Fine, D. (1992). Sexual abuse as a factor in adolescent pregnancy and child maltreatment. *Family Planning Perspectives*, 24(1), 4–19.

Bradbury, B. (2011). *Young motherhood and child outcomes* (SPRC report 1/11). Sydney: Social Policy Research Centre, University of New South Wales.

Branum, A. M. (2006). Teen maternal age and very preterm birth of twins. *Maternal and Child Health Journal*, 10(3), 229–233.

Brase, G. L., and Brase, S. L. (2012). Emotional regulation of fertility decision making: What is the nature and structure of "baby fever"? *Emotion*, 12(5), 1141.

Braun, M., and Glöckner-Rist, A. G. (2011). Perceived consequences of female labor-force participation: A multi-level latent-class analysis across 22 countries. *OBETS: Revista de Ciencias Sociales*, 6, 163–184.

Breen, A. V. (2010). *The construction of self-identity and positive behavioural change in pregnant and parenting young women* (doctoral dissertation). University of Toronto, Ontario, Canada.

Breheny, M., and Stephens, C. (2007a). Irreconcilable differences: Health professionals' constructions of adolescence and motherhood. *Social Science and Medicine*, 64(1), 112–124.

Breheny, M., and Stephens, C. (2007b). Individual responsibility and social constraint: The construction of adolescent motherhood in social scientific research. *Culture, Health and Sexuality*, 9(4), 333–346.

Brien, M. J., and Willis, R. J. (2008). Costs and consequences for the fathers. In S. D. Hoffman and R. A. Maynard (eds.), *Kids having kids: Economic and social consequences of teen pregnancy* (pp. 119–160). Washington, DC: The Urban Institute Press.

Broman, S. H. (1981). Long-term development of children born to teenagers. In K. G. Scott, T. Field, and E. G. Robertson (eds.), *Teenage parents and their offspring* (pp. 195–225). New York: Grune and Stratton.

Bronfenbrenner, U. (1977). Toward an experimental ecology of human development. *American Psychologist*, 32(7), 513–531.

Bronfenbrenner, U. (1986). Alienation and the four worlds of childhood. *Phi Delta Kappan* 67(6), 430–436.

Bronfenbrenner, U., and Ceci, S. J. (1994). Nature-nurture reconceptualized in developmental perspective: A bioecological model. *Psychological Review*, 101(4), 568–586.

Brotherson, S. E., and Duncan, W. C. (2004). Rebinding the ties that bind: Government efforts to preserve and promote marriage. *Family Relations*, 53(5), 459–468.

Brown, J. D., L'Engle, K. L., Pardun, C. J., Guo, G., Kenneavy, K., and Jackson, C. (2006). Sexy media matter: Exposure to sexual content in music, movies, television, and magazines predicts black and white adolescents' sexual behavior. *Pediatrics*, 117(4), 1018–1027.

Brückner, H., and Bearman, P. (2005). After the promise: The STD consequences of adolescent virginity pledges. *Journal of Adolescent Health*, 36(4), 271–278.

Brückner, H., Martin, A., and Bearman, P. S. (2004). Ambivalence and pregnancy: Adolescents' attitudes, contraceptive use and pregnancy. *Perspectives on Sexual and Reproductive Health*, 36(6), 248–257.

Bunting, L., and McAuley, C. (2004). Research review: Teenage pregnancy and parenthood: The role of fathers. *Child and Family Social Work*, 9, 295–303.

Butler, K., Winkworth, G., McArthur, M., and Smyth, J. (2010). *Experiences and aspirations of younger mothers* (report for the Department of Families, Housing, Community Services and Indigenous Affairs). Canberra: Institute of Child Protection Studies, Australian Catholic University.

Carnevale, A. P., Jayasundera, T., and Hanson, A. R. (2012). *Career and technical education: Five ways that pay along the way to the B.A. Executive summary*. Washington, DC: Georgetown University Center on Education and the Workforce.

Casares, W. N., Lahiff, M., Eskenazi, B., and Halpern-Felsher, B. L. (2010). Unpredicted trajectories: The relationship between race/ethnicity, pregnancy during adolescence, and young women's outcomes. *Journal of Adolescent Health*, 47(2), 143–150.

Casey, B. J., Jones, R. M., and Hare, T. A. (2008). The adolescent brain. *Annals of the New York Academy of Science*, 1124, 111–126.

Centers for Disease Control and Prevention (2012). *Sexual experience and contraceptive use among female teens – United States, 1995, 2002, and 2006–2010* [MMWR, 61(17), 297–301]. Retrieved January 6, 2014, from www.cdc.gov/mmwr/pdf/wk/mm6117.pdf.

Chandra, A., Martino, S. C., Collins, R. L., Elliott, M. N., Berry, S. H., Kanouse, D. E., and Miu, A. (2008). Does watching sex on television predict teen pregnancy? Findings from a national longitudinal survey of youth. *Pediatrics*, 122(5), 1047–1054.

Chase-Lansdale, P. L., Brooks-Gunn, J., and Zamsky, E. S. (1994). Young African-American multigenerational families in poverty: Quality of mothering and grandmothering. *Child Development*, 65(2), 373–393.

Cherlin, A., Cross-Barnet, C., Burton, L. M., and Garrett-Peters, R. (2008). Promises they can keep: Low-income women's attitudes toward motherhood, marriage, and divorce. *Journal of Marriage and Family*, 70(4), 919–933.

Chevalier, A., and Viitanen, T. K. (2003). The long-run labour market consequences of teenage motherhood in Britain. *Journal of Population Economics*, 16(2), 323–343.

Chilman, C. S. (1990). Promoting healthy adolescent sexuality. *Family Relations*, 39(2), 123–131.

Choi, H., and Marks, N. F. (2013). Marital quality, socioeconomic status, and physical health. *Journal of Marriage and Family*, 75(4), 903–919.

Chumlea, W. C., Schubert, C. M., Roche, A. F., Kulin, H. E., Lee, P. A., Himes, J. H., and Sun, S. S. (2003). Age at menarche and racial comparisons in US girls. *Pediatrics*, 111(1), 110–113.

Clark, L. F., Miller, K. S., Nagy, S. S., Avery, J., Roth, D. L., Liddon, N., and Mukherjee, S. (2005). Adult identity mentoring: Reducing sexual risk for African-American seventh-grade students. *Journal of Adolescent Health*, 37(4), 337.e1–337.e10.

Clemmens, D. (2003). Adolescent motherhood: A meta-synthesis of qualitative studies. *MCN: The American Journal of Maternal/Child Nursing*, 28(2), 93–99.

Cohen, S. (1972). *Folk devils and moral panics: The creation of the mods and rockers*. London: Granada Publishing.

Collins, R. L., Elliott, M. N., Berry, S. H., Kanouse, D. E., and Hunter, S. B. (2003). Entertainment television as a healthy sex educator: The impact of condom-efficacy information in an episode of *Friends*. *Pediatrics*, 112(5), 1115–1121.

Collins, R. L., Elliott, M. N., Berry, S. H., Kanouse, D. E., Kunkel, D., Hunter, S. B., and Miu, A. (2004). Watching sex on television predicts adolescent initiation of sexual behavior. *Pediatrics*, 114, e280–e289.

Collins, W. A. (2003). More than myth: The developmental significance of romantic relationships during adolescence. *Journal of Research on Adolescence*, 13(1), 1–24.

Connelly, C. D., and Strauss, M. A. (1992). Mother's age and risk for physical abuse. *Child Abuse and Neglect*, 16, 709–718.

Cooper, C. E., McLanahan, S. S., Meadows, S. O., and Brooks-Gunn, J. (2009). Family structure transitions and maternal parenting stress. *Journal of Marriage and Family*, 71(3), 558–574.

Copen, C. E., Daniels, K., Vespa, J., and Mosher, W. D. (2012). *First marriages in the United States: Data from the 2006–2010 National Survey of Family Growth* (National Health Statistics Reports, 49). Hyattsville: National Center for Health Statistics.

Cornelius, M. D., Goldschmidt, L., De Genna, N. M., and Larkby, C. (2012). Long-term effects of prenatal cigarette smoke exposure on behavior dysregulation among 14-year-old offspring of teenage mothers. *Maternal and Child Health Journal*, 16(3), 694–705.

Costa, F. M., Jessor, R., Donovan, J. E., and Fortenberry, J. D. (1995). Early initiation of sexual intercourse: The influence of psychosocial unconventionality. *Journal of Research on Adolescence*, 5(1), 93–121.

Counting It Up (n.d.). Retrieved January 7, 2014, from The National Campaign to Prevent Teen and Unplanned Pregnancy website: www.thenationalcampaign.org/costs/about-faq.aspx.

Counting It Up: The public costs of teen childbearing: Key data (2013). The National Campaign to Prevent Teen and Unplanned Pregnancy. Retrieved June 8, 2014, from http://thenationalcampaign.org/resource/counting-it-key-data-2013.

Courtney, M. E., Dworsky, A., Brown, A., Cary, C., Love, K., and Vorhies, V. (2011). *Midwest evaluation of the adult functioning of former foster youth: Outcomes at age 26*. Chicago: Chapin Hall at the University of Chicago.

Covington, R., Peters, H. E., Sabia, J. J., and Price, J. P. (2011). *Teen fatherhood and educational attainment: Evidence from three cohorts of youth*. Retrieved January 7,

2014, from http://resiliencelaw.org/wordpress2011/wp-content/uploads/2012/04/Teen-Fatherhood-and-Educational-Attainment.pdf.

Coyne, C. A., Långström, N., Rickert, M. E., Lichtenstein, P., and D'Onofrio, B. M. (2013). Maternal age at first birth and offspring criminality: Using the children-of-twins design to test causal hypotheses. *Development and Psychopathology*, 25(1), 17–35.

Crijns, I., Bos, J., Knol, M., Straus, S., and de Jong-van den Berg, L. (2012). Paternal drug use: before and during pregnancy. *Expert Opinion on Drug Safety*, 11(4), 513–518.

Cummings, E. M., Davies, P. T., and Campbell, S. B. (2000). *Developmental psychopathology and family process*. New York: The Guilford Press.

Curtin, S. C., Abma, J. C., Ventura, S. J., and Henshaw, S. K. (2013). *Pregnancy rates for US women continue to drop* (NCHS data brief, no. 136). Hyattsville: National Center for Health Statistics.

Dahinten, V. S., Shapka, J. D., and Willms, J. D. (2007). Adolescent children of adolescent mothers: The impact of family functioning on trajectories of development. *Journal of Youth and Adolescence*, 36(2), 195–212.

Dahl, G. B. (2005). *Early teen marriage and future poverty* (no. w11328). Cambridge, MA: National Bureau of Economic Research. Retrieved January 7, 2014, from www.nber.org/papers/w11328.

Dahl, R. E. (2004). Adolescent brain development: A period of vulnerabilities and opportunities. *Annals of the New York Academy of Sciences*, 1021, 1–22.

Dailard, C. (2002). Abstinence promotion and teen family planning: The misguided drive for equal funding. *The Guttmacher Report on Public Policy*, 5(1), 1–3.

Dake, K. (1992). Myths of nature: Culture and the social construction of risk. *Journal of Social Issues*, 48(4), 21–37.

Dash, L. (1989). *When children want children: An inside look at the crisis of teenage parenthood*. New York: William Morrow and Company, Inc.

Davidson, M. (1983). *Uncommon sense: The life and thought of Ludwig von Bertalanffy*. Los Angeles: J. P. Tarcher.

Debiec, K. E., Paul, K. J., Mitchell, C. M., and Hitti, J. E. (2010). Inadequate prenatal care and risk of preterm delivery among adolescents: A retrospective study over 10 years. *American Journal of Obstetrics and Gynecology*, 203(2), 122.e1-6.

De Genna, N. M., Larkby, C., and Cornelius, M. D. (2013). The dysregulation profile predicts cannabis use in the offspring of teenage mothers. *ISRN Addiction*. Retrieved from the Hindawi Publishing Corporation website: http://dx.doi.org/10.1155/2013/659313.

Denny, G., and Young, M. (2006). An evaluation of an abstinence-only sex education curriculum: An 18-month follow-up. *Journal of School Health*, 76(8), 414–422.

DiCenso, A., Guyatt, G., Willan, A., and Griffith, L. (2002). Interventions to reduce unintended pregnancies among adolescents: Systematic review of randomised controlled trials. *BMJ: British Medical Journal*, 324(7351), 1426.

Dickins, T. E., Johns, S. E., and Chipman, A. (2012). Teenage pregnancy in the United Kingdom: A behavioral ecological perspective. *Journal of Social, Evolutionary, and Cultural Psychology*, 6(3), 344–359.

Dinh, J. (2010, December 22). MTV's "16 and Pregnant" credited for decline in teen pregnancy rates. *MTV*. Retrieved January 7, 2014, from www.mtv.com/news/articles/1654818/mtvs-16-pregnant-credited-decline-teen-pregnancy-rates.jhtml.

Dolgen, L. (2011, May 5). Why I created MTV's "16 and Pregnant." *CNN*. Retrieved January 7, 2014, from www.cnn.com/2011/SHOWBIZ/TV/05/04/teen.mom.dolgen/.

Doniger, A., Riley, J. S., Utter, C. A., and Adams, E. (2001). Impact evaluation of the "Not me, not now" abstinence-oriented, adolescent pregnancy prevention communications program, Monroe County, N.Y. *Journal of Health Communication*, 6(1), 45–60.

Donovan, J. E., Jessor, R., and Costa, F. M. (1991). Adolescent health behavior and conventionality/unconventionality: An extension of problem-behavior theory. *Health Psychology*, 10(1), 52–61.

Drebitko, C. N., Sadler, L. S., Leventhal, J. M., Daley, A. M., and Reynolds, H. (2005). Adolescent girls with negative pregnancy tests. *Journal of Pediatric and Adolescent Gynecology*, 18, 261–267.

Duffy, J., and Levin-Epstein, J. (2002). *Add it up. Teen parents and welfare … undercounted, oversanctioned, underserved*. Washington, DC: Center for Law and Social Policy.

Duncan, S. (2007). What's the problem with teenage parents? And what's the problem with policy? *Critical Social Policy*, 27(3), 307–334.

Durkheim, E. (1960). Sociology and its scientific field. In K. H. Wolff (ed.), *Emile Durkheim, 1858–1917: A collection of essays, with translations and a bibliography* (pp. 354–375). Columbus: The Ohio State University Press.

Dunkel Schetter, C. (2011). Psychological science on pregnancy: Stress processes, biopsychosocial models, and emerging research issues. *Annual Review of Psychology*, 62, 531–558.

Dunkel Schetter, C., and Lobel, M. (2012). Pregnancy and birth outcomes: A multi-level analysis of prenatal stress and birth weight. In A. Baum, T. A. Revenson, and J. Singer (eds.), *Handbook of health psychology* (pp. 431–465). New York: Psychology Press.

Earnshaw, V. A., Rosenthal, L., Lewis, J. B., Stasko, E. C., Tobin, J. N., Lewis, T. T., Reid, A. E., and Ickovics, J. R. (2013). Maternal experiences with everyday discrimination and infant birth weight: A test of mediators and moderators among young, urban women of color. *Annals of Behavioral Medicine*, 45(1), 13–23.

East, P. L., and Felice, M. E. (1996). *Adolescent pregnancy and parenting: Findings from a racially diverse sample*. Mahwah, NJ: Lawrence Erlbaum Associates.

Easterbrooks, M., Chaudhuri, J. H., Bartlett, J. D., and Copeman, A. (2011). Resilience in parenting among young mothers: Family and ecological risks and opportunities. *Children and Youth Services Review*, 33(1), 42–50.

Elliott, S. (2010). Parents' constructions of teen sexuality: Sex panics, contradictory discourses, and social inequality. *Symbolic Interaction*, 33(2), 191–212.

Ellis, B. J., and Boyce, W. T. (2011). Differential susceptibility to the environment: Toward an understanding of sensitivity to developmental experiences and context. *Development and Psychopathology*, 23(1), 1–5.

Ensor, R., and Hughes, C. (2010). With a little help from my friends: Maternal social support, via parenting, promotes willingness to share in preschoolers born to young mothers. *Infant and Child Development*, 19, 127–141.

Ermisch, J. (2003). *Does a "teen-birth" have longer-term impacts on the mother? Suggestive evidence from the British Household Panel Study*. England: Institute for Social and Economic Research, University of Essex.

Eyal, K., and Kunkel, D. (2008). The effects of sex in television drama shows on emerging adults' sexual attitudes and moral judgments. *Journal of Broadcasting and Electronic Media*, 52(2), 161–181.

Falci, C. D., Mortimer, J. T., and Noel, J. (2010). Parental timing and depressive symptoms in early adulthood. *Advances in Life Course Research*, 15(1), 1–10.

Farber, N. (2009). *Adolescent pregnancy: Policy and prevention services*. New York: Springer Publishing Company.

Farrington, D. P., Jolliffe, D., Loeber, R., Stouthamer-Loeber, M., and Kalb, L. M. (2001). The concentration of offenders in families, and family criminality in the prediction of boys' delinquency. *Journal of Adolescence*, 24, 579–596.

Farris, J. R., Bert, S. C., Nicholson, J. S., Glass, K., and Borkowski, J. G. (2013). Effective intervention programming: Improving maternal adjustment through parent education. *Administration and Policy in Mental Health and Mental Health Services Research*, 40, 211–223.

Farris, J. R., Borkowski, J. G., Lefever, J. E. B., and Whitman, T. L. (2013). Two are better than one: The joint influence of maternal preparedness for parenting and children's self-esteem on academic achievement and adjustment. *Early Education and Development*, 24, 346–365.

Farris, J. R., Nicholson, J. S., Borkowski, J. G., and Whitman, T. L. (2011). Onset and progression of disruptive behavior problems among community boys and girls: A prospective longitudinal analysis. *Journal of Emotional and Behavioral Disorders*, 19, 233–246.

Federal Communications Commission (2013). *Consumer guide: Obscene, indecent and profane broadcasts*. Washington, DC: Consumer and Governmental Affairs Bureau. Retrieved January 7, 2014, from http://transition.fcc.gov/cgb/consumerfacts/obscene.pdf.

Ferguson, C. J., and Heene, M. (2012). A vast graveyard of undead theories: Publication bias and psychological science's aversion to the null. *Perspectives on Psychological Science*, 7(6), 555–561.

Fergusson, D. M., Boden, J. M., and Horwood, L. J. (2012). Transition to parenthood and substance use disorders: Findings from a 30-year longitudinal study. *Drug and Alcohol Dependence*, 125(3), 295–300.

Festy, P., and Prioux, F. (2002). *FFS: An evaluation of the Fertility and Family Surveys project*. United Nations Publications. Retrieved January 7, 2014, from www.unece.org/fileadmin/DAM/pau/_docs/ffs/FFS_2000_Prog_EvalReprt.pdf.

Fine, M., and McClelland, S. I. (2006). The politics of teen women's sexuality: Public policy and the adolescent female body. *Emory Law Journal*, 56, 993–1038

Finlay, A. (1996). Teenage pregnancy, romantic love and social science: An uneasy relationship. In V. James and J. Gabe (eds.), *Health and the sociology of emotion* (pp. 79–96). Hoboken: Wiley-Blackwell.

Finlay, K., and Neumark, D. (2010). Is marriage always good for children? Evidence from families affected by incarceration. *Journal of Human Resources*, 45(4), 1046–1088.

Fletcher, J. M. (2012). The effects of teenage childbearing on the short- and long-term health behaviors of mothers. *Journal of Population Economics*, 25, 201–218.

Fletcher, J. M., and Wolfe, B. L. (2009). Education and labor market consequences of teenage childbearing evidence using the timing of pregnancy outcomes and community fixed effects. *Journal of Human Resources*, 44(2), 303–325.

Fletcher, J. M., and Wolfe, B. L. (2012). The effects of teenage fatherhood on young adult outcomes. *Economic Inquiry*, 50(1), 182–201.

Francesconi, M. (2008). Adult outcomes for children of teenage mothers. *The Scandinavian Journal of Economics*, 110(1), 93–117.

Frey, K. A., Navarro, S. M., Kotelchuck, M., and Lu, M. C. (2008). The clinical content of preconception care: Preconception care for men. *American Journal of Obstetrics and Gynecology*, 199(6), S389–S395.

Frimmel, W., Halla, M., and Winter-Ebmer, R. (2012). *Can pro-marriage policies work? An analysis of marginal marriages* (CEPR discussion paper no. DP9081). Retrieved January 7, 2014, from the Social Science Research Network website: http://papers.ssrn.com/sol3/papers.cfm?abstract_id=2153531.

Furstenberg, F. F. (1976). The social consequences of teenage parenthood. *Family Planning Perspectives*, 8(4), 148–164.

Furstenberg, F. F. (2007). Should government promote marriage? *Journal of Policy Analysis and Management*, 26(4), 956–960.

Furstenberg Jr., F. F., Brooks-Gunn, J., and Morgan, S. P. (1987). Adolescent mothers and their children in later life. *Family Planning Perspectives*, 19(4), 142–151.

Furstenberg, F. F., Kennedy, S., McCloyd, V. C., Rumbaut, R., and Settersten Jr., R. A. (2003). *Between adolescence and adulthood: Expectations about the timing of adulthood* (Research Network working paper no. 1). Retrieved January 7, 2014, from The Network on Transitions to Adulthood website: http://transitions.s410.sureserver.com/wp-content/uploads/2011/08/between.pdf.

Gaudie, J., Mitrou, F., Lawrence, D., Stanley, F., Silburn, S., and Zubrick, S. (2010). Antecedents of teenage pregnancy from a 14-year follow-up study using data linkage. *BMC Public Health*, 10(1), 63.

Gavin, A. R., Thompson, E., Rue, T., and Guo, Y. (2012). Maternal early life risk factors for offspring birth weight: Findings from the Add Health study. *Prevention Science*, 13(2), 162–172.

Gavin, L. E., Catalano, R. F., David-Ferdon, C., Gloppen, K. M., and Markham, C. M. (2010). A review of positive youth development programs that promote adolescent sexual and reproductive health. *Journal of Adolescent Health*, 46(3), S75–S91.

Gee, C. B., McNerney, C. M., Reiter, M. J., and Leaman, S. C. (2007). Adolescent and young adult mothers' relationship quality during the transition to parenthood: Associations with father involvement in fragile families. *Journal of Youth and Adolescence*, 36, 213–224.

Gerbner, G., and Gross, L. (1976). Living with television: The violence profile. *Journal of Communication*, 26(2), 172–194.

Geronimus, A. T. (2003). Damned if you do: Culture, identity, privilege, and teenage childbearing in the United States. *Social Science and Medicine*, 57(5), 881–893.

Geronimus, A. T., and Korenman, S. (1993). Maternal youth or family background? On the health disadvantages of infants with teenage mothers. *American Journal of Epidemiology*, 137(2), 213–225.

Geronimus, A. T., Korenman, S., and Hillemeier, M. M. (1994). Does young maternal age adversely affect child development? Evidence from cousin comparisons in the United States. *Population and Development Review*, 20(3), 585–609.

Giedd, J. N. (2008). The teen brain: Insights from neuroimaging. *Journal of Adolescent Health*, 42(4), 335–343.

Girls Incorporated. (2007). *Girls and sexual activity*. New York. Retrieved March 31, 2014, from www.girlsinc.org/sites/default/files/downloads/girlsandsexualactivity.pdf.

Glauser, B. G., and Strauss, A. L. (1967). *The discovery of grounded theory*. Chicago: Aldine.

Goerge, R. M., Harden, A., and Lee, B. J. (2008). Consequences of teen childbearing for child abuse, neglect, and foster care placement. In S. D. Hoffman and R. A. Maynard (eds.), *Kids having kids: Economic costs and social consequences of teen pregnancy* (pp. 257–288). Washington, DC: The Urban Institute Press.

Gogtay, N., Giedd, J. N., Lusk, L., Hayashi, K. M., Greenstein, D., Vaituzis, A. C., Nugent, T. F., Herman, D. G., Clasen, L. S., Toga, A. W., Rapoport, J. L. and Thompson, P. M. (2004). Dynamic mapping of human cortical development during childhood through early adulthood. *Proceedings of the National Academy of Sciences of the United States of America*, 101(21), 8174–8179.

Goodman, A., Kaplan, G., and Walker, I. (2004). *Understanding the effects of early motherhood in Britain: The effects on mothers* (IFS working papers 04/20). London: Institute for Fiscal Studies. Retrieved January 7, 2014, from http://hdl.handle.net/10419/71559.

Graham, H., and McDermott, E. (2006). Qualitative research and the evidence base of policy: Insights from studies of teenage mothers in the UK. *Journal of Social Policy*, 35(1), 21–37.

Grigsby Bates, K. (2010, August 10). MTV's "Teen Mom" makes for teaching moments. *National Public Radio*. Retrieved January 7, 2014, from www.npr.org/templates/story/story.php?storyId=128626258.

Grogger, J. (1997). Incarceration-related costs of early childbearing. In R. A. Maynard (ed.), *Kids having kids: Economic costs and social consequences of teen pregnancy* (pp. 231–256). Washington, DC: The Urban Institute Press.

Grogger, J. (2008). Consequences of teen childbearing for incarceration among adult children: Approach and estimates through 1991. In S. D. Hoffman and R. A. Maynard (eds.), *Kids having kids: Economic costs and social consequences of teen pregnancy* (pp. 289–311). Washington, DC: The Urban Institute Press.

Grote, N. K., Bridge, J. A., Gavin, A. R., Melville, J. L., Iyengar, S., and Katon, W. J. (2010). A meta-analysis of depression during pregnancy and the risk of preterm birth, low birth weight, and intrauterine growth restriction. *Archives of General Psychiatry*, 67(10), 1012–1024.

Guglielmo, L. (ed.) (2013). *MTV and teen pregnancy: Critical essays on 16 and Pregnant and Teen Mom*. Lanham: Scarecrow Press.

Guttentag, C. L., Landry, S. H., Williams, J. M., Baggett, K. M., Noria, C. W., Borkowski, J. G., Swank, P. R., Farris, J. R., Crawford, A., Lanzi, R. G., Carta, J. J., Warren, S. F., and Ramey, S. L. (2014). "My Baby and Me": Effects of an early, comprehensive parenting intervention on at-risk mothers and their children. *Developmental Psychology*, 50, 1482–1496. Advance online publication. doi: 10.1037/a0035682

Hacking, I. (1999). *The social construction of what?* Cambridge, MA: Harvard University Press.

Hamilton, B. E., Martin, J. A., and Ventura, S. J. (2013). *Births: Preliminary data for 2012* (National Vital Statistics Reports, 62(3). Hyattsville: National Center for Health Statistics.

Hansen, K., Hawkes, D., and Joshi, H. (2009). The timing of motherhood, mothers' employment and child outcomes. In J. Stillwell, E. Coast, and D. Kneale (eds.), *Fertility, living arrangements, care and mobility* (pp. 59–80). Netherlands: Springer.

Hao, L., Astone, N. M., and Cherlin, A. J. (2007). Effects of child support and welfare policies on nonmarital teenage childbearing and motherhood. *Population Research and Policy Review*, 26(3), 235–257.

Harden, A., Brunton, G., Fletcher, A., Oakley, A., Burchett, H., and Backhans, M. (2006). *Young people, pregnancy and social exclusion: A systematic synthesis of research evidence to identify effective, appropriate and promising approaches for prevention and support*. London: EPPI-Centre, Social Science Research Unit, Institute of Education, University of London. Retrieved January 7, 2014, from http://eprints.ioe.ac.uk/5927/1/Harden2006Youngpeople.pdf.

Harden, K. P., Lynch, S. K., Turkheimer, E., Emery, R. E., D'Onofrio, B. M., Slutske, W. S., Waldron, M. D., Heath, A. C., Statham, D. J., and Martin, N. G. (2007). A behavior genetic investigation of adolescent motherhood and offspring mental health problems. *Journal of Abnormal Psychology*, 116(4), 667–683.

Hardy, R., Lawlor, D. A., Black, S., Mishra, G. D., and Kuh, D. (2009). Age at birth of first child and coronary heart disease risk factors at age 53 years in men and women: British birth cohort study. *Journal of Epidemiology and Community Health*, 63(2), 99–105.

Harris, K. M., Halpern, C. T., Whitsel, E., Hussey, J., Tabor, J., Entzel, P., and Udry, J. R. (2009). *The National Longitudinal Study of Adolescent Health: Research Design*: www.cpc. unc.edu/projects/addhealth/design, 18–20.

Harris, R. J., and Barlett, C. P. (2009). Effects of sex in the media. In J. Bryant and M. B. Oliver (eds.), *Media effects: Advances in theory and research*, 3rd ed. (pp. 304–324). New York: Routledge.

Hartmann, D., and Swartz, T. T. (2006). The new adulthood? The transition to adulthood from the perspective of transitioning young adults. *Advances in Life Course Research*, 11, 253–286.

Hawkes, D., and Joshi, H. (2012). Age at motherhood and child development: Evidence from the UK Millennium Cohort. *National Institute Economic Review*, 222(1), R52–R66.

Hawkins, J. D., Kosterman, R., Catalano, R. F., Hill, K. G., and Abbott, R. D. (2005). Promoting positive adult functioning through social development intervention in childhood: Long-term effects from the Seattle Social Development Project. *Archives of Pediatrics and Adolescent Medicine*, 159(1), 25–31.

Heilborn, M. L., and Cabral, C. S. (2011). A new look at teenage pregnancy in Brazil. *ISRN Obstetrics and Gynecology*, 1–7. Retrieved January 7, 2014, from the Hindawi Publishing Corporation website: http://dx.doi.org/10.5402/2011/975234.

Henly, J. R. (1997). The complexity of support: The impact of family structure and provisional support on African American and White adolescent mothers' well-being. *American Journal of Community Psychology*, 25(5), 629–655.

Hennessy, M., Bleakley, A., and Fishbein, M. (2012). Measurement models for reasoned action theory. *The Annals of the American Academy of Political and Social Science*, 640(1), 42–57.

Hennessy, M., Bleakley, A., Fishbein, M., and Jordan, A. (2009). Estimating the longitudinal association between adolescent sexual behavior and exposure to sexual media content. *Journal of Sex Research*, 46(6), 586–596.

Henretta, J. C., Grundy, E. M. D., Okell, L. C., and Wadsworth, M. E. J. (2008). Early motherhood and mental health in midlife: A study of British and American cohorts. *Aging and Mental Health*, 12(5), 605–614.

The Heritage Foundation. (n.d.). Retrieved January 7, 2014, from www.heritage.org/ about.

Herman-Giddens, M. E., Slora, E. J., Wasserman, R. C., Bourdony, C. J., Bhapkar, M. V., Koch, G. G., and Hasemeier, C. M. (1997). Secondary sexual characteristics and menses in young girls seen in office practice: A study from the Pediatric Research in Office Settings Network. *Pediatrics*, 99(4), 505–512.

Hetsroni, A. (2007). Three decades of sexual content on prime-time network programming: A longitudinal meta-analytic review. *Journal of Communication*, 57(2), 318–348.

Higgins, J. A., Popkin, R. A., and Santelli, J. S. (2012). Pregnancy ambivalence and contraceptive use among young adults in the United States. *Perspectives on Sexual and Reproductive Health*, 44(4), 236–243.

Hobcraft, J., and Kiernan, K. (2001). Childhood poverty, early motherhood and adult social exclusion. *British Journal of Sociology*, 52(3), 495–517.

Hoefer, C. (2008). Causal determinism. *Stanford encyclopedia of philosophy*. Retrieved January, 6, 2014, from http://plato.stanford.edu/archives/win2009/entries/determinism-causal/.

Hoffman, J. (2011, April 8). Fighting teenage pregnancy with MTV stars as Exhibit A. *The New York Times*. Retrieved June 8, 2014, from http://thenationalcampaign.org/resource/numbers.

Hoffman, S. D. (2006). *By the numbers: The public costs of teen childbearing*. Washington, DC: The National Campaign to Prevent Teen Pregnancy. Retrieved January 7, 2014, from www.thenationalcampaign.org/costs/pdf/report/BTN_National_Report.pdf.

Hoffman, S. D. (2008). Updated estimates of the consequences of teen childbearing for mothers. In S. D. Hoffman and R. A. Maynard (eds.), *Kids having kids: Economic costs and social consequences of teen pregnancy* (pp. 74–92). Washington, DC: The Urban Institute Press.

Hoffman, S. D., and Maynard, R. A. (eds.) (2008). *Kids having kids: Economic costs and social consequences of teen pregnancy*. Washington, DC: The Urban Institute Press.

Hoffman, S. D., and Scher, L. (2008). Consequences of teen childbearing for the life chances of children, 1979–2002. In S. D. Hoffman and R. A. Maynard (eds.), *Kids having kids: Economic costs and social consequences of teen pregnancy* (pp. 342–358). Washington, DC: The Urban Institute Press.

Holmlund, H. (2005). Estimating long-term consequences of teenage childbearing – an examination of the siblings approach. *The Journal of Human Resources*, 40(3), 716–743.

Homma, Y., Wang, N., Saewyc, E., and Kishor, N. (2012). The relationship between sexual abuse and risky sexual behavior among adolescent boys: A meta-analysis. *Journal of Adolescent Health*, 51(1), 18–24.

Horn, I. B., Joseph, J. G., and Cheng, T. L. (2004). Nonabusive physical punishment and child behavior among African-American children: A systematic review. *Journal of the National Medical Association*, 96(9), 1162–1168.

Horvath-Rose, A., and Peters, H. E. (2001). Welfare waivers and non-marital childbearing. In G. J. Duncan and P. L. Chase-Lansdale (eds.), *For better and for worse: Welfare reform and the well-being of children and families* (pp. 222–244). New York: Russell Sage Foundation.

Hotz, V. J., McElroy, S. W., and Sanders, S. G. (2008). Consequences of teen childbearing for mothers through 1993. In S. D. Hoffman and R. A. Maynard (eds.), *Kids having kids: Economic costs and social consequences of teen pregnancy* (pp. 52–74). Washington, DC: The Urban Institute Press.

Howell, M., and Keefe, M. (2007). *The history of federal abstinence-only funding*. Retrieved January 7, 2014, from the Advocates for Youth website: www.advocatesforyouth.org/storage/advfy/documents/fshistoryabonly.pdf.

Hueston, W. J., Geesey, M. E., and Diaz, V. (2008). Prenatal care initiation among pregnant teens in the United States: An analysis over 25 years. *Journal of Adolescent Health*, 42(3), 243–248.

Hunt, G., Joe-Laidler, K., and MacKenzie, K. (2005). Moving into motherhood: Gang girls and controlled risk. *Youth and Society*, 36(3), 333–373.

Hutchinson, M. K., and Montgomery, A. J. (2007). Parent communication and sexual risk among African Americans. *Western Journal of Nursing Research*, 29(6), 691–707.

Jaccard, J., Dodge, T., and Dittus, P. (2003). Do adolescents want to avoid pregnancy? Attitudes towards pregnancy as predictors of pregnancy. *Journal of Adolescent Health*, 33(2), 79–83.

Jacobsen, R. H. (2011). *Long-term performance of young mothers and their children in Denmark: Labour market, health care and prescription drugs*. Copenhagen: Centre for Economic and Business Research. Retrieved January 7, 2014, from http://openarchive.cbs.dk/handle/10398/8377.

Jaffee, S. R. (2002). Pathways to adversity in young adulthood among early childbearers. *Journal of Family Psychology*, 16(1), 38–49.

Jaffee, S., Caspi, A., Moffitt, T. E., Belsky, J. A. Y., and Silva, P. (2001). Why are children born to teen mothers at risk for adverse outcomes in young adulthood? Results from a 20-year longitudinal study. *Development and Psychopathology*, 13(2), 377–397.

Jaffee, S. R., Moffitt, T. E., Caspi, A., and Taylor, A. (2003). Life with (or without) father: The benefits of living with two biological parents depend on the father's antisocial behavior. *Child Development*, 74(1), 109–126.

Jemmott, J. B., Jemmott, L. S., and Fong, G. T. (1998). Abstinence and safer sex HIV risk-reduction interventions for African American adolescents: A randomized controlled trial. *JAMA: The Journal of the American Medical Association*, 279(19), 1529–1536.

Jemmott, J. B., Jemmott, L. S., and Fong, G. T. (2010). Efficacy of a theory-based abstinence-only intervention over 24 months. *Archives of Pediatrics and Adolescent Medicine*, 164(2), 152–159.

Jessor, R., and Jessor, S. L. (1977). *Problem behavior and psychosocial development: A longitudinal study of youth*. New York: Academic Press.

Jessor, S. L., and Jessor, R. (1975). Transition from virginity to nonvirginity among youth: A social-psychological study over time. *Developmental Psychology*, 11(4), 473–484.

Jones, D. J., Lewis, T., Litrownik, A., Thompson, R., Proctor, L. J., Isbell, T., Dubowitz, H., English, D., Jones, B., Nagin, D., and Runyan, D. (2013). Linking childhood sexual abuse and early adolescent risk behavior: The intervening role of internalizing and externalizing problems. *Journal of Abnormal Psychology*, 41, 139–150.

Jonsson, P. (2010, December 21). A force behind the lower teen birthrate: MTV's "16 and Pregnant." *Christian Science Monitor*. Retrieved January 7, 2014, from www.csmonitor.com/USA/Society/2010/1221/A-force-behind-the-lower-teen-birthrate-MTV-s-16-and-Pregnant.

Jurich, J. A., and Myers-Bowman, K. S. (1998). Systems theory and its application to research on human sexuality. *Journal of Sex Research*, 35(1), 72–87.

Kaestner, R., Korenman, S., and O'Neill, J. (2003). Has welfare reform changed teenage behaviors? *Journal of Policy Analysis and Management*, 22(2), 225–248.

Kalil, A., Spencer, M. S., Spieker, S. J., and Gilchrist, L. D. (1998). Effects of grandmother coresidence and quality of family relationships on depressive symptoms in adolescent mothers. *Family Relations*, 47(4), 433–441.

Kalmijn, M., and Kraaykamp, G. (2005). Late or later? A sibling analysis of the effect of maternal age on children's schooling. *Social Science Research*, 34(3), 634–650.

Kaye, K., Suellentrop, K., and Sloup, C. (2009). *The Fog Zone: How misperceptions, magical thinking, and ambivalence put young adults at risk for unplanned pregnancy*. Washington, DC: The National Campaign to Prevent Teen and Unplanned Pregnancy. Retrieved June 8, 2014, from http://thenationalcampaign.org/resource/fog-zone-0.

Kearney, M. S., and Levine, P. B. (2011). *Income inequality and early non-marital childbearing: An economic exploration of the "culture of despair"* (no. w17157). National Bureau of Economic Research.

Kearney, M. S., and Levine, P. B. (2012). Why is the teen birth rate in the United States so high and why does it matter? *The Journal of Economic Perspectives*, 26(2), 141–166.

Kearney, M. S., and Levine, P. B. (2014). *Media influences on social outcomes: The impact of MTV's 16 and pregnant on teen childbearing* (working paper no. 19795). National Bureau of Economic Research. Retrieved April 2, 2014, from www.econ.ucsb.edu/about_us/events/seminar_papers/Kearney.pdf.

Kelly, D. M. (1996). Stigma stories: Four discourses about teen mothers, welfare, and poverty. *Youth and Society*, 27(4), 421–449.

Kennedy, A. C. (2008). Eugenics, "degenerate girls," and social workers during the progressive era. *Affilia*, 23(1), 22–37.

Kim, C., and Rector, R. (2010, February 19). Evidence on the effectiveness of abstinence education: An update. *Backgrounder*, 2372. Retrieved January 7, 2014, from The Heritage Foundation website: www.heritage.org/research/reports/2010/02/evidence-on-the-effectiveness-of-abstinence-education-an-update.

Kingston, D., Heaman, M., Fell, D., and Chalmers, B. (2012). Comparison of adolescent, young adult, and adult women's maternity experiences and practices. *Pediatrics*, 129(5), e1228–e1237.

Kirby, D. (2002). *Do abstinence-only programs delay the initiation of sex among young people and reduce teen pregnancy?* Washington, DC: The National Campaign to Prevent Teen and Unplanned Pregnancy. Retrieved June 8, 2014, from http://groupregnancy.wikispaces.com/file/view/teenpregnancy2.pdf.

Kirby, D. (2007). *Emerging answers 2007: Research findings on programs to reduce teen pregnancy and sexually transmitted diseases.* Washington, DC: The National Campaign to Prevent Teen and Unplanned Pregnancy. Retrieved June 8, 2014, from http://thenationalcampaign.org/resource/emerging-answers-2007%E2%80%94full-report.

Kirby, D. B., Laris, B. A., and Rolleri, L. A. (2007). Sex and HIV education programs: Their impact on sexual behaviors of young people throughout the world. *Journal of Adolescent Health*, 40(3), 206–217.

Kirchengast, S. (2009). Teenage-pregnancies: A biomedical and a sociocultural approach to a current problem. *Current Women's Health Reviews*, 5(1), 1–7.

Kives, S., and Jamieson, M. A. (2001). Desire for pregnancy among adolescents in an antenatal clinic. *Journal of Pediatric and Adolescent Gynecology*, 14(3), 150.

Kline, R. B. (2004). *Beyond significance testing: Reforming data analysis methods in behavioral research.* Washington, DC: American Psychological Association.

Kost, K., and Henshaw, S. (2013). *US teenage pregnancies, births and abortions, 2008: National and State trends by age, race and ethnicity.* New York: Guttmacher Institute. Retrieved June 8, 2014, from www.guttmacher.org/pubs/USTPtrends10.pdf.

Krishnakumar, A., and Black, M. M. (2003). Family processes within three-generation households, and adolescent mothers' satisfaction with father involvement. *Journal of Family Psychology*, 17(4), 488–498.

Krone, K. E. (2005). *Oprah Winfrey.* Minneapolis: Lerner Publications.

Kunkel, D., Eyal, K., Finnerty, K., Biely, E., and Donnerstein, E. (2005). *Sex on TV.* Menlo Park: A Kaiser Family Foundation Report.

Ladd-Taylor, M. (2001). Eugenics, sterilisation and modern marriage in the USA: The strange career of Paul Popenoe. *Gender and History*, 13(2), 298–327.

Lanzi, R. G., Bert, S. C., Jacobs, B. K., and the Centers for the Prevention of Child Neglect (2009). Depression among a sample of first-time adolescent and adult mothers. *Journal of Child and Adolescent Psychiatric Nursing*, 22(4), 194–202.

La Taillade, J. J., Hofferth, S., and Wight, V. R. (2010). Consequences of fatherhood for young men's relationships. *Research in Human Development*, 7(2), 103–122.

Lawlor, D. A., Mortensen, L., and Andersen, A. M. N. (2011). Mechanisms underlying the associations of maternal age with adverse perinatal outcomes: A sibling study of 264,695 Danish women and their firstborn offspring. *International Journal of Epidemiology*, 40(5), 1205–1214.

Lawlor, D. A., and Shaw, M. (2002). Too much too young? Teenage pregnancy is not a public health problem. *International Journal of Epidemiology*, 31(3), 552–553.

Laws, K. R. (2013). Negativland: A home for all findings in psychology. *BMC Psychology*, 1(2). Retrieved January 7, 2014, from www.biomedcentral.com/2050-7283/1/2.

Leadbeater, B. J. R., and Way, N. (2001). *Growing up fast: Transitions to early adulthood of inner-city adolescent mothers*. Mahwah, NJ: Lawrence Erlbaum Associates.

Leeners, B., Stiller, R., Block, E., Görres, G., and Rath, W. (2010). Pregnancy complications in women with childhood sexual abuse experiences. *Journal of Psychosomatic Research*, 69(5), 503–510.

Lehrer, E. L., and Chen, Y. (2011). *Women's age at first marriage and marital instability: Evidence from the 2006–2008 National Survey of Family Growth* (no. 5954). Discussion paper series//Forschungsinstitut zur Zukunft der Arbeit. Retrieved January 7, 2014, from www.econstor.eu/bitstream/10419/55088/1/675946484.pdf.

Lerner, R. M. (2005). *Promoting positive youth development: Theoretical and empirical bases*. Washington, DC: National Research Council. Retrieved January 7, 2014, from http://ase.tufts.edu/iaryd/documents/pubPromotingPositive.pdf.

Lesko, N. (2002). Making adolescence at the turn of the century: Discourse and the exclusion of girls. *Current Issues in Comparative Education*, 2(2), 182–191.

Lesthaeghe, R. (2010). The unfolding story of the second demographic transition. *Population and Development Review*, 36(2), 211–251.

Levin-Epstein, J., and Schwartz, A. (2005). Improving TANF for teens. *Journal of Poverty Law and Policy*, 39, 183–194.

Levine, D., and Painter, G. (2003). The schooling costs of teenage out-of-wedlock childbearing: Analysis with a within-school propensity-score-matching estimator. *Review of Economics and Statistics*, 85, 884–900.

Levine, J. A., Emery, C. R., and Pollack, H. (2007). The well-being of children born to teen mothers. *Journal of Marriage and Family*, 69(1), 105–122.

Lincoln, Y. S., and Guba, E. G. (1985). *Naturalistic inquiry*. Beverly Hills: Sage.

Liu, S. H., and Heiland, F. (2012). Should we get married? The effect of parents' marriage on out-of-wedlock children. *Economic Inquiry*, 50(1), 17–38.

Local Government Association (2013). *Tackling teenage pregnancy: Local government's new public health role*. Retrieved January 7, 2014, from website: www.local.gov.uk/publications/-/journal_content/56/10180/3964823/PUBLICATION.

Lonczak, H. S., Abbott, R. D., Hawkins, J. D., Kosterman, R., and Catalano, R. F. (2002). Effects of the Seattle Social Development Project on sexual behavior, pregnancy, birth, and sexually transmitted disease outcomes by age 21 years. *Archives of Pediatrics and Adolescent Medicine*, 156(5), 438–447.

Lord, C. G., Ross, L., and Lepper, M. R. (1979). Biased assimilation and attitude polarization: The effects of prior theories on subsequently considered evidence. *Journal of Personality and Social Psychology*, 37(11), 2098–2109.

Loughran, D. S., and Zissimopoulos, J. (2007). *Why wait? The effect of marriage and childbearing on the wages of men and women* (working paper WR-482). Santa Monica: RAND Corporation. Retrieved January 7, 2014, from www.rand.org/pubs/working_papers/WR482-1.html.

Lu, M. C., Jones, L., Bond, M. J., Wright, K., Pumpuang, M., Maidenberg, M., Jones, D., Garfield, C., and Rowley, D. L. (2010). Where is the F in MCH? Father involvement in African American families. *Ethnicity and Disease*, 20, 49–61.

Luker, K. (1996). *Dubious conceptions: The politics of teenage pregnancy*. Cambridge, MA: Harvard University Press.

Maccoby, E. E. (1991). Different reproductive strategies in males and females. *Child Development*, 62(4), 676–681.

Macleod, C. (2011). *"Adolescence," pregnancy and abortion: Constructing a threat of degeneration*. New York: Routledge.

McClelland, S. I., and Fine, M. (2008). Embedded science: Critical analysis of abstinence-only evaluation research. *Cultural Studies ⇔ Critical Methodologies*, 8, 50–81.

McDermott, E., Graham, H., and Hamilton, V. (2004). Experiences of being a teenage mother in the UK: A report of a systematic review of qualitative studies. Swindon: Economic and Social Research Council. Retrieved January 7, 2014, from www.sphsu. mrc.ac.uk/Evidence/Research/Review%2010/SR%20Executive%20Summary.pdf.

McLanahan, S. (2007). Should government promote marriage? *Journal of Policy Analysis and Management*, 26(4), 951.

McLaughlin, S. D., and Micklin, M. (1983). The timing of the first birth and changes in personal efficacy. *Journal of Marriage and the Family*, 45(1), 47–55.

Madkour, A. S., Harville, E. W., and Xie, Y. (2014). Neighborhood disadvantage, racial concentration and the birth weight of infants born to adolescent mothers. *Maternal and Child Health Journal*, 18, 663–671.

Magnusson, D. (1998). The logic and implications of a person-oriented approach. In R. B. Cairns, L. R. Bergman, and J. Kagan (eds.), *Methods and models for studying the individual: Essays in honor of Marian Radke-Yarrow* (pp. 33–64). Thousand Oaks: SAGE Publications.

Malabarey, O. T., Balayla, J., Klam, S. L., Shrim, A., and Abenhaim, H. A. (2012). Pregnancies in young adolescent mothers: A population-based study on 37 million births. *Journal of Pediatric and Adolescent Gynecology*, 25(2), 98–102.

Males, M. (2006). Youth health services, development programs, and teenage birth rates in 55 California cities. *Californian Journal of Health Promotion*, 4(1), 46–57.

Manlove, J. S., Terry-Humen, E., Mincieli, L. A., and Moore, K. A. (2008). Outcomes for children of teen mothers from kindergarten through adolescence. In S. D. Hoffman and R. A. Maynard (eds.), *Kids having kids: Economic costs and social consequences of teen pregnancy* (pp. 161–196). Washington, DC: The Urban Institute Press.

Marcus, L. (2011, April 10). What ruined 16 and Pregnant Teen Mom [Web blog post]. Retrieved January 7, 2014, from www.huffingtonpost.com/lilit-marcus/16-and-pregnant-teen-mom_b_859197.html.

Marie, D., Fergusson, D. M., and Boden, J. M. (2011). Cultural identity and pregnancy/parenthood by age 20: Evidence from a New Zealand birth cohort. *Social Policy Journal of New Zealand*, 37, 19–36.

Markovitz, B. P., Cook, R., Flick, L. H. and Leet, T. L. (2005). Socioeconomic factors and adolescent pregnancy outcomes: Distinctions between neonatal and post-neonatal deaths? *BMC Public Health*, 5(79), doi: 10.1186/1471–2458–5–79.

Martin, J. A., Hamilton, B. E., Ventura, S. J., Osterman, M. J. K., and Matthews, T. J. (2013). *Births: Final data for 2011* (National Vital Statistics Reports, 62(1). Hyattsville: National Center for Health Statistics.

Martin, J. A., Hamilton, B. E., Ventura, S. J., Osterman, M. J. K., Wilson, E. C., and Matthews, T. J. (2012). *Births: Final data for 2010* (National Vital Statistics Reports, 61(1)). Hyattsville: National Center for Health Statistics.

Mattson, S. N., Roesch, S. C., Glass, L., Deweese, B. N., Coles, C. D., Kable, J. A., May, P. A., Kalberg, W. O., Sowell, E. R., Adnams, C. M., Jones, K. L., and Riley, E. P. (2012). Further development of a neurobehavioral profile of fetal alcohol spectrum disorders. *Alcoholism: Clinical and Experimental Research*, 37(3), 517–528.

Mawer, C. (1999). Preventing teenage pregnancies, supporting teenage mothers: Target is ambitious but probably achievable. *BMJ: British Medical Journal*, 318, 1713–1714.

Maykut, P. and Morehouse, R. (1994). *Beginning qualitative research: A philosophical and practical guide*. London: Falmer Press Teachers' Library.

Maynard, R. A. (ed.). (1996). *Kids having kids: A Robin Hood Foundation special report on the costs of adolescent childbearing*. New York: The Robin Hood Foundation. Retrieved January 6, 2014, from www.uvm.edu/~nnfruvm/robnhood.html.

Maynard, R. A. (1997). The costs of adolescent childbearing. In R. A. Maynard (ed.), *Kids having kids: Economic costs and social consequences of teen pregnancy* (pp. 285–338). Washington, DC: The Urban Institute Press.

Maynard, R. A., and Hoffman, S. D. (2008). The costs of adolescent childbearing. In S. D. Hoffman and R. A. Maynard (eds.), *Kids having kids: Economic costs and social consequences of teen pregnancy* (pp. 359–401). Washington, DC: The Urban Institute Press.

Meadows, P. (2010). *National evaluation of Sure Start local programmes: An economic perspective* (Research Report DFE-RR073). Institute for the Study of Children, Families and Social Issues, University of London. Prepared for the Department of Education, UK, London. Retrieved January 7, 2014, from www.calderdaleforward.org.uk/workspace/uploads/files/sure-start-evaluation-4f746138050c2.pdf.

Meckler, M., and Baillie, J. (2003). The truth about social construction in administrative science. *Journal of Management Inquiry*, 12(3), 273–284.

Midgley, G. (2006). Systemic intervention for public health. *American Journal of Public Health*, 96(3), 466–472.

Miller, W. B., Barber, J. S., and Gatny, H. H. (2013). The effects of ambivalent fertility desires on pregnancy risk in young women in the USA. *Population Studies*, 67(1), 25–38.

Miller, W. B., Bard, D. E., Pasta, D. J., and Rodgers, J. L. (2010). Biodemographic modeling of the links between fertility motivation and fertility outcomes in the NLSY79. *Demography*, 47(2), 393–414.

Mission, values and guiding principles (n.d.) Retrieved January 6, 2014, from the Guttmacher Institute website: www.guttmacher.org/about/mission.html.

Moffitt, R. A., Reville, R. T., Winkler, A. E., and Burstain, J. M. (2009). *Cohabitation and marriage rules in state TANF programs*. Washington, DC: US Department of Health and Human Services. Retrieved January 7, 2014, from http://aspe.hhs.gov/hsp/09/CohabitationMarriageRules/.

Mollborn, S. (2010). Predictors and consequences of adolescent norms against teenage pregnancy. *Sociological Quarterly*, 51(2), 303–328.

Montano, D. E., and Kasprzyk, D. (2008). Theory of reasoned action, theory of planned behavior, and the integrated behavioral model. In K. Glanz, B. K. Rimer, and K. Viswanath (eds.), *Health Behavior and Health Education: Theory, Research, and Practice*, 4th ed. (pp. 67–96). San Francisco: Jossey-Bass.

Mosher, W. D., Jones, J., and Abma, J. C. (2012). *Intended and unintended births in the United States: 1982–2010* (National Health Statistics Reports, 55). Hyattsville: National Center for Health Statistics.

MTV's *16 and Pregnant* (n.d.). Retrieved January 7, 2014, from www.mtv.com/shows/16_and_pregnant/season_4/series.jhtml.

Munro, G. D., Stansbury, J. A., and Tsai, J. (2012). A causal role for negative affect: Misattribution in biased evaluations of scientific information. *Self and Identity*, 11, 1–15.

Murcott, A. (1980). The social construction of teenage pregnancy: A problem in the ideologies of childhood and reproduction. *Sociology of Health and Illness*, 2(1), 1–23.

Murphy, C. (2012). Teen Momism on MTV: Postfeminist subjectivities in *16 and Pregnant*. Networking Knowledge. *Journal of the MeCCSA-PGN*, 5(1), 84–99.

Murphy, C. C., Schei, B., Myhr, T. L., and Du Mont, J. (2001). Abuse: A risk factor for low birth weight? A systematic review and meta-analysis. *Canadian Medical Association Journal*, 164(11), 1567–1572.

Murray on Senate floor: Attacks on women's health appalling, an insult to women everywhere (2012, February 17) [news release]. Retrieved from www.murray.senate.gov/public/index.cfm/newsreleases?ID=21ec1ba5-07fa-48fc-86d4-455b1350ed22.

Nathanson, C. A. (1991). *Dangerous passage: The social control of sexuality in women's adolescence*. Philadelphia: Temple University Press.

Ng, A. S., and Kaye, K. (2012). *Why it matters: Teen childbearing, education, and economic wellbeing*. Retrieved June 8, 2014, from The National Campaign to Prevent Teen and Unplanned Pregnancy website: http://thenationalcampaign.org/resource/why-it-matters-teen-childbearing-education-and-economic-wellbeing.

Nicholson, J. S., Deboeck, P., Farris, J. R., Boker, S. M., and Borkowski, J. G. (2011). Maternal depressive symptomatology and child behavior: Transactional relationship with simultaneous bidirectional coupling. *Developmental Psychology*, 47, 1312–1323.

Nicholson, J. S., Farris, J. R., Gandy, J., Loy, A., Bamji, Z., Eichelberger, J., Homick, J., Johnson, C., and Lemons, C. (2014, March). The role of the media in constructing beliefs: An evaluation of MTV's *16 and Pregnant* and *Teen Mom* series. In J. S. Nicholson (Chair), *Common beliefs about teen moms: More myth than truth?* Symposium conducted at the biennial meeting of the Society for Research on Adolescence, Austin, TX.

Noll, J. G., Shenk, C. E., and Putnam, K. T. (2009). Childhood sexual abuse and adolescent pregnancy: A meta-analytic update. *Journal of Pediatric Psychology*, 34(4), 366–378.

Oberlander, S. E., Agostini, W. R. M., Houston, A. M., and Black, M. M. (2010). A seven-year investigation of marital expectations and marriage among urban, low-income, African American adolescent mothers. *Journal of Family Psychology*, 24(1), 31–40.

Oberlander, S. E., and Black, M. M. (2011). African American adolescent mothers' early caregiving involvement and children's behavior and academic performance at age 7. *Journal of Clinical Child and Adolescent Psychology*, 40(5), 756–764.

Oberlander, S. E., Black, M. M., and Starr, R. H. (2007). African American adolescent mothers and grandmothers: A multigenerational approach to parenting. *American Journal of Community Psychology*, 39, 37–46.

OECD (2011), *Education at a glance*. OECD Publishing. Retrieved January 7, 2014, from www.oecd.org/edu/eag2011.

Oesterle, S., Hawkins, J. D., Hill, K. G., and Bailey, J. A. (2010). Men's and women's pathways to adulthood and their adolescent precursors. *Journal of Marriage and Family*, 72(5), 1436–1453.

Office of National Statistics (2012). Retrieved January 7, 2014, from http://www.ons.gov.uk/ons/rel/vsob1/birth-summary-tables–england-and-wales/2012/rft-births-summary-tables-2012.xls

Offner, P. (2003). *Teenagers and welfare reform*. Retrieved January 7, 2014, from The Urban Institute website: www.urban.org/uploadedPDF/410808_teenagers_and_welfare_reform.pdf.

Okoroh, E. M., Coonrod, D. V., Chapple, K., and Drachman, D. (2012). Are neonatal morbidities associated with no prenatal care different from those associated with inadequate prenatal care? *Open Journal of Obstetrics and Gynecology*, 2(2), 89–97.

Osterman, M. J. K, Martin, J. A., Mathews, T. J., and Hamilton, B. E. (2011). *Expanded data from the new birth certificate* (National Vital Statistics Reports, 59(7). Hyattsville: National Center for Health Statistics.

Oxford, M. L., Gilchrist, L. D., Lohr, M. J., Gillmore, M. R., Morrison, D. M., and Spieker, S. J. (2005). Life course heterogeneity in the transition from adolescence to adulthood among adolescent mothers. *Journal of Research on Adolescence*, 15(4), 479–504.

Palin, B. (2011). *Not afraid of life: My journey so far*. New York: HarperCollins.

Pardun, C. J., L'Engle, K. L., and Brown, J. D. (2005). Linking exposure to outcomes: Early adolescents' consumption of sexual content in six media. *Mass Communication and Society*, 8(2), 75–91.

Paul, J. (1968). The return of punitive sterilization proposals: Current attacks on illegitimacy and the AFDC program. *Law and Society Review*, 3(1), 77–106.

Pedrosa, A. A., Pires, R., Carvalho, P., Canavarro, M. C., and Dattilio, F. (2011). Ecological contexts in adolescent pregnancy: The role of individual, sociodemographic, familial and relational variables in understanding risk of occurrence and adjustment patterns. *Contemporary Family Therapy*, 33(2), 107–127.

Pettigrew, M., Whitehead, M., Macintyre, S. J., Graham, H., and Egan, M. (2004). Evidence for public health policy on inequalities 1: The reality according to policymakers. *Journal of Epidemiology and Community Health*, 5, 811–816.

Phipps, M.G., and Nunes, A. P. (2012). Assessing pregnancy intention and associated risks in pregnant adolescents. *Maternal and Child Health Journal*, 16(9), 1820–1827.

Phoenix, A. (1991). *Young mothers?* Cambridge: Polity Press.

Pluess, M., and Belsky, J. (2010). Differential susceptibility to parenting and quality child care. *Developmental Psychology*, 46(2), 379–390.

Public Cost: FAQ. (n.d.) Retrieved June 8, 2014, from *The National Campaign to Prevent Teen and Unplanned Pregnancy* website: http://thenationalcampaign.org/why-it-matters/public-costs/faqs.

Pungello, E. P., Kainz, K., Burchinal, M., Wasik, B. H., Sparling, J. J., Ramey, C. T., and Campbell, F. A. (2010). Early educational intervention, early cumulative risk, and the early home environment as predictors of young adult outcomes within a high-risk sample. *Child Development*, 81(1), 410–426.

Raymo, J., Lim, S., Perelli-Harris, B., Carlson, M. J., and Iwasawa, M. (2011). Educational differences in early childbearing: A cross-national comparative study. In *The changing transition to adulthood in Japan: Current demographic research and policy implications* (pp. 73–104). Tokyo: National Institute of Population and Social Security Research.

Rector, R., and Johnson, K. A. (2005a). *Teenage sexual abstinence and academic achievement*. Retrieved January 7, 2014, from The Heritage Foundation website: www.heritage.org/research/reports/2005/10/teenage-sexual-abstinence-and-academic-achievement.

Rector, R., and Johnson, K. A. (2005b). *Adolescent virginity pledges, condom use, and sexually transmitted diseases among young adults*. Retrieved January 7, 2014, from The Heritage Foundation website: www.heritage.org/research/reports/2005/06/adolescent-virginity-pledges-condom-use-and-sexually-transmitted-diseases-among-young-adults.

Rector, R. E., Pardue, M. G., and Martin, S. (2004). *What do parents want taught in sex education programs?* Retrieved January 7, 2014, from The Heritage Foundation website: www.heritage.org/research/reports/2004/01/what-do-parents-want-taught-in-sex-education-programs.

Reinberg, S. (2012, May 3). More teen girls using contraceptives: CDC. *Health Day*. Retrieved January 7, 2014, from http://consumer.healthday.com/women-s-health-information-34/birth-health-news-61/more-teen-girls-using-contraceptives-cdc-664433.html.

Resnick, M. D., Bearman, P. S., Blum, R. W., Bauman, K. E., Harris, K. M., Jones, J., Tabor, J., Beuhring, T., Sieving, R. E., Shew, M., Ireland, M., Bearinger, L. H., and Udry, J. R. (1997). Protecting adolescents from harm. *JAMA: The Journal of the American Medical Association*, 278(10), 823–832.

Rhode, D. L., and Lawson, A. (1993). Introduction. In A. Lawson and D. L. Rhode (eds.), *The politics of pregnancy: Adolescent sexuality and public policy* (pp. 23–45). New Haven: Yale University Press.

Rideout, V. J., Foehr, U. G., and Roberts, D. F. (2010, January). *Generation M²: Media in the lives of 8- to 18-year-olds.* Menlo Park: The Henry J. Kaiser Family Foundation. Retrieved January 7, 2014, from http://kff.org/other/report/generation-m2-media-in-the-lives-of-8-to-18-year-olds/.

Roeper, R. (2011, May 17). Making celebs of teen moms has drawbacks. *Chicago Sun-Times.com*. Retrieved January 7, 2014, from www.suntimes.com/news/roeper/5431883-417/making-celebs-of-teen-moms-has-drawbacks.html.

Rosenbaum, P. R., and Rubin, D. B. (1985). Constructing a control group using multivariate matched sampling methods that incorporate the propensity score. *The American Statistician*, 39(1), 33–38.

Rosengard, C., Pollock, L., Weitzen, S., Meers, A., and Phipps, M. G. (2006). Concepts of the advantages and disadvantages of teenage childbearing among pregnant adolescents: A qualitative analysis. *Pediatrics*, 118(2), 503–510.

Rosman, E. A., and Yoshikawa, H. (2001). Effects of welfare reform on children of adolescent mothers: Moderation by maternal depression, father involvement, and grandmother involvement. *Women and Health*, 32(3), 253–290.

Ross, L. (1977). The intuitive psychologist and his shortcomings: Distortions in the attribution process. *Advances in Experimental Social Psychology*, 10, 173–220.

Roth, T. L., and Sweatt, J. D. (2011). Epigenetic mechanisms and environmental shaping of the brain during sensitive periods of development. *Journal of Child Psychology and Psychiatry*, 52(4), 398–408.

Rotkirch, A., Basten, S., Väisänen, H., and Jokela, M. (2011). Baby longing and men's reproductive motivation. *Vienna Yearbook of Population Research*, 9, 283–306.

Ryan, P. J. (2007). Six Blacks from home: Childhood, motherhood, and eugenics in America. *Journal of Policy History*, 19(3), 253–281.

Santelli, J. S., Lindberg, L. D., Orr, M. G., Finer, L. B., and Speizer, I. (2009). Toward a multidimensional measure of pregnancy intentions: Evidence from the United States. *Studies in Family Planning*, 40(2), 87–100.

Santelli, J., Ott, M. A., Lyon, M., Rogers, J., Summers, D., and Schleifer, R. (2006). Abstinence and abstinence-only education: A review of US policies and programs. *The Journal of Adolescent Health*, 38(1), 72–81.

Sapolsky, B. S., and Tabarlet, J. O. (1991). Sex in primetime television: 1979 versus 1989. *Journal of Broadcasting and Electronic Media*, 35(4), 505–516.

Sapphire's story: How "Push" became "Precious" (2009). Retrieved January 6, 2014, from www.npr.org/templates/story/story.php?storyId=120176695.

Saul, R. (1998). Whatever happened to the Adolescent Family Life Act? *The Guttmacher Report on Public Policy*, 1(2), 5–11.

Savage, S. (2002). The flaw of averages. *Harvard Business Review*, 80(11), 20–21.

Scafidi, B. (2008). *The taxpayer costs of divorce and unwed childbearing: First-ever estimates for the nation and all fifty states.* New York: Institute for American Values. Retrieved 8 June, 2014, from http://americanvalues.org/catalog/pdfs/COFF.pdf.

Scher, L. S. (2008). What do we know about the effectiveness of programs aimed at reducing teen sexual risk-taking? In S. D. Hoffman and R. A. Maynard (eds.), *Kids having kids: Economic costs and social consequences of teen pregnancy* (pp. 403–433). Washington, DC: The Urban Institute Press.

Scher, L. S., and Hoffman, S. D. (2008). Consequences of teen childbearing for incarceration among adult children: Updated estimates through 2002. In S. D. Hoffman and R. A. Maynard (eds.), *Kids having kids: Economic costs and social consequences of teen pregnancy* (pp. 311–321). Washington, DC: The Urban Institute Press.

Scher, L., Maynard, R., and Stagner, M. (2006). Interventions intended to reduce pregnancy-related outcomes among adolescents. Campbell Systematic Reviews, doi: 10.4073/csr.2006.12. Retrieved January 7, 2014, from www.campbellcollaboration.org/lib/download/103/.

Schlossman, S., and Wallach, S. (1978). The crime of precocious sexuality: Female juvenile delinquency in the progressive era. *Harvard Educational Review*, 48(1), 65–94.

Seiler, N. (2002). *Is teen marriage a solution?* Washington, DC: Center for Law and Social Policy. Retrieved January 7, 2014, from www.clasp.org/resources-and-publications/archive/0087.pdf.

Selman, P. (2003). Scapegoating and moral panics: Teenage pregnancy in Britain and the United States. In S. Cunningham-Burley and L. Jamieson (eds.), *Families and the state: Changing relationships* (pp. 159–186). Basingstoke: Palgrave Macmillan.

Shanahan, J., and Morgan, M. (1999). *Television and its viewers: Cultivation theory and research*. New York: Cambridge University Press.

Shapiro, D. L., and Marcy, H. M. (2002). *Knocking on the door: Barriers to welfare and other assistance for teen parents. A three-city research study*. Chicago: Center for Impact Research. Retrieved January 7, 2014, from the Center for Impact Research website: www.impactresearch.org/documents/cirknockdoor.pdf.

Shaw, A. (2010). Media representations of adolescent pregnancy: The problem with choice. *Atlantis*, 32(2), 55–65.

Sheeder, J., Teal, S. B., Crane, L. A., and Stevens-Simon, C. (2010). Adolescent childbearing ambivalence: Is it the sum of its parts? *Journal of Pediatric and Adolescent Gynecology*, 23(2), 86–92.

Shields, C. (2008). *Aristotle*. Stanford encyclopedia of philosophy. Retrieved from the Center for the Study of Language and Information, Stanford University, website: http://plato.stanford.edu/entries/aristotle/.

Shrum, L. J., and Lee, J. (2012). Television's persuasive narratives: How television influences values, attitudes, and beliefs. In L. J. Shrum (ed.), *The psychology of entertainment media: Blurring the lines between entertainment and persuasion*, 2nd ed. (pp. 147–167). New York: Taylor and Francis.

Sigle-Rushton, W. (2005). Young fatherhood and subsequent disadvantage in the United Kingdom. *Journal of Marriage and Family*, 67, 735–753.

Singh, S., Sedgh, G., and Hussain, R. (2010). Unintended pregnancy: Worldwide levels, trends, and outcomes. *Studies in Family Planning*, 41(4), 241–250.

Singh, S., Wulf, D., Hussain, R., Bankole, A., and Sedgh, G. (2009). *Abortion worldwide: A decade of uneven progress*. New York: Guttmacher Institute.

Singhal, A., and Rogers, E. M. (2001). The entertainment–education strategy in campaigns. In R. E. Rice and C. Atkins (eds.), *Public communication campaigns*, 3rd ed. (pp. 343–356). Thousand Oaks: Sage Publications.

Slater, M. D. (2007). Reinforcing spirals: The mutual influence of media selectivity and media effects, and their impact on individual behavior and social identity. *Communication Theory*, 17(3), 281–303.

Smith, E. F. (2012). They don't teach this in high school: An examination of the portrayal of teenage pregnancy in the MTV television show *16 and Pregnant*. *Proceedings of the New York State Communication Association*, 2010(1), 10.

Smith, S., and Weed, K. (2013, June). *Does the reality television show* 16 and Pregnant *portray the reality of being a teen mom?* Poster presented at the South Carolina Campaign to Prevent Teen and Unwanted Pregnancy Summer Institute, Columbia, SC.

SmithBattle, L. (2007). Legacies of advantage and disadvantage: The case of teen mothers. *Public Health Nursing*, 24(5), 409–420.

SmithBattle, L. (2012). Moving policies upstream to mitigate the social determinants of early childbearing. *Public Health Nursing*, 29(5), 444–454.

SmithBattle, L. (2013). Reducing the stigmatization of teen mothers. MCN. *American Journal of Maternal Child Nursing*, 38(4), 235–241.

Social Exclusion Unit (SEU) (1999). *Teenage pregnancy* (Cm 4342). London: HMSO.

Solomon-Fears, C. (2013). *Teenage pregnancy prevention: Statistics and programs*. Washington, DC: Congressional Research Service, Library of Congress. Retrieved January 7, 2014, from www.fas.org/sgp/crs/misc/RS20301.pdf.

Somers, C. L., and Paulson, S. E. (2000). Students' perceptions of parent–adolescent closeness and communication about sexuality: relations with sexual knowledge, attitudes, and behaviors. *Journal of Adolescence*, 23(5), 629–644.

Somers, C. L., and Vollmar, W. L. (2006). Parent–adolescent relationships and adolescent sexuality: Closeness, communication, and comfort among diverse US adolescent samples. *Social Behavior and Personality*, 34(4), 451–460.

Sonfield, A., Kost, K., Gold, R. B., and Finer, L. B. (2011). The public costs of births resulting from unintended pregnancies: National and state-level estimates. *Perspectives on Sexual and Reproductive Health*, 43(2), 94–102.

Spence, N. J. (2008). The long-term consequences of childbearing: Physical and psychological well-being of mothers in later life. *Research on Aging*, 30(6), 722–751.

Spieker, S. J., and Bensley, L. (1994). Roles of living arrangements and grandmother social support in adolescent mothering and infant attachment. *Developmental Psychology*, 30, 102–111.

Status of the lawsuits challenging the Affordable Care Act's birth control coverage benefit (2014, January). National Women's Law Center, Washington, DC. Retrieved April 2, 2014, from www.nwlc.org/status-lawsuits-challenging-affordable-care-act%E2%80%99s-birth-control-coverage-benefit.

Steinberg, L. (2010). Commentary: A behavioral scientist looks at the science of adolescent brain development. *Brain and Cognition*, 72(1), 160–164.

Steinberg, L., and Monahan, K. C. (2010). Adolescents' exposure to sexy media does not hasten the initiation of sexual intercourse. *Developmental Psychology*, 47(2), 562–576.

Strange, K. (2011). A longitudinal analysis of the relationship between fertility timing and schooling. *Demography*, 48, 931–956.

Strayhorn, J. M., and Strayhorn, J. C. (2009). Religiosity and teen birth rate in the United States. *Reproductive Health*, 6(14), 1–7.

Suellentrop, K., Brown, J., and Ortiz, R. (2010, October). *Evaluating the impact of* MTV's 16 and Pregnant *on teen viewers' attitudes about teen pregnancy* (Science Says 45). Retrieved June 8, 2014, from The National Campaign to Prevent Teen and Unplanned Pregnancy website: http://thenationalcampaign.org/resource/science-says-45.

Taylor, J. L. (2009). Midlife impacts of adolescent parenthood. *Journal of Family Issues*, 30(4), 484–510.

Taylor, L. D. (2005). Effects of visual and verbal sexual television content and perceived realism on attitudes and beliefs. *Journal of Sex Research*, 42(2), 130–137.

Teen Births (2013). *Child Trends Data Bank*. Retrieved January 7, 2014, from www.childtrends.org/wp-content/uploads/2012/11/13_Teen_Birth.pdf.

Teenage Pregnancy (2012). *March of Dimes Pregnancy and Newborn Health Education Center*. Retrieved January 7, 2014, from www.marchofdimes.com/glue/files/teenage-pregnancy.pdf.

Thompson, R. A., Flood, M. F., and Goodvin, R. (2006). Social support and developmental psychopathology. *Developmental Psychopathology*, 3, 1–37.

Tolman, D. L., and McClelland, S. I. (2011). Normative sexuality development in adolescence: A decade in review 2000–2009. *Journal of Research on Adolescence*, 21(1), 242–255.

Toomey, R. B., Umaña-Taylor, A. J., Jahromi, L. B., and Updegraff, K. A. (2013). Measuring social support from mother figures in the transition from pregnancy to parenthood among Mexican-origin adolescent mothers. *Hispanic Journal of Behavioral Sciences*, 35(2), 194–212.

Trenholm, C., Devaney, B., Fortson, K., Quay, L., Wheeler, J., and Clark, M. (2007). *Impacts of four Title V, Section 510 abstinence education programs*. Princeton: Mathematica Policy Research, Inc. Retrieved January 7, 2014, from www.mathematica-mpr.com/publications/PDFs/impactabstinence.pdf.

Trenholm, C., Devaney, B., Fortson, K., Quay, L., Wheeler, J., and Clark, M. (2008). Impacts of abstinence education on teen sexual activity, risk of pregnancy, and risk of sexually transmitted diseases. *Journal of Policy Analysis and Management*, 27(2), 255–276.

Trickett, P. K., Noll, J. G., and Putnam, F. W. (2011). The impact of sexual abuse on female development: Lessons from a multigenerational, longitudinal research study. *Development and Psychopathology*, 23(2), 453–476.

Tuffin, K., Rouch, G., and Frewin, K. (2010). Constructing adolescent fatherhood: Responsibilities and intergenerational repair. *Culture, Health and Sexuality*, 12(5), 485–498.

Turning to fairness. Insurance discrimination against women today and the Affordable Care Act (2012, March). National Women's Law Center, Washington, DC. Retrieved April 2, 2014, from www.nwlc.org/resource/report-turning-fairness-insurance-discrimination-against-women-today-and-affordable-care-ac.

United Nations, Department of Economic and Social Affairs, Population Division (2013). *World fertility data 2012* (POP/DB/FERT/REV2012). Retrieved January 7, 2014, from www.un.org/en/development/desa/population/publications/dataset/fertility/wfd2012/MainFrame.html.

Urban, J. B., Osgood, N. D., and Mabry, P. L. (2011). Developmental systems science: Exploring the application of systems science methods to developmental science questions. *Research in Human Development*, 8(1), 1–25.

US Department of Health and Human Services (2010). *HHS awards evidence-based teen pregnancy prevention grants* (news release). Retrieved January 7, 2014, from www.hhs.gov/news/press/2010pres/09/20100930a.html.

US Weekly (2010, August 30). *Inside their struggle*. Retrieved January 7, 2014, from www.usmagazine.com/celebrity-news/pictures/the-year-in-us-weekly-20102911/11627.

Vieira, C. L., Coeli, C. M., Pinheiro, R. S., Brandão, E. R., Camargo Jr., K. R., and Aguiar, F. P. (2012). Modifying effect of prenatal care on the association between young maternal age and adverse birth outcomes. *Journal of Pediatric and Adolescent Gynecology*, 25(3), 185–189.

Voight, J. D., Hans, S. L., and Bernstein, V. J. (1996). Support networks of adolescent mothers: Effects on parenting experience and behavior. *Infant Mental Health Journal*, 17, 58–73.

Wadhwa, P. D., Entringer, S., Buss, C., and Lu, M. C. (2011). The contribution of maternal stress to preterm birth: Issues and considerations. *Clinics in Perinatology*, 38(3), 351–384.

Walker, I., and Zhu, Y. (2009). *The causal effect of teen motherhood on worklessness* (School of Economics discussion papers KDPE 0917). Canterbury: University of Kent. Retrieved January 7, 2014, from ftp://ftp.ukc.ac.uk/pub/ejr/RePEc/ukc/ukcedp/0917.pdf.

Wallerstein, N., and Duran, B. (2010). Community-based participatory research contributions to intervention research: The intersection of science and practice to improve health equity. *American Journal of Public Health*, 100(S1), S40–S46.

Ward, L. M. (2003). Understanding the role of entertainment media in the sexual socialization of American youth: A review of empirical research. *Developmental Review*, 23(3), 347–388.

Warner, T. D., Giordano, P. C., Manning, W. D., and Longmore, M. A. (2011). Everybody's doin' it (right?): Neighborhood norms and sexual activity in adolescence. *Social Science Research*, 40(6), 1676–1690.

Webbink, D., Martin, N. G., and Visscher, P. M. (2008). Does teenage childbearing increase smoking, drinking and body size? *Journal of Health Economics*, 27, 888–903.

Weed, K., Keogh, D., and Borkowski, J. G., (2000). Predictors of resiliency in adolescent mothers. *Journal of Applied Developmental Psychology*, 21(2), 207–231.

Weed, K., and LeMay, R. (2012, October). *Mothers' perceived impact of teen pregnancy: Are perceived positive outcomes real?* Poster presented at the Carolina Women's Health Research Forum, Columbia, SC.

Weed, K., Nicholson, J., and Richter, T (2013, June). *Perceptions of teen pregnancy and parenting.* Poster presented at the South Carolina Campaign to Prevent Teen and Unwanted Pregnancy Summer Institute, Columbia, SC.

Weed, K., and Noria, C. (2011, March). Breaking the cycle: Resilient children with vulnerable adolescent mothers. In J. R. Farris and K. Valentino (Chairs), *Breaking the cycle: Developmental pathways of children born to adolescent mothers.* Symposium presented at the Society for Research in Child Development Biennial Meeting, Montreal, Quebec, Canada.

Weed, S. E., Ericksen, I. H., and Birch, P. J. (2005). *An evaluation of the Heritage Keepers abstinence education program.* Presented at the Abstinence Education Evaluation Conference: Strengthening Programs Through Scientific Evaluation, Baltimore, MD. Retrieved on January 7, 2014, from http://instituteresearch.com/docs/Heritage_ Keepers_Eval_(Weed,_Ericksen,_and_Birch,_2005).pdf.

Weed, S. E., Ericksen, I. H., Birch, P. J., White, J. M., Evans, M. T., and Anderson, N. E. (2007). *"Abstinence" or "Comprehensive" sex education? – The* Mathematica *study in context.* Retrieved January 7, 2014, from The Institute for Research and Evaluation website: www.abstinenceassociation.org/docs/Abstinence_vs_Comprehensive_Sex_ Ed.pdf.

Weed, S. E., Ericksen, I. H., Lewis, A., Grant, G. E., and Wibberly, K. H. (2008). An abstinence program's impact on cognitive mediators and sexual initiation. *American Journal of Health Behavior*, 32(1), 60–73.

Wegman, M. E. (2001). Infant mortality in the 20th century, dramatic but uneven progress. *The Journal of Nutrition*, 131(2), 401S–408S.

Werner, E. E., and Smith, R. S. (1992). *Overcoming the odds: High-risk children from birth to adulthood*. Ithaca: Cornell University Press.

When children have children (2012, May). *Facts for Families*, 31. Washington, DC: American Academy of Child and Adolescent Psychiatry. Retrieved January 6, 2014, from www.aacap.org/aacap/Families_and_Youth/Facts_for_Families/Facts_for_Families_Pages/When_Children_Have_Children_31.aspx.

Whitman, T. L., Borkowski, J. G., Keogh, D., and Weed, K. (2001). *Interwoven lives: Adolescent mothers and their children*. Mahwah, NJ: Erlbaum.

Wiggins, M., Oakley, A., Sawtell, M., Austerberry, H., Clemens, F., and Elbourne, D. (2005). *Teenage parenthood and social exclusion: A multi-method study: Summary report of findings*. London: Social Science Research Unit Report, Institute of Education. Retrieved June 8, 2014, http://webarchive.nationalarchives.gov.uk/20080925155335/http://dcsf.gov.uk/research/data/uploadfiles/RW57.pdf.

Witt, M. A. (2012). *Anglos' and Latinos' self-regulation to standards for education and parenthood* (unpublished doctoral dissertation). Duke University, North Carolina.

Wood, R. G., Avellar, S., and Goesling, B. (2008). *Pathways to adulthood and marriage: Teenagers' attitudes, expectations, and relationship patterns*. Retrieved January 7, 2014, from the Mathematica Policy Research website: www.mathematica-mpr.net/publications/PDFs/pathwaystoadulthoodrpt.pdf.

Woodward, L. J., Fergusson, D. M., and Horwood, L. J. (2006). Gender differences in the transition to early parenthood. *Development and Psychopathology*, 18, 275–294.

World Health Organization (2012). Adolescent pregnancy. Retrieved January 7, 2014, from www.who.int/mediacentre/factsheets/fs364/en/.

Wright, P. J. (2009). Sexual socialization messages in mainstream entertainment mass media: A review and synthesis. *Sexuality and Culture*, 13(4), 181–200.

Wright, P. J. (2011). Mass media effects on youth sexual behavior: Assessing the claim for causality. *Communication Yearbook*, 35, 343–386.

Wright, P. J., Randall, A. K., and Arroyo, A. (2013). Father–daughter communication about sex moderates the association between exposure to MTV's *16 and Pregnant/Teen Mom* and female students' pregnancy-risk behavior. *Sexuality and Culture*, 17(1), 50–66.

Yoo, S. H., Hayford, S. R., and Guzzo, K. B. (2012). *Ambivalence towards pregnancy: Is it a singular or multifaceted concept?* (2012 working paper series). Retrieved January 7, 2014, from The Center for Family and Demographic Research website: www2.bgsu.edu/downloads/cas/file110196.pdf.

Zolna, M., and Lindberg, L. (2012). *Unintended pregnancy: Incidence and outcomes among young adult unmarried women in the United States, 2001 and 2008*. Retrieved January 7, 2014, from the Guttmacher Institute website: www.guttmacher.org/pubs/unintended-pregnancy-US-2001-2008.pdf.

Zubrick, S. R., Silburn, S. R., Gurrin, L., Teoh, H., Shepherd, C., Carlton, J., and Lawrence, D. (1997). *Western Australian Child Health Survey: Education, health and competence*. Perth, Western Australia: Australian Bureau of Statistics and the TVW Telethon Institute for Child Health Research.

Index